MANIPULATION
of the SPINE, THORAX
and PELVIS

For Elsevier:
Senior Content Strategist: Rita Demetriou-Swanwick
Senior Content Development Specialist: Nicola Lally
Project Manager: Andrew Riley
Design: Christian Bilbow
Illustrator: MacPS

FOURTH EDITION

MANIPULATION
of the SPINE, THORAX
and PELVIS

with access to **www.spinethoraxpelvis.com**

Peter Gibbons MB BS DO DM-SMed MHSc
Adjunct Associate Professor, Department of Rehabilitation Sciences,
College of Allied Health,
Oklahoma University Health Science Center, USA

Philip Tehan DO DipPhysio MHSc
Adjunct Associate Professor, College of Health & Biomedicine,
Victoria University, Australia
Adjunct Associate Professor, Department of Rehabilitation Sciences,
College of Allied Health,
Oklahoma University Health Science Center, USA

Foreword by
Timothy W. Flynn, PT PhD OCS FAAOMPT
Professor, School of Physical Therapy, South College, USA
Executive Team, Evidence in Motion, USA

Photographs by
Tim Turner
Effie and Shane Coleman

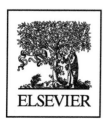

ELSEVIER

Edinburgh London New York Oxford Philadelphia St Louis Sydney Toronto 2016

ELSEVIER

ISBN 978-0-7020-5921-6
eISBN 978-0-7020-6511-8

Notices

Knowledge and best practice in this field are constantly changing. As new research and experience broaden our understanding, changes in research methods, professional practices, or medical treatment may become necessary.

Practitioners and researchers must always rely on their own experience and knowledge in evaluating and using any information, methods, compounds, or experiments described herein. In using such information or methods they should be mindful of their own safety and the safety of others, including parties for whom they have a professional responsibility.

With respect to any drug or pharmaceutical products identified, readers are advised to check the most current information provided (i) on procedures featured or (ii) by the manufacturer of each product to be administered, to verify the recommended dose or formula, the method and duration of administration, and contraindications. It is the responsibility of practitioners, relying on their own experience and knowledge of their patients, to make diagnoses, to determine dosages and the best treatment for each individual patient, and to take all appropriate safety precautions.

To the fullest extent of the law, neither the Publisher nor the authors, contributors, or editors, assume any liability for any injury and/or damage to persons or property as a matter of products liability, negligence or otherwise, or from any use or operation of any methods, products, instructions, or ideas contained in the material herein.

The Publisher

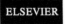

your source for books,
journals and multimedia
in the health sciences

www.elsevierhealth.com

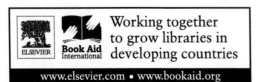

Working together to grow libraries in developing countries

www.elsevier.com • www.bookaid.org

The publisher's policy is to use paper manufactured from sustainable forests

Foreword

It is my distinct honor to provide the Foreword to the fourth edition of *Manipulation of the Spine, Thorax, and Pelvis*. The Foreword to the first 3 editions of this superb text was written by the late Dr. Philip Greenman, DO, FAAO. It was not only his teaching, but also his belief in my abilities and his personal mentorship that facilitated my career in the research and practice of manipulative medicine. It is with deep gratitude to his legacy that we are all able to build upon the practice of manipulative medicine.

As a modern world we have failed to treat spinal pain in a consistent and effective manner. In fact we continue down a path of overutilization of medical imaging, pharmaceutical treatments, spinal injections, and spinal surgeries. These typically invasive and frequently harmful treatments have not slowed the prevalence of spinal pain but have increased the number of lives lived in chronic pain. If there is a silver lining it is that there is a steady stream of research demonstrating that manual or manipulative therapy, exercise, and patient education delivered by caring and compassionate practitioners is not only safe and effective but delivered at a lower financial burden to the individual and society.

Expertise in manipulative therapy requires that the practitioner be committed to excelling in the craft of manual medicine. The main purpose of this text is to provide the framework for the development and refinement of expertise in spinal manipulation. As a teacher of manual therapy I frequently ask my students when they have an oral or physical examination do they prefer a dentist or clinician to have gentle caring hands or rough aggressive hands? I have yet to find students that prefer the latter. This text focuses on teaching practitioners to develop gentle therapeutic hands coupled with comfortable and relaxed patient positions. In addition, the text addresses the important issues surrounding patient consent and discusses safety issues in the broader context of relative risk. The text closes with a final word to the practitioner to be reflective on how they are performing manipulative techniques and thus focuses on continuous improvement and refinement of their skills.

In summary, I urge manual therapy practitioners to not only read the text and view the videos, but also to take the time to develop gentle hands, exceptional body awareness, and caring words, which are all part of the art and science of manipulation.

Timothy W. Flynn PT, PhD, OCS, FAAOMPT
Professor, School of Physical Therapy, South College, USA
Executive Team, Evidence in Motion, USA

Preface

This fourth edition of *Manipulation of the Spine, Thorax and Pelvis* has been produced at a time of increasing knowledge related to the use of manipulative techniques in clinical practice and has been updated accordingly. The move towards an evidence-based and patient-centred approach to healthcare requires the modern practitioner to utilize the best available evidence to inform clinical practice and to be cognizant of the legal and ethical requirements for informed consent, and the fourth edition reflects these requirements of practice.

Patient comfort and safety remain major considerations when selecting a treatment approach. Some manipulative approaches use full leverage, end-range and barrier techniques, which can be uncomfortable for the patient. This text presents an approach that uses minimal leverages necessary to achieve a cavitation in a safe and effective manner and which is comfortable for the patient.

Evidence seems to be lacking for a strong association between neck manipulation and stroke but is also absent for no association. Current biomechanical evidence is insufficient to establish the claim that cervical spine HVLA thrust techniques cause cervical artery dissection and subsequent stroke. On the basis of current knowledge, the absolute risk of stoke following neck manipulation is unknown but likely to be very small and to have been significantly overestimated in the past. The evidence supports the view that patients may present to practitioners with neck pain and/or headache attributable to a dissection in progress, and this requires a change in focus to the early detection of a patient with a dissecting cervical artery. Research evidence would suggest that cervical spine pretreatment screening for arterial dysfunction is not valid and lacks clinical utility. The text has been updated to embrace current research findings relating to cervical artery dysfunction and the association between neck manipulation and stroke.

Our goal continues to be presentation of a text that will provide the necessary information relating to all aspects of the delivery of HVLA thrust techniques in one comprehensive volume so that practitioners can use these techniques safely and in the appropriate circumstances. Research evidence supports the view that the risks associated with spinal manipulation are low, with an increasing body of evidence demonstrating clinical efficacy, particularly when applied in a multimodal approach. Since the third edition, additional research and guidelines that support the use of HVLA thrust techniques have been published, and these have been incorporated into the fourth edition. The evidence base for the use of spinal manipulation in patients with disc lesions and radiculopathy has been updated and expanded. This edition also reviews the evidence for the use of spinal manipulation in the treatment of pregnant women and children.

For a commonly used treatment approach, it is surprising that there are such limited resources to support learning and skill refinement in HVLA thrust techniques. Most of the learning of HVLA thrust techniques has been dependent on personal instruction and demonstration. There are still only a handful of books and manuals on osteopathic techniques, and few of these relate solely to thrust techniques.

The material presented in this text was developed in response to the learning needs of undergraduate and postgraduate students over a 40-year period. The novice has to acquire basic skills, and experienced practitioners should reflect upon their performance and constantly refine each thrust technique. It has been our experience that the structured, step-by-step format used in the text and the visual reinforcement offered by the accompanying video material have been successful in assisting both initial development and subsequent refinement of the psychomotor skills necessary for the effective delivery of HVLA thrust techniques. Experience has shown that the video images have proved useful for both students and practitioners.

Peter Gibbons, Philip Tehan
Melbourne 2016

Acknowledgements

As in the first three editions, we are grateful to those colleagues who knowingly or unknowingly assisted in the development of the book. We also acknowledge that the constant questioning by undergraduate and postgraduate students has contributed significantly to the development of the material in the text.

Tim Turner has provided the photographs for all editions, with Effie and Shane Coleman providing additional photographs and video for the fourth edition. We would like to thank them for their patience and understanding during the many photography sessions. We are indebted to Andrea Robertson for her good humour and endurance during the long sessions spent as the model for the photographs and videos and also to Sarah Sturges and Alastair Tehan who acted as models for additional material appearing in the fourth edition. We greatly appreciate the assistance of Dr Frank Burke (Consultant Radiologist) in providing access to imaging facilities and advice regarding the fluoroscopic images of the lumbar spine and to Dr John Kwon for providing fluoroscopic images of the cervical spine that appear on the videos. The teaching potential of the text has been greatly enhanced by the visual material and their contribution. We would like to thank Brett Vaughan and Ouita Spalding for assistance with the literature search and manuscript preparation for this edition and to Victoria University for providing the venue for photographs and filming.

A special thanks is extended to Rita Demetriou-Swanwick and Nicola Lally at Elsevier for their help, support and encouragement for the fourth edition.

Most importantly, our greatest debt of gratitude goes to Jill Tehan and Christine Leek whose tireless support made the writing and updating of this book possible.

Contents

 The website – www.spinethoraxpelvis.com – accompanying this text includes video sequences of all the techniques described in Part B (with the exception of the last technique described in Chapter 11.) These are indicated in the text by the following symbol.

The website is designed to be used as an adjunct to the text and not as a stand-alone product.

Contents

Companion website: www.spinethoraxpelvis.com

* video bank

* image bank

HVLA thrust techniques – an osteopathic perspective

1

Introduction

Manipulative techniques for the spine, thorax and pelvis are commonly utilized for the treatment of pain and dysfunction. Proficiency in their use requires training, practice and development of palpatory and psychomotor skills. The purpose of this book is to provide a resource that will aid development of the knowledge and skills necessary to perform high-velocity low-amplitude (HVLA) thrust techniques in practice. It is written not just for the novice manipulator but also for any practitioner who uses thrust techniques. Although the book presents an osteopathic perspective, it does not promote or endorse any particular treatment model or approach.

The term 'manipulation' is often used to describe a range of manual therapy techniques. This text focuses specifically upon HVLA thrust procedures, where the practitioner applies a rapid thrust or impulse. The aim of HVLA thrust techniques is to achieve joint cavitation, which is accompanied by a 'popping' or 'cracking' sound. This audible release distinguishes HVLA thrust techniques from other osteopathic manipulative techniques. HVLA thrust techniques are also known by a number of different names, e.g. adjustment, high-velocity thrust, mobilization with impulse and grade V mobilization.

The book is divided into three parts. Part A comprises seven chapters that provide an osteopathic perspective on the use of HVLA

thrust techniques and reviews indications, research evidence, kinematics, safety and consent.

An overview of the osteopathic history, principles and practice that underpin osteopathic manipulative technique and treatment is presented in Chapter 2. Chapter 3 reviews spinal kinematics and coupled motion of the spine. Practitioners require knowledge of biomechanics and coupled motion characteristics in order to apply the principles of spinal locking used in HVLA thrust techniques. The osteopathic profession has developed a classification of spinal motions. Chapter 4 describes Type 1 and Type 2 movements and the relevance of coupled motion to spinal positioning and joint locking with consideration of the modifications necessary when treating the stiffer and more mobile spine. A minimal leverage approach that emphasizes patient comfort and avoids end range or motion restriction barrier thrust techniques is outlined.

Complications of, and contraindications to, HVLA thrust techniques are outlined in Chapter 5. The relative risks of thrust and non-thrust techniques and the association between cervical spine HVLA thrust techniques and cervical artery dissection are reviewed. The clinical history, presentation and examination findings for patients presenting with symptoms and signs consistent with cervical artery dissection are presented. Premanipulative assessment for upper cervical instability is described and the use of testing protocols is reviewed in light of the published literature.

Chapter 6 reviews the literature relating to cavitation and the evidence related to the efficacy of spinal manipulation and outlines a clinical decision-making process that will assist practitioners to determine when a HVLA thrust technique might be used in clinical practice. Evidence for the use of HVLA thrust techniques in patients with disc lesions is outlined and the available evidence for the use of thrust techniques in pregnancy and for children is reviewed.

Consent is a key concept in the provision of healthcare, and this is reviewed in Chapter 7, with particular emphasis on explaining potential risks involved in the manipulation of all regions of the spine.

Part B outlines in detail specific HVLA thrust techniques for the spine, rib cage and pelvis. This part combines photographs and descriptive text that is supported by video images of HVLA thrust techniques.

HVLA thrust techniques can be described in terms of bone movement or joint gliding. In this text, all 41 techniques utilizing the principle of joint gliding are outlined. This approach has been shown to be effective in the teaching of HVLA thrust techniques to both undergraduate and postgraduate students.

The text has been designed to provide a logical step-by-step format that has consistency throughout the book. Each technique is described from the moment the patient is positioned on the couch, through a series of steps up to and including segmental localization and delivery of the thrust. Each individual technique is logically organized under a number of specific headings:

- Contact point(s)
- Applicator(s)
- Patient positioning
- Operator stance
- Positioning for thrust
- Adjustments to achieve appropriate pre-thrust tension

- Immediately pre-thrust
- Delivering thrust.

Individuals use a variety of methods to acquire complex psychomotor skills, and structured and repeated practice is a key element in the development and maintenance of proficiency. Experiencing these both as an operator and as a model can enhance the learning of HVLA thrust techniques.

The art of manipulation is very individual, requiring HVLA thrust techniques to be adapted to the needs of both practitioner and patient. Although some modification to the described techniques will occur with developing proficiency, the underlying principles remain the same. These principles can be summarized as follows:

1. Exclude contraindications
2. Obtain informed consent
3. Ensure patient comfort
4. Ensure operator comfort and optimal posture
5. Use spinal locking
6. Identify appropriate pre-thrust tissue tension
7. Apply HVLA thrust.

If these principles are applied, HVLA thrust techniques provide a safe and effective treatment option.

A common experience in the evolution of proficiency in thrust techniques is a sense of frustration and impatience when skill development is slow or variable. Experienced practitioners can similarly experience difficulties achieving cavitation in certain circumstances. Part C provides a troubleshooting and self-evaluation guide to identify problems that may limit the effective application of HVLA thrust techniques.

Integral to the practice of osteopathic medicine is an understanding of the interrelationship of mind, body and environment. Osteopathic treatment encompasses more than joint manipulation alone, and this manual represents only part of the art and science of osteopathic medicine.

2

Osteopathic history, principles and practice

THE ORIGINS AND EARLY DEVELOPMENT OF OSTEOPATHY

Andrew Taylor Still (Fig. 2.1), founder of the osteopathic approach, was born in 1828 in the American state of Virginia. Like most American physicians of the time, he learned medicine by apprenticeship.[1] The term *osteopathy* was articulated by Still in about 1889,[2] and he believed that it was an independent system of medicine, but his ideas initially met with considerable opposition. See Table 2.1 for key dates in the early history of osteopathy.

THE FIRST OSTEOPATHIC SCHOOLS

The American School of Osteopathy in Kirksville was formed by Still in 1892.[3] The school graduated its first students 2 years later, and in 1896 the state of Vermont was the first to recognize the profession of osteopathy. Between 1896 and 1899, 13 osteopathic colleges were opened in the United States.[4] Still died in 1917, and at that time there were approximately 5000 osteopathic practitioners in America,[5] and many others had moved to different parts of the world.

Australia

Osteopathy was introduced to Australia in 1909. The initial development of the profession centred largely in Victoria, and by 1939 there were 13 overseas-trained osteopaths working in that state.[6]

United Kingdom

John Martin Littlejohn, a Scotsman who immigrated to America in 1892 and who studied at the American School of Osteopathy, was the first person to introduce osteopathy in the UK. He returned to live in England in 1913 and opened the British School of Osteopathy in London in 1917.[7]

Europe

By the 1930s osteopathic practice had spread into mainland Europe. Many of the European practitioners who studied osteopathy were qualified physiotherapists, who would avoid legal and regulatory sanctions by using osteopathic techniques within their existing practice.

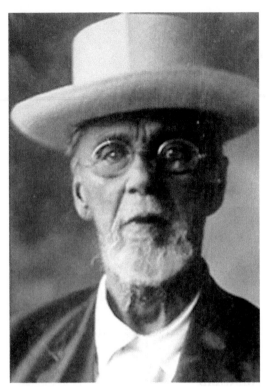

Figure 2.1 A.T. Still.

Table 2.1 Key dates in the early history of osteopathy

1828	A.T. Still was born.
1892	A.T. Still opened the American School of Osteopathy in Kirksville, Missouri.
1917	A.T. Still died.
1909	Osteopathy was introduced to Australia.
1917	John Martin Littlejohn opened the British School of Osteopathy.
1930s	Osteopathy was introduced to mainland Europe.

Box 2.1 Osteopathic principles

- The human being is a dynamic unit of function.
- The body possesses self-regulatory mechanisms that are self-healing in nature.
- Structure and function are interrelated at all levels.
- Rational treatment is based on these principles.

CURRENT OSTEOPATHIC HEALTHCARE WORLDWIDE

Osteopathic healthcare is now provided in every continent except Antarctica and is practised in more than 50 countries. Globally, two professional streams have emerged – osteopathic physicians (practicing osteopathic medicine) and osteopaths (practicing osteopathy). All osteopathic physicians hold medical degrees and are licensed to practise the full range of medical care, including prescribing medicines and performing surgery.[4] Osteopaths are generally not licensed to prescribe medicines, perform surgery or assist in childbirth but are able to practise manual and manipulative procedures within the framework of each country.[7] The training pathways and regulatory structures differ for the two professional streams and have developed in different ways and at different speeds influenced by the specific cultural, economic, legal and political factors of individual countries.[8]

PRINCIPLES UNDERPINNING OSTEOPATHIC HEALTHCARE

In 1953, a Special Committee on Osteopathic Principles and Osteopathic Technique at the Kirksville College of Osteopathy and Surgery published a list of four osteopathic principles,[9] which are listed in Box 2.1.

A list of basic tenets and principles for patient care was published in 2002.[10] (Box 2.2). These osteopathic tenets and principles, in conjunction with current medical knowledge, inform the care given to

Box 2.2 Basic tenets and principles for patient care

Basic Tenets
- A person is the product of dynamic interaction between body, mind and spirit.
- An inherent property of this dynamic interaction is the capacity of the individual for the maintenance of health and recovery from disease.
- Many forces, both intrinsic and extrinsic to the person, can challenge this inherent capacity and contribute to the onset of illness.
- The musculoskeletal system significantly influences the individual's ability to restore this inherent capacity and therefore to resist disease processes.

Principles for Patient Care
- The patient is the primary focus of healthcare.
- The patient has the primary responsibility for his or her health.
- An effective treatment program for patient care is founded on these tenets and:
  - incorporates evidence-based guidelines,
  - optimizes the patient's natural healing capacity,
  - addresses the primary cause of disease, and
  - emphasizes health maintenance and disease prevention.

Box 2.3 Clinical decision making

- Exclude contraindications.
- Determine influence of psychosocial factors.
- Identify the presence of a treatable lesion – somatic dysfunction.
- Perform risk/benefit analysis.
- Identify patient preference for treatment approach.
- Refer for further assessment, if indicated, or decide upon appropriate treatment which may include co-management.

patients by both osteopathic physicians and osteopaths.

OSTEOPATHIC ASSESSMENT AND DIAGNOSIS

Osteopathic physicians and osteopaths assess and treat the 'whole person' rather than just focusing on specific symptoms or illnesses. All patients undergo structural and functional assessments on the basis that the primary cause of symptoms or dysfunction may be remote from the symptomatic area.[4] Osteopathic practitioners use all the standard clinical processes in history taking and examination, including imaging or laboratory tests, when clinically indicated. A common template for clinical decision making used by osteopathic physicians and osteopaths is outlined in Box 2.3.

PALPATION AND OSTEOPATHIC DIAGNOSIS

An emphasis on the neuromusculoskeletal system as being integral to the body's function and a person's health is important when considering osteopathic assessment and diagnosis. Palpation is fundamental to osteopathic structural and functional diagnoses, but a number of studies have reported poor reliability of clinical tests involving palpation. The development of a high level of palpatory skill requires practice and patience.[11]

Research has explored both interexaminer and intraexaminer reliability of various diagnostic palpatory procedures. Interexaminer reliability consists of one assessment of all subjects by each of two or more raters, blinded to each other's observations, and allows assessment of rater agreement. Intraexaminer reliability is determined by repeated measurements of single individuals to evaluate rater self-consistency.

Osteopaths have shown reasonable levels of interexaminer agreement for passive gross motion testing on selected subjects with consistent findings of regional motion asymmetry.[12,13] One osteopathic study demonstrated low agreement of findings for patients with acute spinal complaints when practitioners used their own diagnostic procedures.[14] Level of agreement can be improved by negotiating and selecting specific tests for detecting patient improvement.[15] Standardization of testing procedures can improve both interexaminer and intraexaminer reliability.[16]

In asymptomatic somatic dysfunction, high levels of interexaminer and intraobserver agreement for palpatory findings have yet to be demonstrated. Many studies and systematic reviews indicate that interexaminer and intraexaminer reliability for palpatory motion testing without pain provocation is poor.[17-28]

Poor interexaminer reliability has also been reported for palpating static spinal asymmetry.[29,30] A number of studies have reported only fair to poor reliability for palpation of tissue texture abnormalities.[31-34]

Poor reliability of clinical tests involving palpation may be partially explained by errors in location of bony landmarks[35] and differences in palpation technique.[36] Consensus training has been demonstrated to improve interobserver reliability in the palpatory tests of lumbar spine tissue texture and tenderness,[37] and examiners have been able to maintain and improve interobserver reliability of four lumbar diagnostic palpatory tests over a 4-month period.[38] Palpation as a diagnostic tool has been reported to demonstrate high levels of sensitivity and specificity in detecting symptomatic intervertebral segments.[39,40] A further study refuted some of these findings, demonstrating that manual examination had high sensitivity but poor specificity for identifying cervical zygapophysial joint pain.[41]

Whilst the reliability of palpation has been extensively investigated, its validity remains relatively underresearched. The validity of pain provocation and motion palpation tests to accurately distinguish symptomatic from nonsymptomatic segments in the cervical spine has been questioned,[41] and it has been reported that manual palpation of specific lumbopelvic bony points has limited validity.[42]

A systematic review of the manual examination of the spine identified that reproducibility of palpation for pain response was consistently better than for motion palpation.[43] Increasing evidence is emerging that clusters of provocation and motion palpation tests have better reliability and validity than single tests for assessing the sacroiliac joints.[28,44-46]

Somatic Dysfunction

The accepted definition for somatic dysfunction in the 'Glossary of osteopathic terminology' is as follows:

> Somatic dysfunction is an impaired or altered function of related components of the somatic (body framework) system: skeletal, arthrodial and myofascial structures, and related vascular, lymphatic and neural elements.[47]

The template for clinical decision making outlined in Box 2.3 is used by practitioners from a range of health professions, but the concept of 'somatic dysfunction' to identify the presence of a treatable lesion has its origins in osteopathy and is still advocated in current osteopathic texts.[48-50]

Traditionally, diagnosis of somatic dysfunction was made on the basis of a number of positive findings. Specific criteria in identifying areas of dysfunction were developed and related to the observational and palpatory findings represented as the acronym TART (tissue tenderness, asymmetry, range of motion and tissue texture changes).[47-50]

Pain provocation and reproduction of familiar symptoms should also be used to localize somatic dysfunction. The presence of

---

Box 2.4 Diagnosis of somatic dysfunction

- S   relates to symptom reproduction
- T   relates to tissue tenderness
- A   relates to asymmetry
- R   relates to range of motion
- T   relates to tissue texture changes

---

somatic dysfunction and/or pathology should be determined not only by physical examination but also by information gained from a thorough patient history taking and patient feedback during assessment. This depth of diagnostic deliberation is essential if one is to select which case may or may not be amenable to treatment and which treatment approach might be the most effective while offering the patient a reasoned prognosis. We would advocate that the convention for the diagnosis of somatic dysfunction – TART – should be expanded to include patient feedback relating to pain provocation and the reproduction of familiar symptoms.

Somatic Dysfunction is Identified by the S-T-A-R-T of Diagnosis (Box 2.4)

S relates to symptom reproduction

Although somatic dysfunction can be asymptomatic, it commonly exists within the context of a patient presenting with symptoms. Pain provocation and the reporting of reproduction of familiar symptoms are therefore essential components of the physical examination.

T relates to tissue tenderness

Undue tissue tenderness is often present and must be differentiated from reproduction of the patient's familiar pain.

A relates to asymmetry

DiGiovanna links the criteria of asymmetry to a positional focus stating that the

'position of the vertebra or other bone is asymmetrical'.[48] Greenman broadens the concept of asymmetry by including functional in addition to structural asymmetry.[49]

R relates to range of motion

Alteration in range of motion can apply to a single joint, several joints or a region of the musculoskeletal system. The abnormality may be either restricted or increased mobility and includes assessment of quality of movement and 'end feel'.

T relates to tissue texture changes

The identification of tissue texture changes is important in the diagnosis of somatic dysfunction. Palpable changes may be noted in superficial, intermediate and deep tissues. It is important for clinicians to recognize normal from abnormal.

The diagnosis of somatic dysfunction should not be based upon a single finding but should be determined by the clinician identifying a number of positive findings that are consistent with the patient's clinical presentation (Box 2.5).

For example, a patient with cervicogenic headaches with related somatic dysfunction might present with restricted active and passive range of movement in the cervical spine; segmental assessment may identify localized movement restriction; palpation may identify muscular hypertonicity and/or undue local tenderness; and examination may reproduce the patient's familiar symptoms.

OSTEOPATHIC TREATMENT OBJECTIVES AND CO-MANAGEMENT

Box 2.6 is a list of objectives in the diagnosis and treatment of spinal disorders. The use of pharmaceutical interventions is supported, where clinically indicated, by

Box 2.5 Diagnosis of somatic dysfunction

• Not be based upon a single finding
• Determined by identifying a number of positive findings consistent with the patient's clinical presentation

Box 2.6 Objectives in the diagnosis and treatment of spinal disorders

• Focused history and clinical examination to classify patients into one of the following categories:
  • mechanical pain with no neurological involvement
  • mechanical pain associated with neurological involvement
  • spinal pain due to serious pathology (red flags)
• Assessment of psychosocial risk factors and barriers to return to normal activity
• Provide information to reassure patients about their condition
• Provide patients with information on effective self-care options
• Provide patients with advice to remain active
• Give priority to treatments of known efficacy.

Box 2.7 Osteopathic manipulative techniques

• Soft tissue
• Articulation
• High-velocity low-amplitude (HVLA) thrust
• Body adjustment
• Myofascial
• Muscle energy
• Counterstrain
• Functional
• Positional release
• Craniosacral
• Biodynamics
• Balanced ligamentous
• Visceral
• Lymphatic
• Chapman reflexes
• Triggerpoint

best practice models. The importance of providing lifestyle and general health advice, including dietary and exercise prescription, is recognized. Relevant psychosocial and emotional factors need to be identified with referral to appropriately qualified health professionals, where clinically indicated.

OSTEOPATHIC MANIPULATIVE PRESCRIPTION

Once a practitioner has established treatment objectives, consideration must be given to the specific treatment of somatic dysfunction. Many factors will influence the final composition of the manipulative

prescription, as is the case when a physician considers a patient's age, weight, drug and allergy history, and other factors when prescribing medication. The osteopath similarly takes account of factors such as the patient's age, the acuteness or chronicity of the presenting complaint, general health, response to previous treatment and the osteopath's own training and expertise in the delivery of specific treatment approaches. This list is not exhaustive, and many other factors can influence the final selection of manipulative techniques and the frequency of treatment.

When formulating the manipulative prescription, osteopathic physicians and osteopaths have a wide range of techniques to draw upon (Box 2.7).

Some osteopathic techniques are named according to the activating forces used (e.g. muscle energy, articulation, or high-velocity low-amplitude (HVLA) thrust), whereas other techniques (e.g. strain/counterstrain, myofascial release and osteopathy in the cranial field) refer to a concept of treatment. Techniques are also classified as either direct or indirect techniques. Direct techniques involve the application of force to engage the restrictive barrier, whereas indirect techniques utilize identification of 'freedom' or 'ease' of movement by moving away from the restrictive barrier. Ideally, practitioners should embrace a range of different techniques and not favour any one specific approach. A study of members of the Australian Osteopathic Association identified that high-velocity manipulation was one of the most commonly used forms of osteopathic manipulative treatment.[51]

MULTIMODAL TREATMENT APPROACH

Rarely are HVLA thrust techniques used by osteopathic physicians and osteopaths as a stand-alone treatment approach for the management of spinal pain and dysfunction. Usually HVLA thrust techniques are combined with other osteopathic manipulative techniques (Box 2.7), e.g. soft tissue, articulation and muscle energy.

A number of studies support a multimodal approach to treatment, particularly in the cervical spine, where manipulation, mobilization and exercise regimes are combined in the treatment of spinal pain and dysfunction.[52-63]

References

1 Laughlin GM. Asks if AT Still was even a doctor. Osteopathic Physician 1909;15(Jan):8.

2 Peterson BE. Major events in osteopathic history. In: Chila A ed. Foundations of Osteopathic Medicine, 3rd edn. Philadelphia, PA: Wolters Kluwer Health/Lippincott Williams & Wilkins; 2010 [Ch. 2].

3 Walter GW. The First School of Osteopathic Medicine: A Chronicle, 1892–1992. Kirksville, MO: Thomas Jefferson University Press at Northeast Missouri State University; 1992.

4 Osteopathic International Alliance. Osteopathy and Osteopathic Medicine. A Global View of Practice, Patients, Education and the Contribution to Healthcare Delivery. Chicago, IL: Osteopathic International Alliance; 2013.

5 American Osteopathic Association. Important Dates in Osteopathic History. Chicago, IL: American Osteopathic Association; 2013. <http://history.osteopathic.org/timeline-shtml>.

6 Hawkins P, O'Neill A. Osteopathy in Australia. Bundoora, Victoria: P.I.T. Press; 1990.

7 European Federation of Osteopaths. History of Osteopathy. Brussels, Belgium: EFO; 2013. <http://www.efo.eu/portal/index.php?option=com_content&view=article&id=68&Itemid=74>.

8 Carreiro JE, Fossum C. International osteopathic medicine and osteopathy. In: Chila A ed. Foundations of Osteopathic Medicine, 3rd edn. Philadelphia, PA: Wolters Kluwer Health/Lippincott Williams & Wilkins; 2010 [Ch. 4].

9 Special Committee on Osteopathic Principles and Osteopathic Technique. The osteopathic concept: An interpretation. J Osteopath 1953;7–10.

10 Rogers FJ, D'Alonzo GF, Glover J, et al. Proposed tenets of osteopathic medicine and principles for patient care. J Am Osteopath Assoc 2002;102:63–5.

11 Ehrenfeuchter WC, Kappler RE. Palpatory examination. In: Chila A ed. Foundations of Osteopathic Medicine, 3rd edn. Philadelphia, PA: Wolters Kluwer Health/Lippincott Williams & Wilkins; 2010 [Ch. 33].

12 Johnston WL, Elkiss ML, Marino RV, et al. Passive gross motion testing: Part II. A study of interexaminer agreement. J Am Osteopath Assoc 1982;81(5):65–9.

13 Johnston WL, Beal MC, Blum GA, et al. Passive gross motion testing: Part III. Examiner agreement on selected subjects. J Am Osteopath Assoc 1982;81(5):70–4.

14 McConnell DG, Beal MC, Dinnar U, et al. Low agreement of findings in neuromusculoskeletal examinations by a group of osteopathic physicians using their own procedures. J Am Osteopath Assoc 1980;79(7):59–68.

15 Beal MC, Goodridge JP, Johnston WL, et al. Interexaminer agreement on patient improvement after negotiated selection of tests. J Am Osteopath Assoc 1980;79(7):45–53.

16 Marcotte J, Normand M, Black P. The kinematics of motion palpation and its effect on the reliability for cervical spine rotation. J Manipulative Physiol Ther 2002;25(7):471.

17 Van Duersen LLJM, Patijn J, Ockhuysen AL, et al. The value of some clinical tests of the sacroiliac joint. Man Med 1990;5:96–9.

18 Laslett M, Williams M. The reliability of selected pain provocation tests for sacroiliac

joint pathology. In: Leeming A, Mooney V, Dorman T, et al. eds. The Integrated Function of the Lumbar Spine and Sacroiliac Joint. Rotterdam: ECO; 1995:485–498.

19 Gonnella C, Paris S, Kutner M. Reliability in evaluating passive intervertebral motion. Phys Ther 1982;62:436–44.

20 Matyas T, Bach T. The reliability of selected techniques in clinical arthrokinematics. Aust J Physiother 1985;31(5):175–95.

21 Harvey D, Byfield D. Preliminary studies with a mechanical model for the evaluation of spinal motion palpation. Clin Biomech 1991;6:79–82.

22 Lewit K, Liebenson C. Palpation–problems and implications. J Manipulative Physiol Ther 1993;16(9):586–90.

23 Panzer DM. The reliability of lumbar motion palpation. J Manipulative Physiol Ther 1992;15(8):518–24.

24 Love RM, Brodeur R. Inter- and intra-examiner reliability of motion palpation for the thoracolumbar spine. J Manipulative Physiol Ther 1987;10(1):1–4.

25 Smedmark V, Wallin M, Arvidsson I. Inter-examiner reliability in assessing passive intervertebral motion of the cervical spine. Man Ther 2000;5(2):97–101.

26 Hestboek L, Leboeuf-Yde C. Are chiropractic tests for the lumbo-pelvic spine reliable and valid? A systematic critical literature review. J Manipulative Physiol Ther 2000;23(4):258–75.

27 Van Trijffel E, Anderegg Q, Bossuyt P, et al. Inter-examiner reliability of passive assessment of intervertebral motion in the cervical and lumbar spine: A systematic review. Man Ther 2005;10(4):256–69.

28 Robinson H, Brox J, Robinson R, et al. The reliability of selected motion and pain provocation tests for the sacroiliac joint. Man Ther 2007;12(1):72–9.

29 Sutton C, Nono L, Johnston R, et al. The effects of experience on the inter-reliability of osteopaths to detect changes in posterior superior iliac spine levels using a hidden heel wedge. J Bodyw Mov Ther 2013;17(2):143–50.

30 Spring F, Gibbons P, Tehan P. Intra-examiner and inter-examiner reliability of a positional diagnostic screen for the lumbar spine. J Osteopathic Med 2001;4:47–55.

31 Seffinger MA, Najm WI, Mishra SI, et al. Reliability of spinal palpation for diagnosis of back and neck pain. Spine 2004;29:E413–25.

32 Boline PD, Haas M, Meyer JJ, et al. Interexaminer reliability of eight evaluative dimensions of lumbar segmental abnormality: Part II. J Manip Physiol Ther 1993;16:363–74.

33 Stochkendahl MJ, Christensen HW, Hartvigsen J, et al. Manual examination of the spine: A systematic critical literature review of reproducibility. J Manip Physiol Ther 2006;29:475–85.

34 Paulet T, Fryer G. Inter-examiner reliability of palpation for tissue texture abnormality in the thoracic paraspinal region. Int J Osteopath Med 2009;12(3):92–6.

35 O'Haire C, Gibbons P. Inter-examiner and intra-examiner agreement for assessing sacroiliac anatomical landmarks using palpation and observation: A pilot study. Man Ther 2000;5(1):13–20.

36 Holmgren U, Waling K. Inter-examiner reliability of four static palpation tests used for assessing pelvic dysfunction. Man Ther 2008;13(1):50–6.

37 Degenhardt BF, Snider K, Snider E, et al. Interobserver reliability of osteopathic palpatory diagnostic tests of the lumbar spine: Improvements from consensus training. J Am Osteopath Assoc 2005;105(10):465–73.

38 Degenhardt BF, Johnson JC, Snider KT, et al. Maintenance and improvement of interobserver reliability of osteopathic palpatory tests over a 4 month period. J Am Osteopath Assoc 2010;110(10):579–86.

39 Jull G, Bogduk N, Marsland A. The accuracy of manual diagnosis for cervical zygapophysial joint pain syndromes. Med J Aust 1988;148:233–6.

40 Jull G, Zito G, Trott P, et al. Inter-examiner reliability to detect painful upper cervical joint dysfunction. Aust J Physiother 1997;43(2):125–9.

41 King W, Lau P, Lees R, et al. The validity of manual examination in assessing patients with neck pain. Spine J 2007;7(1):22–6.

42 Kilby J, Heneghan NR, Maybury M. Manual palpation of lumbo-pelvic landmarks: A validity study. Man Ther 2012;17(3):259–62.

43 Stochkendahl M, Christensen H, Hartvigsen J, et al. Manual examination of the spine: A systematic critical literature review of reproducibility. J Manipulative Physiol Ther 2006;29(6):475–85.

44 Cibulka M, Koldenhoff R. Clinical usefulness of a cluster of sacroiliac joint tests in patients with and without low back pain. J Orthop Sports Phys Ther 1999;29(2):83–9.

45 Arab A, Abdollahi I, Joghataei M, et al. Inter- and intra-examiner reliability of single

and composites of selected motion palpation and pain provocation tests for sacroiliac joint. Man Ther 2009;14(2):213–21.

46 Laslett M. Diagnosis of sacroiliac joint pain: Validity of individual provocation tests and composites of tests. Man Ther 2005;10(3):207–18.

47 The Glossary Review Committee of the Educational Council on Osteopathic Principles. Glossary of osteopathic terminology. In: Allen TW ed. AOA Yearbook and Directory of Osteopathic Physicians. Chicago, IL: American Osteopathic Association; 1993 [Glossary].

48 DiGiovanna EL, Schiowitz S, Dowling DJ. An Osteopathic Approach to Diagnosis and Treatment, 3rd edn. Philadelphia, PA: Lippincott Williams & Wilkins; 2005.

49 DeStefano L. Greenman's Principles of Manual Medicine, 4th edn. Philadelphia, PA: Lippincott Williams & Wilkins; 2010.

50 Hohner JG, Tyler CC. Thrust (high velocity/low amplitude) approach; "the pop". In: Chila A ed. Foundations of Osteopathic Medicine, 3rd edn. Philadelphia, PA: Wolters Kluwer Health/ Lippincott Williams & Wilkins; 2010 [Ch. 45].

51 Orrock P. Profile of members of the Australian Osteopathic Association: Part 1–The practitioners. Int J Osteopath Med 2009;12(1):14–24.

52 Jull G, Trott P, Potter H, et al. A randomized controlled trial of exercise and manipulative therapy for cervicogenic headache. Spine 2002;27(17):1835–43.

53 Gross A, Kay T, Kennedy C, et al. Clinical practice guideline on the use of manipulation or mobilization in the treatment of adults with mechanical neck disorders. Man Ther 2002;7(4):193–205.

54 Gross A, Hoving J, Haines T, et al. A Cochrane review of manipulation and mobilization for mechanical neck disorders. Spine 2004;29(14):1541–8.

55 Gross A, Goldsmith A, Hoving J, et al. Conservative management of mechanical neck disorders: A systematic review. J Rheumatol 2007;34(5):1083–102.

56 Hurwitz E, Carragee EJ, Van Der Velde G, et al. Treatment of neck pain: Noninvasive interventions: Results of the Bone and Joint Decade 2000-2010 Task Force on Neck Pain and Its Associated Disorders. Eur Spine J 2008;17(Suppl. 1):123–52.

57 Leaver AM, Refshauge KM, Maher CG, et al. Conservative interventions provide short-term relief for non-specific neck pain: A systematic review. J Physiother 2010;56(2):73–85.

58 Miller J, Gross A, D'Sylva J, et al. Manual therapy and exercise for neck pain: A systematic review. Man Ther 2010;15(4):334–54.

59 Boyles R, Toy P, Mellon J, et al. Effectiveness of manual physical therapy in the treatment of cervical radiculopathy: A systematic review. J Man Manip Ther 2011;19(3):135–42.

60 Forbush SW, Cox T, Wilson E. Treatment of patients with degenerative cervical radiculopathy using a multi-modal conservative approach in a geriatric population: A case series. J Orthop Sports Phys Ther 2011;41(10):723–33.

61 Licciardone J, Kearns CM, Minotti DE. Outcomes of osteopathic manual treatment for chronic low back pain according to baseline pain severity: Results from the Osteopathic Trial. Man Ther 2013;18(6):533–40.

62 Bryans R, Decina P, Descarreaux M, et al. Evidence-based guidelines for the chiropractic treatment of adults with neck pain. J Manipulative Physiol Ther 2014 37(1):42–63.

63 Maiers M, Bronfort G, Evans R, et al. Spinal manipulative therapy and exercise for seniors with chronic neck pain. Spine J 2014;14(9):1879–89.

3

Kinematics and coupled motion of the spine

Clinicians use palpatory assessment of individual intervertebral segments before the application of a thrust technique. The osteopathic profession has used Fryette's model of the physiological movements of the spine to assist in the diagnosis of somatic dysfunction and the application of treatment techniques. Fryette[1] outlined his research into the physiological movements of the vertebral column in 1918. He presented a model that indicated coupled motion occurred in the spine and displayed different coupling characteristics dependent on spinal segmental level and posture. The muscle energy approach is one system of segmental spinal lesion diagnosis and treatment predicated upon Fryette's Laws.[2] Practitioners utilizing muscle energy technique (MET) use these laws of coupled motion as a predictive model both to formulate a mechanical diagnosis and to select the precisely controlled position required in the application of both muscle energy and thrust techniques. Current literature challenges the validity of Fryette's Laws.[3]

BIOMECHANICS

Convention dictates that intervertebral motion is described in relation to motion of the superior vertebra upon the inferior vertebra. Motion is further defined in relation to the anterior surface of the vertebral body; an example would be the direction of vertebral rotation, which is described in relation to the direction in which the anterior surface of the vertebra moves rather than the posterior elements.

In the clinical setting, vertebral motion is described by using standard anatomical cardinal planes and axes of the body. Spinal motion can be described as rotation around, and translation along, an axis as the vertebral body moves along one of the cardinal planes. By convention the vertical axis is labelled the y-axis; the horizontal axis is labelled the x-axis; and the antero-posterior axis is the z-axis (Fig. 3.1).[4]

In biomechanical terms, flexion is anterior (sagittal) rotation of the superior vertebra around the x-axis, while there is accompanying forward (sagittal) translation of the vertebral body along the z-axis. In extension, the opposite occurs, and the superior vertebra rotates posteriorly around the x-axis and translates posteriorly along the z-axis. In sidebending, there is bone rotation around the antero-posterior z-axis, but sidebending is rarely a pure movement and is generally accompanied by vertebral rotation. The combination, and association, of one movement with others is termed 'coupled motion'. The concept of coupled motion is not recent. As early as 1905, Lovett[5] published his observations of coupled motion of the spine.

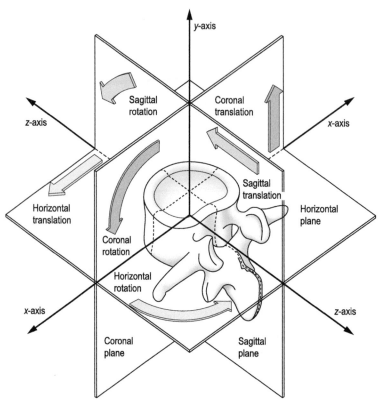

Figure 3.1 Axes of motion. (Reproduced with permission from Bogduk.[4])

COUPLED MOTION

Coupled motion is described by White and Panjabi[6] as a 'phenomenon of consistent association of one motion (translation or rotation) about an axis with another motion about a second axis'. Bogduk and Twomey[4] describe *coupled movements* as 'movements that occur in an unintended or unexpected direction during the execution of a desired motion'. Stokes et al[7] simply state coupling to be when 'a primary (or intentional) movement results in a joint also moving in other directions'. Where rotation occurs in a consistent manner as an accompaniment to sidebending it has been termed *conjunct rotation*.[8,9] Therefore, in rotation the vertebra should rotate around the vertical *y*-axis, but translation will be complex depending on the extent and direction of coupling

movements. Coupling will cause shifting axes of motion.

Greenman[10] maintains that rotation of the spinal column is always coupled with sidebending with the exception of the atlanto-axial joint. The coupled rotation can be in the same direction as sidebending (e.g. sidebending right, rotation right) or in opposite directions (e.g. sidebending right, rotation left). The osteopathic profession developed the convention of naming the coupled movements as *Type 1* and *Type 2* movements (Figs. 3.2 and 3.3).[11]

These concepts of vertebral motion are attributed to Fryette. Fryette acknowledges the contribution made to his understanding of spinal movement by Lovett. Lovett had undertaken research on cadavers in order to understand the structure and aetiology of scoliotic curves.

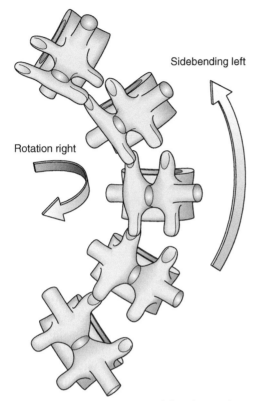

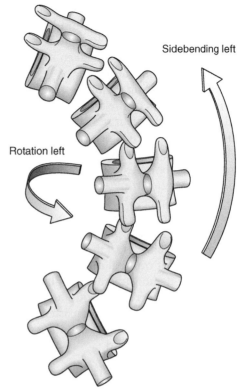

Figure 3.2 Type 1 movement. Sidebending and rotation occur to opposite sides. (Reproduced with permission from Gibbons and Tehan.[11])

Figure 3.3 Type 2 movement. Sidebending and rotation occur to the same side. (Reproduced with permission from Gibbons and Tehan.[11])

Fryette acknowledged that Lovett's findings for the thoracic and lumbar spine were correct in the position Lovett had placed the spine for his cadaveric experiments but maintained they would not be true if the lumbar and thoracic spine were placed in different positions of flexion or extension. Fryette performed his own experiments upon a 'spine mounted in soft rubber' and introduced the concept of neutral (facets not engaged) and nonneutral (facets engaged and controlling vertebral motion) positioning. Fryette defined *neutral* 'to mean the position of any area of the spine in which the facets are idling, in the position between the beginning of flexion and the beginning of extension'. In the cervical spine below C2, the facets are considered always to be in a nonneutral position and are therefore

assumed to control vertebral motion. The thoracic and lumbar regions have the possibility of neutral and nonneutral positioning. Mitchell[2] summarizes Fryette's Laws as follows:

Fryette's Laws

- Law 1. Neutral sidebending produces rotation to the other side, or, in other words, the sidebending group rotates itself towards the convexity of the sidebend, with maximum rotation at the apex.
- Law 2. Nonneutral (vertebra hyperflexed or hyperextended) rotation and sidebending go to the same side, individual joints acting at one time.
- Law 3. Introducing motion to a vertebral joint in one plane automatically reduces its mobility in the other two planes.

Research into coupled movement has been undertaken on cadavers and live subjects. Cadaver research has allowed precise measurements to be taken of coupling behaviour but has the disadvantage of being unable to reflect the activity of muscles or the accurate effects of load on different postures. Plain radiography has been superseded by biplanar radiographic studies, three-dimensional computed tomography (CT), digital videofluoroscopy and magnetic resonance imaging (MRI).

Reviews of the literature conclude that coupled motion exists, but there is conflicting evidence as to the specific characteristics of coupled motion.[12-15] Many authors have demonstrated a coupling relationship between sideflexion and rotation[9,16-34] but there is inconsistent reporting of the direction of coupling between spinal levels and individuals.[14,15,27,28,35-37]

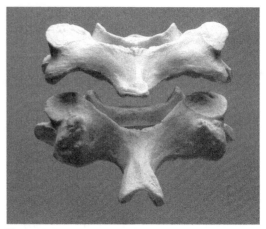

Figure 3.4

Cervical spine (Fig. 3.4)

Stoddard[16] demonstrated radiologically that sidebending in the cervical spine is always accompanied by rotation to the same side regardless of cervical posture. Stoddard's observations in relation to the cervical spine are consistent with Lovett's findings and Fryette's Laws. These findings are further supported by research undertaken using biplanar X-ray analysis,[21] three-dimensional CT imaging[33] and stereophotogrammetry.[25] In 20 normal male volunteers, when the head was rotated, lateral bending occurred by coupling in the same direction at each segment below the C3 vertebra. Interestingly coupling was not restricted to lateral bending. At the same time, flexion took place by coupling at each segment below the C5–6 vertebra and extension above the C4–5 level. Twenty healthy volunteers underwent three-dimensional CT imaging in neutral and maximum axial rotation positions. Axial rotation between the C0–1

and C1–2 segments was coupled with lateral flexion to the opposite side and extension. In the cervical spine, below C2, axial rotation was found to be maximal at the C4–5 segment and coupled with lateral flexion to the same side. Extension was associated at the segments C2 to C5, whereas flexion occurred at the segments C5 to C7.[33] In a study of active range of motion in the cervical spine during daily functional tasks, Bennett et al[26] noted that the normal coupling pattern for the cervical spine is rotation and sidebending to the same side. Three-dimensional MRI confirms that the coupling of lateral bending and axial rotation was in the same direction in the cervical spine below C2.[28] Malmstrom et al[27] confirmed this coupling behaviour in asymptomatic subjects up to the age of 70 years with decreasing coupling in all cardinal planes with increasing age. Elderly subjects (70–79 years of age) exhibited a change in coupling behaviour with rotation being coupled with contralateral lateral flexion. However, Lansade et al[38] reported that age and gender had no significant influence on coupled movements in the cervical spine in a study of 140 asymptomatic volunteers aged 20 to 93 years.

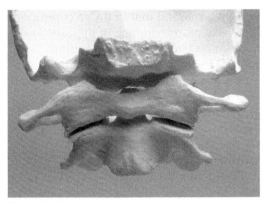

Figure 3.5

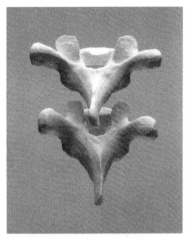

Figure 3.6

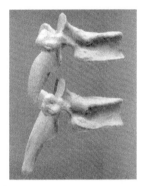

Figure 3.7

Craniocervical junction (Fig. 3.5)

The anatomy of the upper cervical spine differs significantly from the cervical spine below C2. Coupling behaviour has been reported in relation to the upper cervical spine[25,33,39–41] but has not been as extensively investigated as in other regions of the spine. Stereophotogrammetry revealed consistent coupling of axial rotation and lateral bending to the opposite side at C0–1 and C1–2, and vice versa.[25] Three-dimensional MRI[41] and three-dimensional CT[33] have confirmed the relationship between axial rotation and lateral bending to the opposite side. This is the reverse of the coupling behaviour in the cervical spine below C2.

Cervicothoracic junction (Fig. 3.6)

There is little information available in relation to the kinematics and coupling behaviour in the junctional region between the flexible cervical spine and the more rigid thoracic region. Osteopathic texts indicate that the prevailing view in relation to coupling in this region is that from C2 to C7 the coupling of axial rotation and lateral flexion is to the same side, whilst below C7 the coupling of axial rotation and lateral flexion can be either to the same or to the opposite side.[10,42] CT imaging has identified that the cervicothoracic junction is twice as stiff as the rest of the cervical spine. Reliable quantitative data for coupling behaviour of axial rotation and lateral flexion in the cervicothoracic spine remains unreported.[43]

Thoracic spine (Fig. 3.7) and lumbar spine (Fig. 3.8)

Although there is agreement as to the direction of axial rotation and lateral flexion coupling in the cervical spine below C2 (i.e. sidebending and rotation occurring to the same side), the patterns for coupling in the thoracic and lumbar spine are less clear. Fujimori et al conducted an in vivo three-dimensional study of the thoracic spine with 13 healthy volunteers. The thoracic spine was studied in three positions; neutral, right and left maximum trunk

19

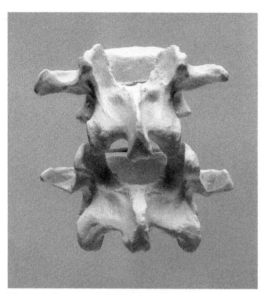

Figure 3.8

rotation. At the upper thoracic segments, lateral bending was coupled with axial rotation in the same direction, but at the middle and lower thoracic segments lateral bending occurred both in the same and opposite direction to axial rotation.[32] In another in vivo three-dimensional study of the thoracic spine with 15 healthy male volunteers, Fujimori et al observed that coupled axial rotation was generally observed in the same direction as lateral bending. However, high variability was found between the T2 and T6 segments. The thoracic spine was studied in three supine positions; neutral, right maximum lateral bending and left maximum lateral bending.[34]

Stoddard's findings in the lumbar spine were that 'sidebending is accompanied by rotation to the opposite side if the commencing position is an erect one of extension. If, however, the starting position is full flexion, sidebending is then accompanied by rotation to the same side'.[16] Russell et al, in a study of the range and coupled movements of the lumbar spine using a 3Space Isotrak system on 181 asymptomatic volunteers aged between 20

to 69 years, found that in the erect position there was strong coupling of opposite axial rotation on lateral bending.[24] Despite subjects being told to make lateral flexion as pure a lateral movement as possible, Russell et al also noted a strong coupling of flexion as well as opposite axial rotation on lateral bending. However, other authors do not support these findings and report inconsistent coupling.[9,15,18,20,22,29]

Plamondon et al, using a stereoradiographic method to study lumbar intervertebral motion in vivo, demonstrated that axial rotation and lateral bending were coupled motions but reported there was 'no strict pattern that the vertebra follow in executing a movement'.[20]

Pearcy and Tibrewal, in a three-dimensional radiographic study of normal volunteers with no history of back pain requiring time off work or medical treatment, found that the relationship between axial rotation and lateral bending is not consistent at different levels of the lumbar spine.[18] Some individuals occasionally demonstrate 'movements in the opposite direction to the voluntary movement at individual intervertebral levels, most commonly at L4–5 and L5–S1. In lateral bending, there was a general tendency for L5–S1 to bend in the opposite direction to the voluntary movement'. This unexpected finding is consistent with a study by Weitz.[44]

Panjabi et al, using fresh human cadaveric lumbar spines from L1 to the sacrum, assessed coupled motion under load in different spinal postures using stereophotogrammetry.[22] They concluded that coupling is an inherent property of the lumbar spine as advocated by Lovett[5] but that in vitro coupling patterns are more complex than generally believed. They demonstrated that the presence of muscles is not a requirement for coupled motion but acknowledged that these muscles may significantly alter coupling behaviour. The specific effect of physiological loading and muscle activity upon coupled motion is presently unknown. In a neutral posture, left axial torque produced right lateral bending at the upper lumbar levels and left lateral bending at the lower two levels, with L3–4 being a transition level. They concluded that the 'rotary coupling patterns in the lumbar spine are a function of the intervertebral level and posture'. At the upper lumbar levels, axial torque produced lateral bending to the opposite side, whereas at the lower lumbar levels axial torque produced lateral bending to the same side. It was also noted 'that the spine does not exhibit mechanical reciprocity'; for example, at L4–5, applied left axial torque produced coupled left lateral bending, but applied left lateral bending produced coupled right axial rotation.

The finding of Panjabi et al[22] that at 'L2–3, coupled lateral bending increased from about 0.5° in the fully extended posture to 1.5° in neutral and to about 2° in flexed postures' conflicts with Fryette's Third Law, which indicates that introduction of motion to a vertebral joint in one plane automatically reduces its mobility in the other two planes. In lumbar flexion the coupled lateral bending increased by 0.5° from the neutral to the flexed position.

A number of studies have indicated that coupled movement occurs independently of muscular activity.[9,17,45] In 1977, Pope et al[17] utilized a biplanar radiographic technique to evaluate spinal movements in intact cadaveric and living human subjects. They confirmed that 'vertebral motion occurs as a coupling motion and that axial rotation uniformly is associated with lateral bend'. Frymoyer et al[45] measured spinal mobility using orthogonal radiography on 20 male cadavers and nine male living subjects. They found that complex coupling does occur in the lumbar spine and demonstrated remarkably similar spinal behaviour between the two groups. These studies indicate that coupling occurs independently of muscular activity.

Vicenzino and Twomey[9] used four human male postmortem lumbar spines from L1 to the sacrum, with ligaments intact and muscles removed, to assess conjunct rotation of the spine when sidebending was introduced in both flexed and extended positions. They found that in the flexed position, lateral flexion of the lumbar spine was associated with conjunct rotation to the same side. This is consistent with Fryette's Laws. However, in the extended position, lateral flexion was associated with conjunct rotation to the opposite side, which supports Stoddard's radiographic observations of coupled motion in the extended position.[16] These findings are not consistent with Fryette's Laws, which predict that sidebending and rotation to the same side as the facets are not 'idling' when in the extended position. Vicenzino and Twomey's study reveals that the L5–S1 segment is unique in that conjunct rotation was always in the same direction as sideflexion, independent of flexion or extension positioning.[9] This finding for the L5–S1 segment was supported by Pearcy and Tibrewal, who found that during axial rotation at L5–S1, lateral bending always occurred in the same direction as the axial rotation.[18]

Vicenzino and Twomey[9] drew the conclusion that, as both in vitro and in vivo studies have demonstrated conjunct rotation, the noncontractile components of the lumbar spine may have primary responsibility for the direction of conjunct rotation and that neuromuscular activity may only modify the coupling. The impact of muscular activity on coupled motion in both the normal and dysfunctional intervertebral joint requires further study.

The presence of apophysial joint tropism might influence spinal motion and confound predictive models of vertebral coupling. The incidence of facet tropism has been reported as 20% at all lumbar levels but may increase to 30% at the L5–S1 segment.[4] The incidence of facet tropism is also higher in patient populations attending manual medicine practitioners. It has been estimated that as many as 90% of patients presenting with low back pain and sciatica have articular tropism, with pain occurring on the side of the more obliquely oriented facet.[4] Cyron and Hutton[46] subjected 23 cadaveric lumbar intervertebral joints to a combination of compressive and shear forces. When asymmetric facets were present, the vertebrae that had such facets rotated towards the side of the more oblique facet. They concluded that articular tropism could lead to lumbar instability manifesting itself as joint rotation towards the side of the more oblique facet. This was not a study of coupled motion, and no clear comments can therefore be made about the influence of facet tropism on patterns of coupling, but it does suggest that tropism can influence spinal mechanics.

Disc degeneration and spinal pathology presenting with pain and nerve root signs might also influence spinal coupling. In 1985 Pearcy et al[19] undertook a three-dimensional radiographic analysis of lumbar spinal movements. They studied patients with back pain alone and patients with back pain plus nerve tension signs demonstrated by restricted straight leg raise. Coupled movements were increased only in those patients without nerve tension signs, indicating the possibility of asymmetrical muscle action. It was concluded that 'the disturbance from the normal pattern of coupled movements in the group with back pain alone suggests that the ligaments or muscles were involved unilaterally and thus acted asymmetrically when the patient moved'. The fact that coupled movements were increased in the back pain group suggests that muscular activity, although not essential for coupling, can influence the magnitude of coupled movement. The action of the contractile elements in normal, dysfunctional and pain states requires more study before any definite statements can be made relating to their effect upon coupled

motion. Using percutaneous transpedicular screws and optoelectronic camera measurement, Lund et al demonstrated that chronic low back pain patients had different coupling behaviour from that of the normal population.[47]

It is evident that many factors such as facet tropism, vertebral level, intervertebral disc height, back pain and spinal position might influence the degree and direction of coupling.

Although it appears that Fryette's Laws are open to question and clinicians' concepts of lumbar coupling are inconsistent,[48] there are still only two possibilities for the coupling of sidebending and rotation: to the same side or the opposite side. With this in mind, it appears reasonable to classify spinal movement as Type 1 and Type 2 in relation to coupled sidebending and rotation. What is not clearly established is the influence of flexion and extension in relation to Type 1 and Type 2 movements.

CONCLUSION

Conclusions that can be drawn from the literature are limited for a number of reasons. Cadaver studies exclude the effects of muscular activity and normal physiological loading; the studies were also often single segment analysis and generally of small sample size. Plain radiographic studies have inherent measuring difficulties associated with extrapolating three-dimensional movements from two-dimensional films. The use of biplanar radiographic assessment, CT and MRI has improved the accuracy of measurement and allowed studies to be performed with muscular activity and in more normal physiological conditions; again, however, the groups studied were small. Notwithstanding these observations, there are a number of conclusions that can be drawn:

1. Coupled motion occurs in all regions of the spine.
2. Coupled motion occurs independently of muscular activity, but muscular activity might influence the direction and magnitude of coupled movement.
3. Coupling of sidebending and rotation in the thoracic and lumbar spine is variable in degree and direction.
4. Many variables can influence the degree and direction of coupled movement and include pain, vertebral level, posture and facet tropism.
5. There does not appear to be any simple and consistent relationship between conjunct rotation and intervertebral motion segment level in the thoracic and lumbar spine.

There is evidence to support Lovett's initial observations and Fryette's Laws in relation to sidebending and rotation coupling in the cervical spine, that is, sidebending and rotation occur to the same side.[16,21,25,28] However, the evidence in relation to lumbar and thoracic spine coupling is inconsistent.[9,15,18,20,22,29,32]

Although Fryette's Laws may be useful for predicting coupling behaviour in the cervical spine, caution should be exercised when applying these laws for assessment and treatment of the thoracic and lumbar spine.

There has been limited investigation of the coupling behaviour in the craniocervical and cervicothoracic regions. However, evidence suggests that at C0–1 and C1–2, axial rotation and lateral bending occur to opposite sides.[25,33,41]

References

1 Fryette H. Principles of Osteopathic Technic. Newark, OH: American Academy of Osteopathy; 1954 (Reprint 1990).

2 Mitchell FL. The Muscle Energy Manual. East Lansing, MI: MET Press; 1995.

3 Fryer G. Muscle energy technique: An evidence informed approach. Int J Osteopath Med 2011;14:3–9.

4 Bogduk N, Twomey LT. Clinical Anatomy of the Lumbar Spine and Sacrum, 3rd edn. Melbourne, Australia: Churchill Livingstone; 1997.

5 Lovett RW. The mechanism of the normal spine and its relation to scoliosis. Boston Med Surg J 1905;13:349–58.

6 White A, Panjabi M. Clinical Biomechanics of the Spine. Toronto, Canada: Lippincott Company; 1990.

7 Stokes I, Wilder D, Frymoyer J, et al. Assessment of patients with low-back pain by biplanar radiographic measurement of intervertebral motion. Spine 1981;6(3):233–40.

8 MacConaill M. The geometry and algebra of articular kinematics. Biomed Eng 1966;5:205–11.

9 Vicenzino G, Twomey L. Sideflexion induced lumbar spine conjunct rotation and its influencing factors. Aust J Physiother 1993;39(4):299–306.

10 DeStefano L. Greenman's Principles of Manual Medicine, 4th edn. Philadelphia, PA: Lippincott Williams & Wilkins; 2010.

11 Gibbons P, Tehan P. Muscle energy concepts and coupled motion of the spine. Man Ther 1998;3(2):95–101.

12 Brown L. An introduction to the treatment and examination of the spine by combined movements. Physiotherapy 1988;74(7):347–53.

13 Brown L. Treatment and examination of the spine by combined movements–2. Physiotherapy 1990;76(2):666–74.

14 Legaspi O, Edmond S. Does the evidence support the existence of lumbar spine coupled motion? A critical review of the literature. J Orthop Sports Phys Ther 2007;37(4):169–78.

15 Sizer P, Brismee J-M, Cook C. Coupling behaviour of the thoracic spine: A systematic review of literature. J Manipulative Physiol Ther 2007;30(5):390–9.

16 Stoddard A. Manual of Osteopathic Practice. London, UK: Hutchinson Medical Publications; 1969.

17 Pope M, Wilder D, Matteri R, et al. Experimental measurements of vertebral motion under load. Orthop Clin North Am 1977;8(1):155–67.

18 Pearcy M, Tibrewal S. Axial rotation and lateral bending in the normal lumbar spine measured

by three-dimensional radiography. Spine 1984;9(6):582–7.

19 Pearcy M, Portek I, Shepherd J. The effect of low back pain on lumbar spinal movements measured by three-dimensional X-ray analysis. Spine 1985;10(2):150–3.

20 Plamondon A, Gagnon M, Maurais G. Application of a stereoradiographic method for the study of intervertebral motion. Spine 1988;13(9):1027–32.

21 Mimura M, Moriya H, Watanabe T, et al. Three dimensional motion analysis of the cervical spine with special reference to the axial rotation. Spine 1989;14(11):1135–9.

22 Panjabi M, Yamamoto I, Oxland T, et al. How does posture affect coupling in the lumbar spine? Spine 1989;14(9):1002–11.

23 Nagerl H, Kubein-Meesenburg D, Fanghanel J. Elements of a general theory of joints. Anat Anz 1992;174(1):66–75.

24 Russell P, Pearcy M, Unsworth A. Measurement of the range and coupled movements observed in the lumbar spine. Br J Rheumatol 1993;32(6):490–7.

25 Panjabi M, Crisco J, Vasavada A, et al. Mechanical properties of the human cervical spine as shown by three-dimensional load–displacement curves. Spine 2001;26(24):2692–700.

26 Bennett SE, Schenk R, Simmons E. Active range of motion utilized in the cervical spine to perform daily functional tasks. J Spinal Disord Tech 2002;15(4):307–11.

27 Malmstrom E-M, Karlberg M, Fransson P, et al. Primary and coupled cervical movements. The effect of age, gender, and body mass index. A 3-dimensional movement analysis of a population without symptoms of neck disorders. Spine 2006;31(2):E44–50.

28 Ishii T, Mukai Y, Hosono N, et al. Kinematics of the cervical spine in lateral bending. In vivo three-dimensional analysis. Spine 2006;31(2):155–60.

29 Edmondston S, Aggerholm M, Elfving S, et al. Influence of posture on the range of axial rotation and coupled lateral flexion of the thoracic spine. J Manipulative Physiol Ther 2007;30(3):193–9.

30 Fujii R, Sakaura H, Mukai Y, et al. Kinematics of the lumbar spine in trunk rotation: In vivo three-dimensional analysis using magnetic resonance imaging. Eur Spine J 2007;16(11):1867–74.

31 Lee BW, Lee JE, Lee SH, et al. Kinematic analysis of the lumbar spine by digital

videofluoroscopy in 18 asymptomatic subjects and 9 patients with herniated nucleus pulposus. J Manipulative Physiol Ther 2011;34(4):221–30.

32 Fujimori T, Iwasaki M, Nagamoto Y, et al. Kinematics of the thoracic spine in trunk rotation: In vivo 3-dimensional analysis. Spine 2012;37(21):E1318–28.

33 Salem W, Lenders C, Mathieu J, et al. In-vivo three-dimensional kinematics of the cervical spine during maximal axial rotation. Man Ther 2013;18(4):339–44.

34 Fujimori T, Iwasaki M, Nagamoto Y, et al. Kinematics of the thoracic spine in trunk lateral bending: In vivo 3-dimensional analysis. Spine J 2014;14(9):1991–9.

35 Cook C. Coupling behavior of the lumbar spine: A literature review. J Man Manip Ther 2003;11(3):137–45.

36 Edmondston SJ, Henne SE, Loh W, et al. Influence of cranio-cervical posture on three-dimensional motion of the cervical spine. Man Ther 2005;10:44–51.

37 Cook C, Hegedus E, Showalter C, et al. Coupling behaviour of the cervical spine: A systematic review of the literature. J Manipulative Physiol Ther 2006;29:570–5.

38 Lansade C, Laporte S, Thoreux P, et al. Three-dimensional analysis of the cervical spine kinematics: Effect of age and gender in healthy subjects. Spine 2009;34(26):2900–6.

39 Panjabi M, Oda T, Crisco J, et al. Posture affects motion coupling patterns of the upper cervical spine. J Orthop Res 1993;11(4):525–36.

40 Amiri M, Jull G, Bullock-Saxton J. Measurement of upper cervical flexion and extension with the 3-space fast-track measurement system: A repeatability study. J Man Manip Ther 2003;11(4):198–203.

41 Ishii T, Mukai Y, Hosono N, et al. Kinematics of the upper cervical spine in rotation. In vivo three- dimensional analysis. Spine 2004;29(7):E139–44.

42 Ehrenfeuchter WC. Segmental motion testing. In: Chila A ed. Foundations of Osteopathic Medicine, 3rd edn. Philadelphia, PA: Wolters Kluwer Health/Lippincott Williams & Wilkins; 2010 [Ch. 35].

43 Simon S, Davis M, Odhner D, et al. CT imaging techniques for describing motions of the cervicothoracic junction and cervical spine during flexion, extension, and cervical traction. Spine 2006;31(1):44–50.

44 Weitz E. The lateral bending sign. Spine 1981;6(4):388–97.

45 Frymoyer JW, Frymoyer WW, Wilder DG, et al. The mechanical and kinematic analysis of the lumbar spine in normal living human subjects in vivo. J Biomech 1979;12:165–72.

46 Cyron BM, Hutton WC. Articular tropism and stability of the lumbar spine. Spine 1980;5(2):168–72.

47 Lund T, Nydegger T, Ing D, et al. Three-dimensional motion patterns during active bending in patients with chronic low back pain. Spine 2002;27(17):1865–74.

48 Cook C, Showalter C. A survey on the importance of lumbar coupling biomechanics in physiotherapy practice. Man Ther 2004;9(3):164–72.

4

Minimal leverage positioning for HVLA thrust techniques

Note: Minimal leverage positioning on the website should be viewed in conjunction with Chapter 4.

SPINAL POSITIONING

Spinal locking has been described as being necessary for long-lever high-velocity low-amplitude (HVLA) thrust techniques to localize forces and achieve cavitation at a specific vertebral segment.[1-7] Short-lever HVLA thrust techniques do not require locking of adjacent spinal segments.

Positioning can be achieved by either facet apposition or the utilization of ligamentous myofascial tension (Box 4.1).[1-5,7] The principle used in both these approaches is to position the spine in such a way that leverage is localized to one joint without undue strain being placed upon adjacent segments.

The osteopathic profession developed a nomenclature to classify spinal motion based upon the coupling of sidebending and rotation movements. This coupling behaviour will vary depending on spinal positioning:

- Type 1 movement–sidebending and rotation occur in opposite directions (Fig. 4.1[8])
- Type 2 movement–sidebending and rotation occur in the same direction (Fig. 4.2[8]).

The principle of facet apposition positioning is to apply leverages to the spine that cause the facet joints of uninvolved segments to be apposed and consequently locked. To achieve locking by facet apposition, the spine is placed in a position opposite to that of normal coupling behaviour. This approach is commonly used in more mobile parts of the spine, e.g. the cervical and lumbar spine or where patients have mobile and flexible spines.

The principle of ligamentous myofascial positioning is to use the normal physiological movements to localize the leverages to one vertebral segment. To achieve locking by ligamentous myofascial tension, the spine is placed in a position of normal coupling behaviour, and this positioning can be unidirectional or multidirectional. This

Box 4.1 Positioning for HVLA thrust techniques

Facet Apposition	Position OPPOSITE to normal coupling behaviour.	Commonly used in flexible regions, e.g. cervical/lumbar spine and with more flexible patients.
Ligamentous Myofascial	Position WITH normal coupling behaviour.	Commonly used in stiffer regions, e.g. thoracic spine and with less flexible patients.

HVLA, high-velocity, low-amplitude.

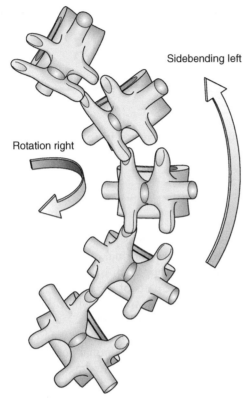

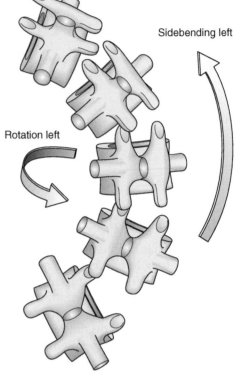

Figure 4.1 Type 1 movement. Sidebending and rotation occur to opposite sides. (Reproduced with permission from Gibbons and Tehan.[8])

Figure 4.2 Type 2 movement. Sidebending and rotation occur to the same side. (Reproduced with permission from Gibbons and Tehan.[8])

approach is commonly used in less mobile parts of the spine, e.g. the thoracic spine, or where patients have stiffer and less flexible spines.

In both these positioning approaches, the vertebral segment at which you wish to produce cavitation should be left free to move and never be locked.

Minimal Leverage Versus Barrier Positioning

Some authors describe the correct positioning for HVLA thrust techniques as placing the segment you wish to cavitate at the restricted motion barrier.[7,9,10] This barrier approach to prethrust positioning can result in full end-range leverages being used in positions that are often uncomfortable for the patient.

Box 4.2 Patient comfort and safety
Minimal leverage approach and NOT end-range or at motion restriction barrier.

Having consideration for patient comfort and safety (Box 4.2), an alternative minimal leverage approach to prethrust positioning is recommended. The positioning is not at end-range or at the motion restriction barrier. The goal is to use the least amount of leverage that will enable the practitioner to safely and effectively achieve a cavitation at the targeted segment in a position that is comfortable for the patient.

When students or practitioners start learning how to apply HVLA thrust

Table 4.1

Spinal level	Coupled motion	Facet apposition locking
C0–1 (occipito-atlantal)	Type 1	Type 2
C1–2 (atlanto-axial)	Complex-primary rotation	Not applicable
C2–7	Type 2	Type 1

techniques, they may find it necessary to use increased leverages, but the prethrust positioning should never be at end-range. With time and practice, the ability to apply quicker velocity thrusts enables practitioners to use even less leverage in the prethrust positioning.

SPINAL POSITIONING

When applying HVLA thrust techniques, it is important to understand that the model presented relates to spinal positioning and is not a model for evaluation and diagnosis of somatic dysfunction.

Cervical Spine

A number of authors describe the normal coupling at the occipito-atlantal (C0–1) segment as axial rotation and lateral bending to the opposite side (i.e. Type 1 movement).[7,11–13] The principle of facet apposition locking does not apply to HVLA thrust techniques directed to the C0–1 segment. However, facet apposition locking can be utilized for HVLA thrust techniques directed to most other cervical levels (Table 4.1).

The type of coupled movement available at the C1–2 segment is complex. This segment has a predominant role in total cervical rotation.[14–17] Up to 77% of total cervical rotation occurs at the atlanto-axial joint, with a mean rotation range of 40.5° to either side.[14,16] The great range of rotation at the atlanto-axial joint can be attributed to facet plane, the loose nature of the ligamentous fibrous capsule and the absence

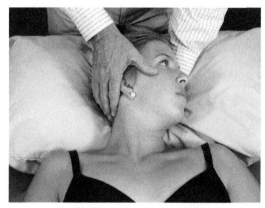

Figure 4.3 Full left cervical spine rotation.

of ligamentum flavum above C2.[17] Only a small amount of rotation occurs at the joints above and below the atlanto-axial joint.[18–20]

Below C2, normal coupling behaviour in the cervical spine is Type 2 (i.e. sidebending and rotation occur to the same side).[7,11,21–25] The average range of cervical spine rotation from neutral position is 80° (Fig. 4.3).[26] For patient comfort and safety, the practitioner should limit the total range of cervical spine rotation when applying thrust techniques. Below C2 this is achieved by combining cervical spine rotation with opposite sidebending (Fig. 4.4). To generate facet apposition locking for HVLA thrust techniques, the operator must introduce a Type 1 movement, which is sidebending of the cervical spine in one direction and rotation in the opposite direction (e.g. sidebending right with rotation left). This positioning stiffens the segments above the joint to be cavitated and enables a thrust to

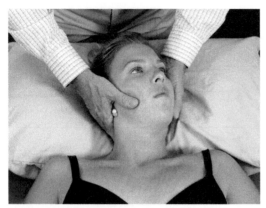

Figure 4.4 Introduction of right sidebending limits the range of available left cervical spine rotation.

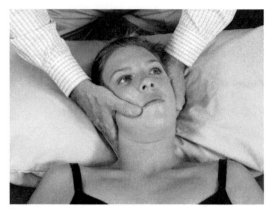

Figure 4.6 Primary sidebending (facet apposition) positioning for down-slope gliding.

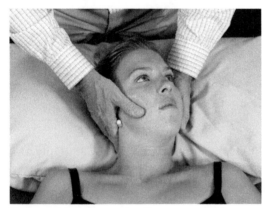

Figure 4.5 Primary rotation (facet apposition) positioning for up-slope gliding.

Box 4.3 Modifications for the stiffer cervical spine

Primary rotation positioning (up-slope)	Lessen or remove secondary sidebending leverage.
Primary sidebending positioning (down-slope)	Lessen or remove secondary rotation leverage.

be applied to one vertebral segment. The amount or degree of sidebending and rotation can be varied to obtain facet locking. The intent should be to have a primary and secondary leverage. The principal or primary leverage can be either sidebending or rotation.

There are two types of prethrust facet apposition positioning that can be used between C2 and C7:

1. **Primary rotation facet apposition positioning** for up-slope gliding. A primary leverage of rotation in one direction with a small amount of secondary leverage of sidebending to the opposite direction (Fig. 4.5).

2. **Primary sidebending (facet apposition) positioning** for down-slope gliding. A primary leverage of sidebending in one direction with a small amount of secondary leverage of rotation to the opposite direction (Fig. 4.6).

Modifications in prethrust positioning may be necessary both for the stiffer and less flexible cervical spine (Box 4.3) and the more mobile or very flexible cervical spine (Box 4.4). Refer to the videos on the website to view these modifications in more detail.

Rationale for Choice of Positioning

The rationale underpinning patient positioning when applying HVLA thrust techniques is to use a model of coupling behaviour that facilitates effective localization of forces to a specific segment of the spine before the application of a thrust. The joint to be thrust should remain free to move and not be locked by the prethrust positioning.

The choice of whether to use the primary rotation or primary sidebending prethrust positioning is initially determined by patient comfort. If a patient has limited cervical spine rotation, then the primary sidebending position is often more comfortable for the patient. If a patient has limited cervical spine sidebending, then the primary rotation position is often more comfortable for the patient. If both positions are comfortable for the patient, the primary rotation (up-slope) positioning is often used when palpation reveals segmental flexion or rotation motion restriction, and the primary sidebending (down-slope) positioning is often used when palpation reveals segmental extension or sidebending motion restriction. If no prethrust positioning is comfortable for the patient, then cervical spine HVLA thrust techniques (C2–7) are contraindicated.

The principles of both facet apposition and ligamentous myofascial positioning that apply to the cervical spine are also utilized for HVLA thrust techniques to the cervicothoracic junction (C7–T3). If cervicothoracic region techniques require facet apposition locking via the cervical spine, this is achieved by introducing Type 1 movements to the cervical spine.

Thoracic and Lumbar Spine

Current research relating to coupled movements of sidebending and rotation in the thoracic and lumbar spine is inconsistent. Although research does not validate any single model for spinal positioning and locking in the thoracic and lumbar spine, the model in Table 4.2 is useful for teaching HVLA thrust techniques.

Evidence supports the view that spinal posture and positioning alter coupling behaviour.[27–30] This has implications for joint locking and positioning in the thoracic and lumbar spine. In relation to patient positioning, the locking procedures will be different depending on whether the patient's spine is placed in a flexed or a neutral/extended position, with evidence indicating that small changes in flexion or extension can significantly alter coupling behaviour.[30]

Box 4.4 Modifications for the flexible cervical spine

Primary rotation positioning (up-slope)	Incorporate lateral translation as well as secondary sidebending leverage.
Primary sidebending positioning (down-slope)	Incorporate lateral translation as well as primary sidebending leverage.

Table 4.2

	Coupled motion	Facet apposition locking
Spinal level		
C7–T3	Type 1 or Type 2	Type 2 or Type 1
T3–L5	Type 1 or Type 2	Type 2 or Type 1
Position of spine T3–L5		
Flexion	Type 2	Type 1–sidebending and rotation to the opposite side
Neutral/extension	Type 1	Type 2–sidebending and rotation to the same side

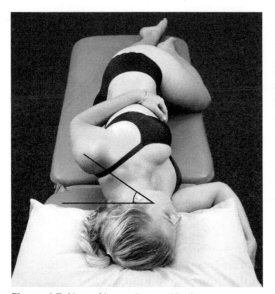

Figure 4.7 Neutral/extension positioning.

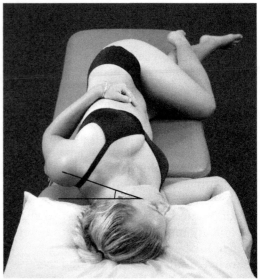

Figure 4.8 Note increased rotation with introduction of trunk flexion from below.

There is some evidence to support the view that in the flexed position, the coupling of sidebending and rotation is to the same side,[27,29] whereas in the neutral/extended position, the coupling of sidebending and rotation occurs to opposite sides.[27,28,31] The model outlined in Table 4.2 incorporates the available evidence and is useful in the teaching and application of HVLA thrust techniques. Because the evidence for coupling behaviour is inconsistent, it must be understood that this is a model for facet apposition positioning and cannot be relied upon in all circumstances.

Because the thoracic spine and rib cage have limited mobility compared with the cervical and lumbar spinal segments, ligamentous myofascial positioning is commonly used for thoracic spine and rib HVLA thrust techniques between T4 and T10.

For patient comfort and safety, the practitioner should limit the total amount of trunk rotation and torsion when using HVLA thrust techniques between T10 and S1. In most instances, this can be achieved by using the facet apposition model with an

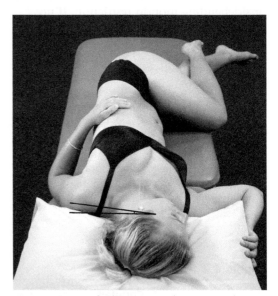

Figure 4.9 Note further increased rotation with introduction of trunk flexion from both above and below.

understanding of coupled motion in the neutral/extension and flexion positions. HVLA thrust techniques can be applied in either a neutral/extension or in a flexed position. In the example of neutral/extension positioning (Fig. 4.7), the practitioner uses spinal positioning and locking to limit the total range of trunk rotation. If the practitioner introduces trunk flexion either from below (Fig. 4.8) or from above and below (Fig. 4.9), an increased range of trunk rotation is then required to achieve the necessary locking before the application of an HVLA thrust technique.

In the example of flexion positioning (Fig. 4.10), the practitioner uses spinal positioning and locking to limit the total range of trunk rotation. If the practitioner removes the rolled towel under the patient's lumbar spine, an increased range of trunk rotation is then required to achieve the necessary locking (Fig. 4.11) before the application of an HVLA thrust technique. Minimizing the amount of trunk rotation in prethrust positioning for sidelying HVLA thrust techniques between T10 and S1 has two benefits. Firstly, this approach lessens the risk of strain and discomfort to the patient's rib cage and spine. Secondly, the practitioner is able to deliver a thrust with a more upright, less bent-forward posture, which enables better utilization of the practitioner's body weight when applying the thrust.

There are two types of prethrust facet apposition positioning that can be used for sidelying HVLA thrust techniques between T10 and S1.

Neutral/extension (facet apposition) positioning

The patient's lumbar and thoracic spine is positioned in a neutral/extended posture (Fig. 4.12). Using the model outlined, the normal coupling behaviour of sidebending and rotation in the neutral/extension position is Type 1 movement. Facet apposition locking will be achieved by introducing a Type 2 movement (i.e. sidebending and rotation to the same side).

The spine in the neutral/extension position is slung between the pelvis and shoulder girdle and creates a long 'C' curve

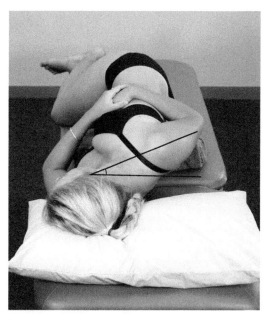

Figure 4.10 Flexion positioning.

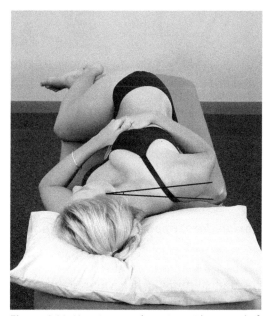

Figure 4.11 Note increased rotation with removal of rolled towel.

with the trunk sidebending to the patient's right when the patient lies on the left side.

Trunk rotation to the right is introduced by gently moving the patient's upper shoulder away from the operator. Rotation and

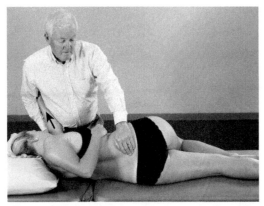

Figure 4.12 Neutral/extension positioning. Direction of body movement (patient).

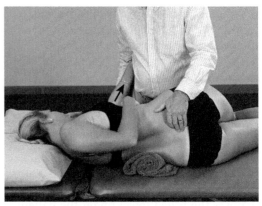

Figure 4.14 Flexion positioning. Direction of body movement (patient).

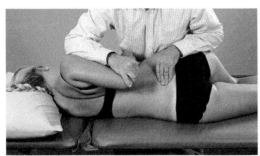

Figure 4.13 Neutral/extension positioning. Type 2 locking. Rotation and sidebending to the same side, i.e. sidebending right and rotation right.

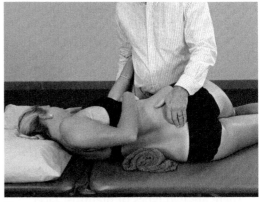

Figure 4.15 Flexion positioning. Type 1 locking. Rotation and sidebending to opposite sides, i.e. sidebending left and rotation right.

sidebending to the same side achieve facet apposition locking in the neutral or extended position, in this instance with sidebending and rotation to the right (Fig. 4.13).

Flexion (facet apposition) positioning

The patient's lumbar and thoracic spine is positioned in a flexed posture (Fig. 4.14). The normal coupling behaviour of sidebending and rotation in the flexed position is Type 2 movement. Facet apposition locking will be achieved by introducing a Type 1 movement (i.e. sidebending and rotation to opposite sides).

To achieve facet apposition locking of the spine, in the flexed posture, the trunk must be rotated and sidebent to opposite sides. The operator introduces trunk sidebending

to the left by placing a rolled towel under the patient's lumbar spine. Trunk rotation to the right is introduced by gently moving the patient's upper shoulder away from the operator (Fig. 4.15).

As practitioners gain experience in applying sidelying HVLA thrust techniques (T10–S1), they can dispense with the rolled towel for flexion positioning and achieve sidebending opposite to the direction of rotation by using manually applied forces to the thorax and pelvis (Fig. 4.16).

Modifications in prethrust positioning may be necessary both for the stiffer and less flexible (Box 4.5) and the more mobile

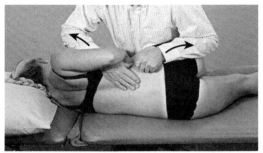

Figure 4.16 Flexion positioning. Type 1 locking. Rotation and sidebending to opposite sides, i.e. sidebending left and rotation right using manually applied forces to the thorax and pelvis. Direction of manually applied forces.

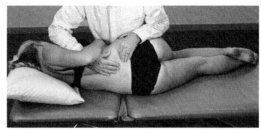

Figure 4.17 Modification for the stiffer thoracolumbar spine.

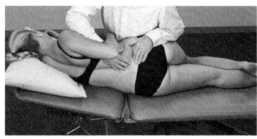

Figure 4.18 Modification for the flexible thoracolumbar spine. Neutral/extension positioning

Box 4.5 Modification for the stiffer thoracolumbar spine (T10–S1)

Use ligamentous myofascial positioning, e.g. flexion positioning without a rolled towel or without manually applied opposite sidebending (Fig. 4.17).

Box 4.6 Modification for the flexible thoracolumbar spine (T10–S1)

In sidelying, use facet apposition positioning with an increase of the sidebending leverage, e.g. neutral/extension positioning with part of the treatment couch elevated (Fig. 4.18).

or very flexible (Box 4.6) thoracolumbar spine (T10–S1). Refer to the videos on the website to view these modifications in more detail.

Many factors such as facet tropism, vertebral level, intervertebral disc height, back pain and spinal position can affect coupling behaviour, and there will be occasions when the model outlined needs to be modified to suit an individual patient. In such circumstances, the operator will need to adjust patient positioning to facilitate effective localization of forces. To achieve this, the operator must develop the palpatory skills necessary to sense appropriate prethrust tension and leverage before delivering the HVLA thrust.

RATIONALE FOR CHOICE OF POSITIONING

The rationale underpinning patient positioning when applying HVLA thrust techniques is to use a model of coupling behaviour that facilitates effective localization of forces to a specific segment of the spine before the application of a thrust. The joint to be thrust should remain free to move and not be locked by the prethrust positioning. The choice of whether to use neutral/extension or flexion facet apposition positioning is initially determined by patient comfort. For example, some patients present with a forward bent posture and are unable to comfortably assume the neutral/extension prethrust positioning. In such cases flexion positioning would be utilized. In a patient with a stiffer, less mobile thoracolumbar spine (T10–S1), flexion positioning without a rolled towel or without manually applied opposite sidebending is generally the position of choice (Fig.4.17). In a patient with a flexible thoracolumbar spine (T10–S1), facet apposition positioning is generally necessary, and this can be either neutral/extension or flexion dependent on the most comfortable positioning for the patient. This approach to patient positioning is more comfortable for the patient, increases the likelihood of achieving cavitation and minimizes the risk of posttreatment soreness. If no pre-thrust positioning is comfortable for the patient, then HVLA thrust techniques for the thoracolumbar spine (T10–S1) are contraindicated.

References

1 Nyberg R. Manipulation: Definition, types, application. In: Basmajian J, Nyberg R eds. Rational Manual Therapies. Baltimore, MD: Williams & Wilkins; 1993:21–47.

2 Downing CH. Principles and Practice of Osteopathy. London, UK: Tamor Pierston; 1985.

3 Stoddard A. Manual of Osteopathic Technique, 2nd edn. London, UK: Hutchinson Medical; 1972.

4 Hartman L. Handbook of Osteopathic Technique, 3rd edn. London, UK: Chapman & Hall; 1997.

5 Beal MC. Teaching of basic principles of osteopathic manipulative techniques. In: Beal MC ed. 1989. The Principles of Palpatory Diagnosis and Manipulative Technique. Newark, OH: American Academy of Osteopathy; 1989:162–4.

6 Kappler RE. Direct action techniques. In: Beal MC ed. The Principles of Palpatory Diagnosis and Manipulative Technique. Newark, OH: American Academy of Osteopathy; 1989; 165–8.

7 DeStefano L. Greenman's Principles of Manual Medicine, 4th edn. Philadelphia, PA: Lippincott Williams & Wilkins; 2010.

8 Gibbons P, Tehan P. Muscle energy concepts and coupled motion of the spine. Man Ther 1998;3(2):95–101.

9 DiGiovanna EL, Schiowitz S, Dowling DJ. An Osteopathic Approach to Diagnosis and Treatment, 3rd edn. Philadelphia, PA: Lippincott Williams & Wilkins; 2005.

10 Hohner JG, Tyler CC. Thrust (high velocity/low amplitude) approach; "the pop". In: Chila A ed. Foundations of Osteopathic Medicine, 3rd ed. Philadelphia, PA: Wolters Kluwer Health/Lippincott Williams & Wilkins; 2010: Ch. 45.

11 Panjabi M, Crisco J, Vasavada A, et al. Mechanical properties of the human cervical spine as shown by three-dimensional load–displacement curves. Spine 2001;26(24):2692–700.

12 Ishii T, Mukai Y, Hosono N, et al. Kinematics of the upper cervical spine in rotation. In vivo three-dimensional analysis. Spine 2004;29(7):E139–44.

13 Salem W, Lenders C, Mathieu J, et al. In-vivo three-dimensional kinematics of the cervical spine during maximal axial rotation. Man Ther 2013;18(4):339–44.

14 Penning L, Wilmink JT. Rotation of the cervical spine: A CT study in normal subjects. Spine 1987;12(8):732–8.

15 Mimura M, Moriya H, Watanabe T, et al. Three dimensional motion analysis of the cervical spine with special reference to axial rotation. Spine 1989;14(11):1135–9.

16 Iai H, Moriya H, Takahashi K, et al. Three dimensional motion analysis of upper cervical spine during axial rotation. Spine 1993;18(16): 2388–92.

17 Guth M. A comparison of cervical rotation in age-matched adolescent competitive swimmers and healthy males. J Orthop Sports Phys Ther 1995;21(1):21–7.

18 Penning L. Normal movements of the cervical spine. J Roentgenol 1978;130(2):317–26.

19 White A, Panjabi M. Clinical Biomechanics of the Spine, 2nd edn. Philadelphia, PA: Lippincott; 1990.

20 Porterfield JA, DeRosa C. Mechanical Neck Pain: Perspectives in Functional Anatomy. Sydney, Australia: WB Saunders; 1995.

21 Mimura M, Moriya H, Watanabe T, et al. Three dimensional motion analysis of the cervical spine with special reference to the axial rotation. Spine 1989;14(11):1135–9.

22 Stoddard A. Manual of Osteopathic Practice. London, UK: Hutchinson Medical; 1969.

23 Bennett SE, Schenk R, Simmons E. Active range of motion utilized in the cervical spine to perform daily functional tasks. J Spinal Disord Tech 2002;15(4):307–11.

24 Ishii T, Mukai Y, Hosono N, et al. Kinematics of the cervical spine in lateral bending. In vivo

three-dimensional analysis. Spine 2006;31(2): 155–60.

25 Malmstrom E-M, Karlberg M, Fransson P, et al. Primary and coupled cervical movements. The effect of age, gender, and body mass index. A 3-dimensional movement analysis of a population without symptoms of neck disorders. Spine 2006;31(2):E44–50.

26 American Medical Association. Guides to the Evaluation of Permanent Impairment, 4th edn. Chicago, IL: American Medical Association; 1999.

27 Vicenzino G, Twomey L. Sideflexion induced lumbar spine conjunct rotation and its influencing factors. Aust J Physiother 1993;39(4):299–306.

28 Fryette H. Principles of Osteopathic Technic. Newark, OH: American Academy of Osteopathy; 1954:15–21 (reprinted 1990).

29 Panjabi M, Yamamoto I, Oxland T, et al. How does posture affect coupling in the lumbar spine? Spine 1989;14(9):1002–11.

30 Drake J, Callaghan J. Do flexion/extension postures affect the in vivo passive lumbar spine response to applied axial twist moments? Clin Biomech 2008;23(5):510–19.

31 Russell P, Pearcy M, Unsworth A. Measurement of the range and coupled movements observed in the lumbar spine. Br J Rheumatol 1993;32(6): 490–7.

5

Safety and HVLA thrust techniques

INTRODUCTION

There are risks and benefits associated with any therapeutic intervention. High-velocity low-amplitude (HVLA) thrust techniques are distinguished from other osteopathic techniques because the practitioner applies a rapid thrust or impulse. Thrust or impulse techniques have been considered potentially more dangerous compared with nonimpulse mobilization.

COMPLICATIONS

Incidence

Cervical spine

Most published literature relating to the incidence of injury resulting from manipulative techniques focuses upon serious sequelae resulting from cervical spine manipulation.

There is wide variation in estimated serious adverse reactions arising from cervical manipulation. Various authors have attempted to estimate the incidence of iatrogenic stroke following cervical spine manipulation.[1-14] Estimates vary from one incident in 10 000 cervical spine manipulations to one incident in 5.85 million cervical spine manipulations. Rivett and Milburn[9] estimated the incidence of severe neurovascular compromise to be within the range of 1 in 50 000 to 1 in 5 million cervical spine manipulations. Other authors estimate complications for cervical spine manipulation to be 1.46 times per 1 million manipulations[15] and 1 case of cerebrovascular accident in every 1.3 million cervical treatment sessions increasing to 1 in every 0.9 million for upper cervical manipulation.[6] Boyle et al[14] reported that the incidence of stroke following manipulation is around 6 cases in every 100 000 of the population, while Patijn[8] found an overall rate of 1 complication per 518 886 manipulations. Miley et al[13] estimated the incidence of vertebral artery dissection attributable to cervical spine manipulation as 1.3 cases for every 100 000 persons less than 45 years of age within 1 week of manipulation. The published research does not make clear which types of neck manipulation technique were applied or the competence and training of the practitioner.[16]

Published figures may not accurately reflect the true incidence of serious cervical spine complications.[7-9,17-19] The frequency with which complications arise in patients receiving cervical spine manipulation can only be an estimate as the true number of manipulations performed and the numbers of patients receiving cervical manipulation remain unknown.[20] In relation to vertebral artery dissection, Haldeman et al[21] indicated that a database of multiple millions of cervical manipulations are necessary to

Table 5.1 Description of trivial trauma associated with vertebrobasilar artery dissection/occlusion cases

Type of trivial trauma	Examples	No. of cases
Sporting activities	Basketball, tennis, softball, swimming, callisthenics	18
Leisure activities	Walking, kneeling at prayer, household chores, sexual intercourse	8
Sustained rotation and/or extension	Wallpapering, washing walls and ceilings, archery, yoga	10
Short-lived rotation and/or extension	Turning head while driving, backing out of driveway, looking up	7
Sudden head movements	Sneezing, fair ride, violent coughing, sudden head flexion	7
Miscellaneous, minor trauma	Minor fall, 'banging' head	2
Miscellaneous	Atlanto-axial instability, postpartum, postgastrectomy	6
Total		58

Haldeman et al.[21]

obtain accurate statistics. Such a complication can arise from normal neck movements and trivial trauma and not only from cervical manipulation.[21-29] Haldeman et al[21] reviewed the published literature to assess the risk factors and precipitating neck movements causing vertebrobasilar artery dissection. A total of 367 cases were identified, of which 252 were either of spontaneous onset or related to trivial (Table 5.1) or major trauma. Less than one-third of cases (115) were associated with cervical manipulation.[21] Haneline and Lewkovich[23] undertook a literature search of the MEDLINE database for published articles relating to cervical artery dissection between 1994 and 2003. Twenty studies met the selection criteria, reporting 606 cervical artery dissection cases. The authors concluded that a minority of cases was associated with cervical spine manipulation. A summary of the findings is outlined in Box 5.1. Williams et al[31] indicate that estimates for stroke following neck manipulation will always be difficult to quantify. Selection, referral and recall bias,

Box 5.1 Aetiology of cervical artery dissections

- 54% internal carotid artery dissection
- 46% vertebral artery dissection
- 61% classified as spontaneous
- 30% associated with trauma / trivial trauma
- 9% associated with cervical spinal manipulation

(Reproduced with permission from Haneline et al.[23])

in addition to age-related variables, have the potential to confound estimation of the risk of vertebrobasilar dissection after neck manipulation.[31,32]

Association between cervical spine HVLA thrust techniques and stroke

The majority of the literature associating HVLA thrust techniques with vertebrobasilar and internal carotid artery stroke is from case reports, surveys and expert opinions. However, in the case of rare events like vertebrobasilar and internal carotid artery stroke, the research design that provides the most useful information is the case-control study.

There have been six reported case-control studies that have investigated the association between cervical spine HVLA thrust techniques and cervical artery dissection.[11,29,30,33–35] The four larger case-control studies found an association between cervical spine HVLA thrust techniques and vertebrobasilar artery stroke in patients under 45 years of age. Cassidy et al[29] analyzed every case of vertebrobasilar stroke in the province of Ontario, Canada, over a 9-year period in a population-based case-control and case-crossover design. They identified that primary care physician visits and attendance for chiropractic treatment were both strongly associated with subsequent vertebrobasilar artery stroke compared with age-matched and gender-matched controls. This study raises the possibility that patients with a vertebrobasilar artery dissection in progress seek clinical care before it progresses to a stroke. Smith et al[30] used a case-control study design to review patients under 60 years of age. Cases included 26 strokes related to internal carotid artery dissection, and 24 strokes related to vertebrobasilar artery dissection compared with 100 nondissection-related strokes. They found a strong association between manipulative therapy received in the previous month and stroke related to vertebrobasilar artery dissection but not internal carotid artery dissection. Rothwell et al[11] examined a database in Ontario, Canada, to identify patients with a vertebrobasilar artery stroke. They identified 582 patients admitted to hospital with a vertebrobasilar artery stroke over a 5-year period. Compared with matched controls, they reported a strong association between chiropractic treatment received within the previous week and stroke in patients under 45 years of age. There was no association in older patients. The CADISP (Cervical Artery Dissections and Ischemic Stroke Patients) Study Group analyzed 966 cases of cervical artery dissections and compared them with age-matched and gender-matched patients who had ischaemic stroke from other causes, as well as healthy subjects.[35] Cervical spine manipulative therapy was found to be significantly associated with cervical artery dissection compared with ischaemic stroke from other causes and compared with healthy subjects. Haynes et al,[36] in a systematic review of five case-control studies, reported that conclusive evidence seems to be lacking for a strong association between neck manipulation and stroke and also appears to be absent for no association.

Although some studies support an association between cervical spine HVLA thrust techniques and cervical artery dissection, especially vertebrobasilar artery dissection, it is still difficult to determine causation because patients may seek treatment for symptoms of a cervical artery dissection in progress. Marx et al[37] evaluated a number of cases of arterial dissection between 1996 and 2005 that had been alleged to have occurred as a result of cervical spine manipulation. They reported that there was clear evidence or high probability, in 5 of 7 carotid and 7 of 9 vertebral artery dissections, that the dissection was present before the manipulation. They reported that neither in the 7 carotid artery cases nor in the 9 vertebral artery cases could a causal link be made between the dissection and the manipulation.

A number of authors[36,38,39] have commented that patients with headache and neck pain from a cervical artery dissection may seek treatment from a manual or manipulative practitioner. Treatment may involve HVLA thrust techniques, mobilization or exercise prescription and often a combination of these interventions is used. In such instances, where a cervical artery dissection is not identified, it is possible that any intervention (manipulation/mobilization/exercise) that involves neck movements could be associated with a cervical artery dissection and any subsequent stroke. Haynes et al,[36] in a systematic review assessing the risk of stroke from neck manipulation, recommended that patients should be advised that neck movements, including manipulation, may increase the risk of a rare form of stroke.

The majority of published articles on serious complications of neck manipulation have focused upon vascular consequences, but nonvascular complications have also been documented. A small number of case reports[40-42] describing spinal cord compression associated with neck manipulation have been published. A number of these patients had undiagnosed pathology, e.g. a large disc protrusion, and the case reports do not address factors such as the training of the practitioner or the type of manipulation technique used.

A systematic review of adverse events and manual therapy came to the conclusion that the risk of major adverse events with manual therapy, including cervical spine HVLA thrust techniques, is low.[43] In circumstances where patients are properly screened and practitioners appropriately trained, Carnes et al[43] described no reports of any major adverse event in the randomized controlled trials (RCTs) they reviewed, a number of which included manipulation of the cervical spine.

Thoracic Spine and Rib Cage

Practitioners need to be aware of the possible complications that can be associated with HVLA thrust techniques applied to the thoracic spine and rib cage. Oppenheim et al[40] studied the medical records of patients presenting to a neurosurgical practice over a 6-year period who suffered a qualitative worsening of symptoms immediately after spinal manipulation. Four of the 18 serious complications identified were in the thoracic spine and included myelopathy, quadriparesis, central cord syndrome and paraparesis. Three of the four patients developed signs and symptoms from pathological fractures of the vertebral bodies that had been weakened due to undiagnosed tumours.

Anecdotally, practitioners have reported the occurrence of rib fractures and, less commonly, vertebral body fractures that developed immediately after thoracic spine or rib HVLA thrust techniques. Some of these fractures may have been associated with undiagnosed diminished bone density or tumours, but others are likely to have been linked to the use of inappropriate and high-force HVLA thrust techniques. Rib and vertebral body fractures have not been widely reported as a complication of spinal manipulation in the published literature.

Puentedura et al,[44] in a small RCT involving 24 patients with acute neck pain, compared thoracic spine thrust joint manipulation with cervical spine thrust joint manipulation in patients who met a clinical prediction model.[44] They reported significantly more transient side effects for those patients who received thoracic spine manipulation compared with the patients who received cervical spine manipulation.

Lumbar Spine and Pelvis

Serious complications associated with HVLA thrust techniques applied to the lumbar spine and pelvis are extremely uncommon, and adverse consequences such as worsening lumbar disc herniation or cauda equina syndrome were found to be extremely rare in five systematic reviews of spinal manipulation.[45] Case reports of serious adverse events following lumbopelvic spinal manipulative therapy have been described with cauda equina syndrome and lumbar disc herniation accounting for the majority of cases.[46] Because of the inherent nature of case reports, it is not possible to establish causation. Therefore it is not known whether the serious adverse events identified in the case reports were caused by the lumbopelvic manipulation or whether the association between the manipulation and the adverse event was incidental.

A number of systematic reviews of RCTs, cohort studies and a patient survey did not identify any serious adverse event associated with lumbopelvic spinal manipulative therapy.[43,47–49] Chou et al[45] reported that serious adverse events, e.g. worsening of lumbar disc herniation, associated with lumbar spine manipulation are very rare and less than 1 per 1 million patient visits. In circumstances where patients are likely to be properly screened and practitioners appropriately trained, Chou et al[45] report that there has not been one serious complication associated with manipulation of the lumbar spine and pelvis in 70 controlled clinical trials.

A systematic review of the safety of spinal manipulation in the treatment of lumbar disc herniations reported the risk of a patient suffering a clinically worsened disc herniation or cauda equina syndrome following spinal manipulation to be less than 1 in 3.7 million.[50] Although it is recognized that spinal manipulation applied to the lumbar spine and pelvis is not without some risks, Haldeman has commented that it should be considered one of the safest forms of treatment available for spinal disorders.[51]

Classification of Complications

Complications can be classified as transient, substantive reversible impairment, substantive nonreversible impairment and serious nonreversible impairment.

Transient

- Local pain or discomfort
- Stiffness
- Headache

- Tiredness/fatigue
- Radiating pain or discomfort
  Transient side effects following.
Cervical spine manipulation are relatively common.[52] Less common transient reactions include dizziness or imbalance, extremity weakness, ringing in the ears, depression or anxiety, nausea or vomiting, blurred or impaired vision, confusion or disorientation.[53]

Transient side effects resulting from manipulative treatment may be more common than one might expect and may remain unreported by patients unless information is explicitly requested. Prospective studies report common side effects resulting from spinal manipulation occur between 30% and 61% of patients.[54–58] After manual therapy, including spinal HVLA thrust techniques, almost half of patients experience adverse events that are minor and of short duration.[43] Carnes et al[43] reported that most of these minor events will occur within 24 hours and resolve within 72 hours.

Substantive reversible impairment

Cervical spine

- Disc herniation/prolapse
- Nerve root compression
- Cervical and upper thoracic spine strain.

Thoracic spine

- Rib fracture
- Minor vertebral body compression fracture
- Posterior element fracture without loss of structural integrity
- Shoulder girdle, thoracic spine and rib cage strain.

Lumbar spine

- Minor vertebral body compression fracture
- Posterior element fracture without loss of structural integrity
- Disc herniation/prolapse

- Nerve root compression
- Shoulder girdle, thoracic spine/rib cage and lumbopelvic region strain.

Substantive nonreversible impairment

Cervical spine

- Unresolved disc herniation/prolapse/ extrusion
- Unresolved radiculopathy.

Thoracic spine

- Significant vertebral body compression fracture
- Posterior element fracture with disruption of the spinal canal.

Lumbar spine

- Significant vertebral body compression fracture
- Posterior element fracture with disruption of the spinal canal
- Unresolved disc herniation/prolapse/ extrusion
- Unresolved radiculopathy.

Serious nonreversible impairment

Cervical spine

- Stroke
- Spinal cord compression.

Thoracic spine

- Spinal cord compression.

Lumbar spine

- Cauda equina syndrome.

Causes of Complications

Complications associated with the use of HVLA thrust techniques generally relate to either incorrect patient selection or poor technique.

Incorrect patient selection

- Lack of or incorrect diagnosis
- Lack of awareness of possible complications

- Inadequate palpatory assessment
- Lack of patient consent.

Poor technique

- Excessive force
- Excessive amplitude
- Excessive leverage
- Inappropriate combination of leverage
- Incorrect plane of thrust
- Poor patient positioning
- Poor operator positioning
- Lack of patient feedback.

HVLA THRUST TECHNIQUES AND RELATIVE RISKS

Most of the research and reporting of both transient and more serious complications of manual interventions has focused upon HVLA thrust techniques. The incidence of complications of other manual therapy techniques remains largely unknown. Nonthrust techniques, including spinal mobilization and massage techniques, have also been associated with serious adverse consequences. Spontaneous intracranial hypotension secondary to a dural tear following cervical and thoracic spine mobilization has been reported.[59] One case of cerebrovascular accident that only partially recovered and six cases of brachialgia with neurological deficit have been reported following cervical spine mobilization.[60] A case of retinal artery occlusion followed 'low-force joint mobilization from C2 to C7',[61] and cerebral artery embolism has been attributed to Shiatsu massage.[62] An internal carotid dissection followed use of a handheld electric massager.[63] An attitudinal study of Australian Manipulative Physiotherapists who had undertaken specific postgraduate study in manipulative therapy reported that 84.5% used manipulation in the cervical spine and that most adverse effects associated with examination or treatment of the cervical spine arose as a result of passive mobilizing and examination techniques ahead of high-velocity thrust techniques.[64] A postal survey of 259 Irish Manipulative Physiotherapists reported more serious adverse events with the use of nonhigh-velocity thrust techniques, compared with high-velocity thrust techniques, which included a transient ischaemic attack, a drop attack and one episode of fainting.[65]

Posadzki et al,[66] in an update of a systematic review of the safety of massage therapy, reported that it seems likely that adverse events of massage therapy are rare. However, the authors identified a number of case reports associating massage therapy with severe adverse events, including cervical internal carotid and vertebral artery dissections. Yin et al,[67] in a systematic review of massage therapy, identified case reports of 138 adverse events associated with massage between 2003 and 2013, which included disc herniation, soft tissue trauma, neurological compromise, spinal cord injury and vertebral artery dissection. They reported that massage therapies are not without risks but that the incidence of serious adverse events is low.

Carnes et al,[43] in a meta-analysis of RCTs, reported a similar risk of mild to moderate adverse events associated with manual therapy, which included HVLA thrust techniques, compared with exercise.

Many patients with musculoskeletal conditions are prescribed nonsteroidal antiinflammatory medication. Dabbs and Lauretti[68] reported the incidence of bleeding or perforation following the use of such medication for the treatment of osteoarthritis as being 4 in 1000 patients, with death occurring in 4 out of 10 000 patients. The authors concluded that the use of nonsteroidal antiinflammatory drugs (NSAIDs) compared with cervical manipulation, for the treatment of comparable conditions, poses a significantly greater risk of serious complications and death. A national prospective survey in the United Kingdom of 19 772 patients receiving 50 276 cervical spine manipulations identified that the risk rates

of cervical manipulation were comparable with the use of antiinflammatory medications commonly prescribed for musculoskeletal conditions.[52] Tramer et al[69] estimated that 1 in 1200 patients taking NSAIDs for 2 months or more will die of gastroduodenal complications and would not have died if they had not taken the medication. Carnes et al[43] reported that the relative risk of having a minor or moderate adverse event with manual therapy (high-velocity thrust) was significantly less than the risk of taking NSAIDs. Oliphant estimated lumbar spine manipulation to be safer than NSAIDs among patients with lumbar disc herniation.[50]

Acupuncture is also used for the treatment of musculoskeletal conditions and is recognized to be a very safe therapeutic intervention in the hands of a well trained and competent practitioner.[70-72] However, a number of serious adverse events resulting from acupuncture have been reported in the literature, including pneumothorax, spinal cord injury, organ trauma and viral hepatitis.[72-76]

Many interventions for the treatment of musculoskeletal conditions are associated with risk, but we do not have risk rates compared with HVLA thrust techniques. Myocardial infarction following exercise prescription, allergic reactions to injection therapies, and burns from heat, cold and electrotherapy are all well recognized as potential complications.

RED FLAGS

The term 'red flags' refers to clinical features that may indicate a serious condition requiring urgent evaluation. Examples include tumours, infection, fractures and neurological damage.[77] Screening for red flags, which includes appropriate historical cues and specific physical examination tests, should occur both at the initial consultation and subsequent visits.[54] In a systematic review of red flags to screen for malignancy and fracture in patients with low back pain,

Table 5.2 Alerting features of serious conditions associated with acute neck pain

Feature or risk factor	Condition
Symptoms and signs of infection (e.g. fever, night sweats)	Infection
Risk factors for infection (e.g. underlying disease process, immunosuppression, penetrating wound, exposure to infectious diseases)	
History of trauma	Fracture
Use of corticosteroids	
Past history of malignancy	Tumour
Age > 50 years	
Failure to improve with treatment	
Unexplained weight loss	
Dysphagia, headache, vomiting	
Neurological symptoms in the limbs	Neurological condition
Cerebrovascular symptoms or signs, anticoagulant use	Cerebral or spinal haemorrhage
Cardiovascular risk factors, transient ischaemic attack	Vertebral or carotid aneurysm

Source: National Health and Medical Research Council.

Downie et al[78] reported that much of the existing research on red flags has only evaluated single clinical features and suggested that future research might be better directed to evaluating combinations of the clinical features of red flags. The alerting features of serious conditions associated with acute neck pain (Table 5.2), acute thoracic spinal pain (Table 5.3) and acute low back pain (Table 5.4) are described.[77]

CONTRAINDICATIONS

Whenever a practitioner applies a therapeutic intervention, due consideration must be given to the risk–benefit ratio. The benefit to the patient must outweigh any potential risk associated with the intervention. Contraindications have been classified as absolute and relative. The distinction between absolute and relative contraindications is influenced by factors such as the skill, experience and training of the practitioner; the type of technique selected; the amount of leverage and force used; and the age, general health and physique of the patient.

Absolute

- Bone: any pathology that has led to significant bone weakening:
  - Tumour, e.g. metastatic deposits
  - Infection, e.g. tuberculosis
  - Metabolic, e.g. osteomalacia
  - Congenital, e.g. dysplasias
  - Iatrogenic, e.g. long-term corticosteroid medication
  - Inflammatory, e.g. severe rheumatoid arthritis
  - Traumatic, e.g. fracture.
- Neurological
  - Cervical myelopathy
  - Cord compression
  - Cauda equina compression
  - Nerve root compression with increasing neurological deficit.
- Vascular
  - Diagnosed cervical artery dissection
  - Aortic aneurysm
  - Bleeding diatheses, e.g. severe haemophilia.
- Lack of a diagnosis
- Lack of patient consent

Table 5.3 Alerting features of serious conditions associated with acute thoracic spinal pain

Feature or risk factor	Condition
Minor trauma (if >50 years, history of osteoporosis and taking corticosteroids)	Fracture
Major trauma	
Fever	Infection
Night sweats	
Risk factors for infection (e.g. underlying disease process, immunosuppression, penetrating wound)	
Past history of malignancy	Tumour
Age > 50 years	
Failure to improve with treatment	
Unexplained weight loss	
Pain at multiple sites	
Pain at rest	
Night pain	
Chest pain or heaviness	Other serious conditions
Movement, change in posture has no effect on pain	
Abdominal pain	
Shortness of breath, cough	

Source: National Health and Medical Research Council.

Table 5.4 Alerting features of serious conditions associated with acute low back pain

Feature or risk factor	Condition
Symptoms and signs of infection (e.g. fever)	Infection
Risk factors for infection (e.g. underlying disease process, immunosuppression, penetrating wound)	
History of trauma	Fracture
Minor trauma (if age > 50 years, history of osteoporosis and taking corticosteroids)	
Past history of malignancy	Tumour
Age > 50 years	
Failure to improve with treatment	
Unexplained weight loss	
Pain at multiple sites	
Pain at rest	
Absence of aggravating factors	Aortic aneurysm

Source: National Health and Medical Research Council.

- Patient positioning cannot be achieved because of pain or resistance.

Relative

Certain categories of patients have an increased potential for adverse reactions following the application of an HVLA thrust technique. Special consideration should be given before the use of HVLA thrust technique in the following circumstances:

- Adverse reactions to previous manual therapy
- Disc herniation or prolapse
- Inflammatory arthritides
- Pregnancy

- Spondylolysis
- Spondylolisthesis
- Osteoporosis
- Anticoagulant or long-term corticosteroid use
- Advanced degenerative joint disease and spondylosis
- Vertigo
- Psychological dependence upon HVLA thrust technique
- Ligamentous laxity/hypermobility
- Arterial calcification.

The above list is not intended to cover all possible clinical situations. Patients who have pathology may also have coincidental spinal pain and discomfort arising from mechanical dysfunction that may benefit from manipulative treatment.

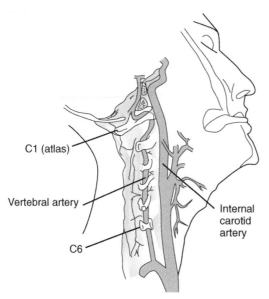

Figure 5.1 Course of the vertebral and internal carotid arteries through the cervical spine. (Reproduced with permission from Elsevier.[79])

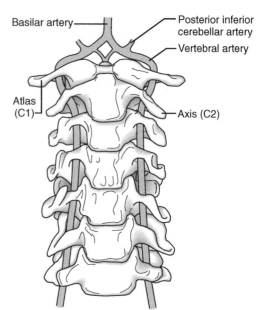

Figure 5.2 Relationship of the cervical spine to the vertebral artery.

VERTEBROBASILAR AND CAROTID ARTERIES

Adverse events can be associated with compromise of the cervical arterial system. Dissection within the cervical arteries is a recognized cause of ischaemic stroke in the young and the middle-aged. Cervical artery dissection should always be considered in the differential diagnosis of patients presenting with headache and/or neck pain.

Both the vertebral and internal carotid arteries should be considered in pretreatment risk assessment. The common carotid artery is easily palpable in the neck above the sternocleidomastoid muscle. It divides into the internal and external carotid arteries at the level of the upper border of the thyroid cartilage. The internal carotid artery[79] (Fig. 5.1) extends directly upwards and through the base of the skull at the carotid canal of the temporal bone to supply the brain. The external carotid artery extends from the bifurcation of the common carotid artery to the neck of the mandible, there dividing into the superficial temporal and maxillary arteries. The carotid arteries supply the blood flow to the anterior part of the brain.

The vertebrobasilar system comprises the two vertebral arteries and their union to form the basilar artery (Fig. 5.2). This system provides approximately 20% of intracranial blood supply.[80] The vertebral and basilar arteries supply the blood flow to the posterior part of the brain. Blood flow in these arteries may be affected by intrinsic and extrinsic factors. Intrinsic factors such as atherosclerosis narrow the vessel lumen, increase turbulence and reduce blood flow. Extrinsic factors compress or impinge upon the external wall of the artery.

Vertebrobasilar Insufficiency

The term 'vertebrobasilar insufficiency' (VBI) encompasses all transient ischaemic attacks (TIAs) of the posterior circulation of the brain. The term 'carotid insufficiency' has been used in the past to describe TIAs of the anterior circulation of the brain but has largely been discarded from current day medical terminology.

Screening Tests for Cervical Artery Dysfunction

For many years practitioners have been advised to use VBI screening tests on patients who presented with head and neck pain in an attempt to identify any patient who might be at risk of having a cervical artery dissection, particularly as a result of cervical spine HVLA thrust techniques. The clinical approach was to screen for signs and symptoms of VBI and then perform one or more head-on-neck VBI positional tests.

Premanipulative testing movements for VBI were advocated as a means of risk management with a view to minimizing harm to the patient.[81] Many physical tests for determining the presence or absence of VBI have been described.[82–87]

Tests for VBI were based upon the premise that cervical spine positioning may reduce the lumen and blood flow in the vertebral arteries.[88–91] In vivo studies lent support to the view that cervical spine positioning may reduce vertebral artery blood flow.[88,89,91–96] Other studies of vertebral artery blood flow did not identify significant change in flow related to cervical spine positioning.[97–101] Most of the studies have examined vertebral artery blood flow. Bowler et al[102] examined 14 healthy subjects to determine the effect of a simulated manipulation position on blood flow in both the internal carotid and the vertebral arteries. They reported that placing the cervical spine in a simulated manipulation position did not adversely affect blood flow through either the internal carotid or the vertebral arteries. In 20 healthy adult participants, Thomas et al[103] examined both vertebral and internal carotid arterial blood flow in a number of positions commonly used in manual therapy, including end-range neck rotation and distraction. They

reported that blood flow to the brain did not appear to be compromised by any of the neck positions that were studied. In an in vivo study investigating vertebral artery blood flow in 10 healthy male participants, Quesnele et al[104] reported no significant changes in blood flow or velocity in the vertebral arteries following an upper cervical spine manipulation. In a systematic review of vertebral and internal carotid artery flow during vascular premanipulative testing, Malo-Urries et al[105] reported no consensus in the published literature on cervical artery blood flow behaviour with different neck movements and positions.

Some published reports linking vertebral artery narrowing or occlusion with cervical spine extension and rotation positioning contributed to the development and use of many premanipulative tests for VBI. It was postulated that a reduction in blood flow as a result of cervical spine positioning would produce detectable symptoms or signs in a patient with VBI. Positive tests were assumed to be a predictor of patients at risk for cerebrovascular complications of manipulation. However, tests for VBI have poor sensitivity and variable specificity.[106,107] The value of these tests in determining VBI has been questioned.[87,108–112]

Screening tests should be both valid and reliable predictors of risk. VBI-testing movements have neither of these qualities, with available scientific evidence failing to show predictive value.[20,38,99,109,113] Screening procedures should also not be harmful. It has been suggested that the tests themselves may hold certain risks and could have a morbid effect on the vertebral artery.[114] Minor adverse effects associated with examination procedures involving rotation, including those related to the use of an established VBI-testing protocol, have been documented.[64]

Research evidence would suggest that cervical spine pretreatment screening tests for arterial dysfunction are not valid and lack clinical utility.[6,38,113,115–117]

Biomechanical Studies

Symons et al[118] attempted to quantify the internal forces on the vertebral artery during neck manipulation and VBI testing on five unembalmed postrigor cadavers. Strains sustained internally by the vertebral artery during neck range of motion testing, VBI screening and HVLA thrust techniques were similar, and all were significantly less than the forces required to disrupt the vertebral artery mechanically. The study concluded that a single typical HVLA thrust technique to the neck is unlikely to cause mechanical disruption of the vertebral artery.[118] Herzog et al[119] analyzed vertebral artery strains during high-speed low amplitude cervical spine manipulation. They reported that vertebral artery strains obtained during neck manipulation are significantly smaller than those obtained during diagnostic and range of motion testing and are much smaller than failure strains. Piper et al[120] quantified mechanical strain in the vertebral artery during cervical spine manipulation and motion of the head and neck in the cardinal planes. They reported that the greatest amount of strain achieved during neck manipulation was comparably lower than vertebral artery strains achieved during passive end-range motions of the head and neck. Current biomechanical evidence is insufficient to establish the claim that HVLA thrust techniques cause vertebrobasilar or internal carotid artery dissection.[39]

Cervical Artery Dissection

Cervical artery dissection occurs when there is haemorrhage within the blood vessel wall. This haemorrhage splits the layers of the vessel wall and results in either an intramural haematoma, which protrudes inward and narrows the vessel lumen, or an aneurysmal dilatation, which causes the external wall to bulge outwards. Most ischaemic symptoms are caused by emboli from the site of the dissection (Fig. 5.3),[121]

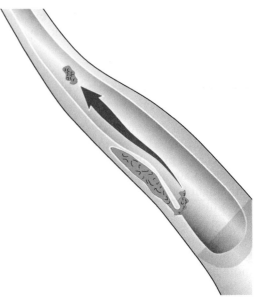

Figure 5.3 Thrombus from a nonocclusive dissection becoming dislodged and embolizing downstream. (Reproduced with permission.)

and the remainder are due to blood vessel narrowing with haemodynamic insufficiency.

Cervical artery dissection can involve the internal carotid or the vertebral arteries. Internal carotid artery dissection is reported to have an annual incidence of 2.5 to 3 per 100 000 patients, and vertebral artery dissection is reported to have an annual incidence of 1 to 1.5 per 100 000 patients.[122]

Clinical History

A number of risk factors are reported to be associated with an increased risk of cervical artery pathology or dissection and should be thoroughly assessed during history taking (Box 5.2).[123,124]

It is critical that clinicians identify those patients who present with signs and/or symptoms of a cervical artery dissection in progress. Patients who present with acute onset neck pain and/or headache may be presenting with a dissecting cervical artery, which may mimic a musculoskeletal complaint. Later ischaemic manifestations of a cervical artery dissection such as cranial nerve dysfunction and brain ischaemia may be latent and develop hours, days or even weeks after onset.

Clinical Presentation

Internal carotid artery dissection

Biller et al[39] reported that a number of patients with an internal carotid artery dissection present with pain on one side of the head, face and neck accompanied by a partial Horner's syndrome. They recommend that in the absence of any other sign or symptom, unilateral Horner's syndrome should be considered to be caused by an internal carotid artery dissection until proven otherwise.

A unilateral headache develops in two-thirds of patients, most commonly in the frontotemporal region, but it can involve the entire hemicranium or the occipital region.[124] The severity of the headache is described to be variable, but most patients consider the headache to be unlike any other pain.[124] Cranial nerve palsies, pulsatile tinnitus and cerebral or retinal ischaemic symptoms have been described as being associated with a dissection of the internal carotid artery.[39]

Vertebral artery dissection

Patients often present with pain in the back of the head and neck. The first signs and symptoms of vertebral artery dissection are less obvious than those of internal carotid artery dissection and often are initially interpreted as musculoskeletal in nature.[124] It has been reported that pain develops in the posterior aspect of the neck in 50% of patients and a headache commonly occurs in the occipital region, but in rare cases it involves the frontal region or the entire hemicranium.[124] Silbert et al[124] reported that only half of the patients in their study considered their neck pain or headache to be unlike any other. Ischaemic symptoms occur in most patients in whom a vertebral artery dissection is diagnosed and may involve the brainstem, the thalamus, temporo-occipital regions or the cerebellar hemispheres.[39] Thomas et al[34] examined the medical records of patients aged 55 years or less with radiologically confirmed or suspected vertebral or internal carotid artery dissection. The records of 47 dissection patients were retrospectively compared with matched controls who had a stroke from some other cause. The authors reported a range of symptoms (Table 5.5) and clinical signs (Table 5.6) associated with vertebral artery and internal carotid dissection.

Dizziness is a common presenting complaint with multiple aetiologies that must be distinguished from dizziness arising from cervical artery dysfunction, in particular vertebrobasilar artery dissection (Box 5.3).

Table 5.5 Clinical symptoms of cervical artery dissection[34]

Symptoms	VBAD	ICAD
Headache	85%	75%
Neck pain	67%	45%
Dizziness	52%	0.5%
Visual disturbance	33%	35%
Paraesthesia (face)	30%	30%
Paraesthesia (UL)	33%	35%
Paraesthesia (LL)	15%	25%

ICAD, Internal carotid artery dissection; *VBAD*, vertebrobasilar artery dissection; *LL*, lower limb; *UL*, upper limb

Table 5.6 Clinical signs of cervical artery dissection[34]

Clinical signs	VBAD	ICAD
Unsteadiness/ataxia	67%	40%
Weakness (UL)	33%	65%
Weakness (LL)	41%	50%
Dysphasia/dysarthria/ aphasia	44%	45%
Facial palsy	22%	60%
Ptosis	19%	60%
Nausea/vomiting	26%	30%
Dysphagia	26%	0.5%
Drowsiness	4%	20%
Confusion	7%	15%
Loss of consciousness	15%	20%

ICAD, Internal carotid artery dissection; *VBAD*, vertebrobasilar artery dissection; *LL*, lower limb; *UL*, upper limb

Box 5.3 Causes of dizziness

SYSTEMIC CAUSES OF DIZZINESS
- Medication
- Hypotension
- Diabetes
- Thyroid disease
- Cardiac or pulmonary insufficiency

CENTRAL CAUSES OF DIZZINESS
- Demyelinating diseases
- Tumours of brain or spinal cord
- Seizures
- Vertebrobasilar insufficiency
- Posttraumatic (concussion) vertigo

PERIPHERAL CAUSES OF DIZZINESS
- Benign positional vertigo
- Ménière's disease
- Cervical spine dysfunction
- Labyrinthitis
- Vestibulotoxic medication

Clinical Examination

For patients presenting with acute onset neck pain and/or headache, a normal physical examination would include pain-free range of motion testing of the cervical spine (Figs. 5.4–5.9). Such range of motion testing might include both active and passive movements but would be performed with care and to the point of provocation of symptoms only. If a

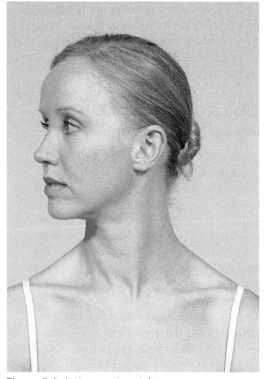

Figure 5.4 Active rotation right.

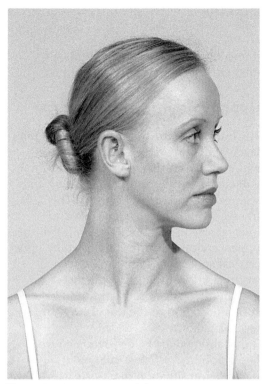

Figure 5.5 Active rotation left.

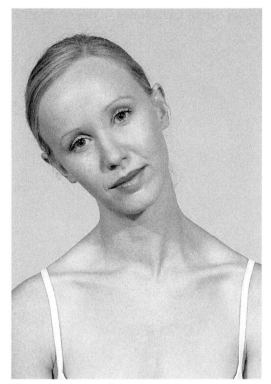

Figure 5.6 Active sidebending right.

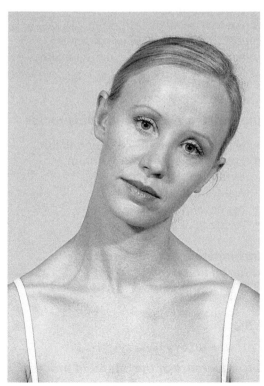

Figure 5.7 Active sidebending left.

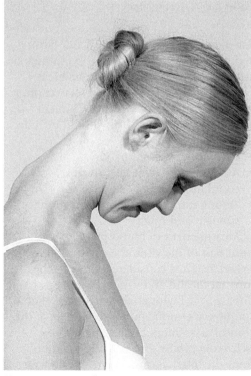

Figure 5.8 Active flexion.

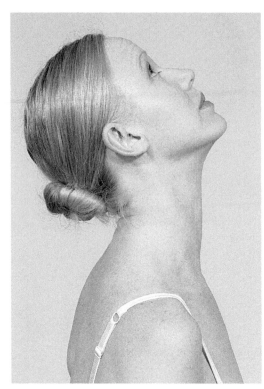

Figure 5.9 Active extension.

patient is positive for historical risk factors and presents with signs and/or symptoms of cervical artery dysfunction or possible vertebral/internal carotid artery dissection, a comprehensive neurological assessment should be undertaken. This should include the following:

- Cranial nerve examination
- Assessment of gait, balance and coordination
- Testing extremity reflexes, sensation, strength and tone.

Measurement of blood pressure should form part of the clinical examination as hypertension is considered a risk factor for internal carotid and vertebral artery disease.[38,125] Taylor et al[125] suggested that a simple eye examination also be part of the clinical assessment because retinal ischaemia can be associated with emboli from the internal carotid artery. Where a cervical artery dissection is suspected, immediate referral to an appropriate medical emergency centre is indicated.

UPPER CERVICAL INSTABILITY

The bony anatomy of the atlanto-axial joint favours mobility rather than stability,[126] with the atlanto-axial joint being more vulnerable to subluxation than other segments of the cervical spine.[127] The transverse and alar ligaments have an integral role in maintaining stability in the upper cervical spine. Instability of the upper cervical spine may compromise related vascular and neurological structures and, in these circumstances, would be a contraindication to the use of HVLA thrust techniques.

Instability must be differentiated from hypermobility.[128,129] Instability is a pathological situation that exists with clinical symptoms or complaints.[128] Causes of upper cervical instability may be a result of incompetence of the odontoid process or the transverse atlantal ligament. These causes can be classified as congenital, inflammatory, neoplastic and traumatic.

Congenital
Incompetence of the odontoid process

- Separate odontoid–'os odontoideum'
- Free apical segment–'ossiculum terminale'
- Agenesis of odontoid base
- Agenesis of apical segment
- Agenesis of odontoid process.

Incompetence of the transverse atlantal ligament

- Idiopathic
- Down's syndrome.

Inflammatory
Incompetence of the odontoid process

- Osteomyelitis.

Incompetence of the transverse atlantal ligament

- Bacterial infection
- Viral infection
- Granulomatous change
- Rheumatoid arthritis
- Ankylosing spondylitis.

Neoplastic

Incompetence of the odontoid process

- Primary tumour of bone
- Metastatic tumour of bone.

Traumatic

Incompetence of the odontoid process

- Acute bony injury
- Chronic bony change.

Incompetence of the transverse atlantal ligament

- Acute ligamentous damage associated with fracture and trauma
- Chronic ligamentous change.

Symptoms and Signs of Upper Cervical Instability

Symptomatic instability of the upper cervical spine is rare. Instability occurs most frequently in patients with rheumatoid arthritis (Fig. 5.10)[130,131] and is also well documented in Down's syndrome[132–135] and in patients subsequent to retropharyngeal inflammatory processes.[136] Ligamentous laxity following an infectious process in the head or neck occurs most frequently in children, but it is a rare complication. Adult cases have also been reported.[136] Between 7% and 30% of all individuals with Down's syndrome show atlanto-axial instability with most of the patients with radiographic evidence of instability being asymptomatic.[137] Upper cervical ligamentous injuries and instability can also result from trauma.[138,139]

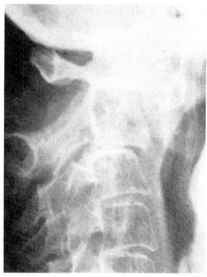

Figure 5.10 Cervical instability as a result of rheumatoid arthritis. Note forward displacement of C1 upon C2 and widening of the atlanto-dental interval. (Reproduced with permission from Elsevier from Adams and Hamblen, 2001.[130])

The ability to recognize symptoms and signs that may indicate upper cervical instability is essential for safe practice. These symptoms are extremely variable and might include:[129]

- Neck pain
- Limitation of neck movements
- Torticollis
- Neurological symptoms
- Headache
- Dizziness
- Buzzing in the ears
- Dysphagia
- Neurological signs
- Hyperreflexia
- Gait disturbances
- Spasticity
- Pareses.

The above symptoms and signs might also indicate the presence of cervical artery dysfunction or spinal cord compression unrelated to upper cervical instability. As a result, it is necessary to establish whether the symptoms or signs are related to instability of the upper cervical spine or to other causes.

There are four cardinal symptoms and signs that may indicate the presence of upper cervical instability:[140]

1. Overt loss of balance in relation to head movements.
2. Facial lip paraesthesia, reproduced by active or passive neck movements.
3. Bilateral or quadrilateral limb paraesthesia either constant or reproduced by neck movements.
4. Nystagmus produced by active or passive neck movements.

Currently the most reliable method for detecting increased movement in the upper cervical spine is by the use of imaging techniques. The atlanto-dental interval is the distance between the most anterior point of the dens of the axis and the back of the anterior arch of the atlas. This is measured on lateral radiographs of the cervical spine in flexion, neutral and extension positions. An atlanto-dental interval > 2.5–3 mm in adults and > 4.5–5 mm in children indicates atlanto-axial instability.[137] Cineradiography has also been shown to be a valuable adjunctive technique in the diagnosis of cervical instability.[141] Functional plain radiographs remain the primary imaging method to evaluate upper cervical spine instability, but computerized tomography (CT) in the flexed position has been reported to be useful in any preoperative imaging workup,[142] with magnetic resonance imaging (MRI) also offering benefits because of the ability to provide direct sagittal projection.[137]

CT and MRI provide complementary information when combined with flexion and extension radiographs. However, caution should be used when using flexion and extension views in cases of acute cervical trauma.[139]

A number of physical tests have been described for the examination of instability of the upper cervical region.[137,140,143–145]

Although these tests are used in clinical practice, the results should be interpreted with caution as there is little research evidence confirming their clinical utility.

Tests have been described for both the transverse atlantal and the alar ligaments. However, caution must be exercised when interpreting these tests if a practitioner relies solely upon the amount of palpable displacement and end feel.[137] When screening for upper cervical instability, consideration should also be given to symptom reproduction or modification. It has been reported that tests of passive intervertebral movement in the upper cervical spine in whiplash-associated disorders corresponded reasonably well with MRI assessment, suggesting potential clinical utility.[146] In a study of 16 individuals, as assessed by MRI, end-range stress tests were performed with the patient in the supine position. The authors reported that the anterior shear and distraction tests for craniocervical instability showed a measurable direct effect on the transverse ligament and tectorial membrane consistent with their theorized mechanism for clinical use.[147] This study confirmed the construct validity of the anterior shear and distraction tests. Osmotherly et al,[148] using MRI, reported that sidebending and rotation stress tests of the alar ligament showed a measurable increase in the length of the contralateral alar ligament, thus confirming the construct validity of these alar ligament stress tests.

Transverse Atlantal Ligament Stress Test

The Sharp–Purser test was designed to demonstrate anterior instability at the atlanto-axial segment in patients with rheumatoid arthritis and ankylosing spondylitis.[143,145] A modified Sharp–Purser test analyzes the onset of symptoms and signs following head and neck flexion and the reduction of signs and symptoms

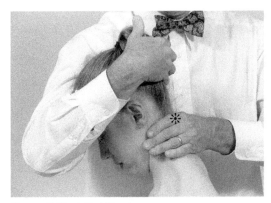

Figure 5.11 ✳ Stabilization.

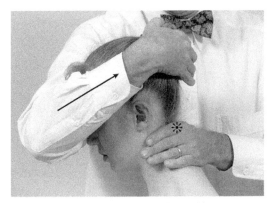

Figure 5.12 ✳ Stabilization. ➡ Plane of force (operator).

accompanying posterior translation of the occiput and atlas on the axis.

Patient position

Sitting with the head and neck relaxed in a semiflexed position.

Operator position

Standing to the right of the patient with your right arm cradling the patient's forehead. The spinous process and vertebral arch of the axis is stabilized with the thumb and index finger of your left hand (Fig. 5.11).

Stress applied

The occiput and atlas are translated posteriorly by applying pressure on the forehead with your right arm (Fig. 5.12).

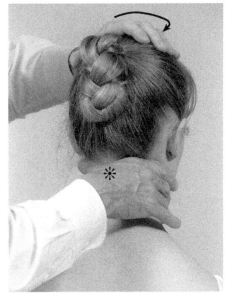

Figure 5.13 ✳ Stabilization. ⇨ Direction of body movement.

Positive test

A positive test occurs with:
1. First onset of symptoms and signs with head and neck flexion.
2. Reduction of symptoms and signs with posterior translation of the occiput and atlas on the axis.
3. Palpable hypermobility of anterior/ posterior translation.

Alar Ligament Stress Tests

There are many tests that purport to stress the alar ligaments and identify alar ligament instability. A comprehensive testing regime might include the following three tests:
1. Patient sitting with the neck in a neutral position. Ensure that there is no sidebending of the head and neck. The operator stabilizes the spinous process and vertebral arch of the axis with thumb and index finger. Passively rotate the occiput and atlas to the right (Fig. 5.13). There should be no more than 20–30° rotation. Repeat the procedure to the left. A positive test is characterized by the onset of symptoms or signs and/or a

57

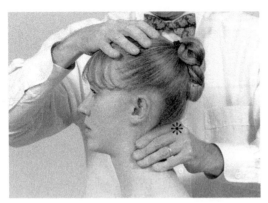

Figure 5.14 ✳ Stabilization.

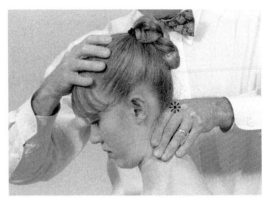

Figure 5.16 ✳ Stabilization.

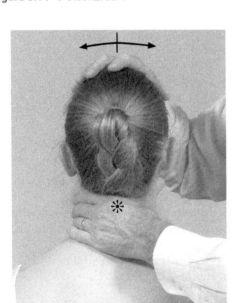

Figure 5.15 ✳ Stabilization. ⇨ Direction of body movement.

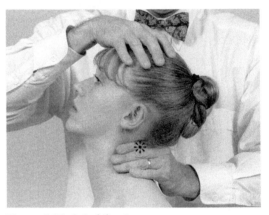

Figure 5.17 ✳ Stabilization.

There should be minimal movement in either direction. This test must be repeated with the neck in flexion (Fig. 5.16) and extension (Fig. 5.17). A positive test is characterized by the onset of symptoms or signs and/or an increased range of passive sidebending in all positions of neutral, flexion and extension.

range of passive rotation greater than 30° at the upper cervical segments.

2. Patient sitting with the neck in a neutral position. Ensure the head is straight and there is no rotation of the neck. The operator stabilizes the spinous process and vertebral arch of the axis with thumb and index finger while placing the other hand on the patient's vertex (Fig. 5.14). Attempt to passively sidebend the head to the left and then the right (Fig. 5.15).

3. Patient supine with the head and neck beyond the end of the couch and in a neutral position. Ensure the head is straight and there is no rotation of the neck. The operator stabilizes the spinous process and vertebral arch of the axis with thumb and index finger while placing the other hand on the patient's vertex (Fig. 5.18). Both hands support

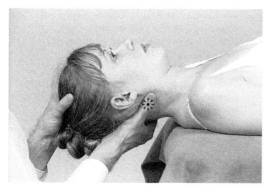

Figure 5.18 ✳ Stabilization.

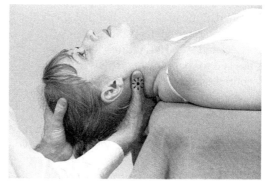

Figure 5.20 ✳ Stabilization.

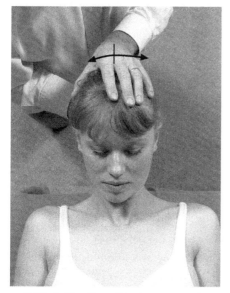

Figure 5.19 ⇨ Direction of body movement.

premise that patients at risk from manipulation to the upper cervical spine may be identified using physical examination techniques. There is a need for continuing research to investigate the reliability, validity and clinical utility of upper cervical instability tests.

TRAINING AND SKILL DEVELOPMENT

The safe application of HVLA thrust techniques is also critically linked to comprehensive training and skill development in the delivery of minimal leverage/non end-range techniques.

the weight of the patient's head. Attempt to passively sidebend the head to the left and then the right. There should be minimal movement in either direction. This test must be repeated with the neck in flexion (Fig. 5.19) and extension (Fig. 5.20).

A positive test is characterized by the onset of symptoms or signs and/or an increased range of passive sidebending in all positions of neutral, flexion and extension.

Transverse atlantal and alar ligament stress tests have been developed on the

CONCLUSION

The risk of major adverse events with manual therapy, including cervical spine HVLA thrust techniques, is low.[43] In circumstances where patients are properly screened and practitioners appropriately trained, Carnes et al[43] reported no major adverse event in the RCTs they reviewed, a number of which included HVLA thrust techniques applied to the cervical spine.

Chou et al[45] reported that serious adverse events associated with lumbar spine HVLA thrust techniques are very rare. In circumstances where patients are properly screened and practitioners appropriately trained, Chou et al[45] reported that there has not been one serious complication associated with HVLA thrust techniques applied to the spine and pelvis in 70 controlled clinical trials.

Patients who present with acute onset neck pain and/or headache may be presenting with a dissection of the vertebral or internal carotid arteries, which may mimic a musculoskeletal complaint. Later ischaemic manifestations such as cranial nerve dysfunction and brain ischaemia may be latent and develop some time after the initial symptoms.

Appropriate training in the use of manipulative thrust techniques and subsequent skill refinement through regular practice are key elements for safe practice and professional competence.[149]

References

1 Carey P. A report on the occurrence of cerebral vascular accidents in chiropractic practice. J Can Chiropractic Assoc 1993;37:104–6.

2 Dabbs V, Lauretti W. A risk assessment of cervical manipulation vs NSAIDs for the treatment of neck pain. J Manipulative Physiol Ther 1995;18:530–6.

3 Dvorak J, Loustalot D, Baumgartner H, et al. Frequency of complications of manipulations of the spine. A survey among the members of the Swiss medical society of manual medicine. Eur Spine J 1993;2:136–9.

4 Haldeman S, Kohlbeck F, McGregor M. Unpredictability of cerebrovascular ischemia associated with cervical spine manipulation therapy: A review of sixty four cases after cervical spine manipulation. Spine 2002;27(1): 49–55.

5 Haynes M. Stroke following cervical manipulation in Perth. Chiropractic J Aust 1994;24:42–6.

6 Klougart N, Leboeuf-Yde C, Rasmussen LR. Safety in chiropractic practice, Part 1: The occurrence of cerebrovascular accidents after manipulation to the neck in Denmark from 1978–1988. J Manipulative Physiol Ther 1996;19:371–7.

7 Lee KP, Carlini WG, McCormick GF, et al. Neurologic complications following chiropractic manipulation: A survey of California neurologists. Neurology 1995;45:1213–15.

8 Patijn J. Complications in manual medicine: A review of the literature. J Man Med 1991;6: 89–92.

9 Rivett DA, Milburn PA. A prospective study of cervical spine manipulation. J Man Med 1996;4:166–70.

10 Rivett D, Reid D. Risk of stroke for cervical spine manipulation in New Zealand. N Z J Physiother 1998;26:14–17.

11 Rothwell DM, Bondy SJ, Williams JI. Chiropractic manipulation and stroke: A population-based case-control study. Stroke 2001;32:1054–60.

12 Lee VH, Brown RD, Mandrekker JN, et al. Incidence and outcome of cervical artery dissections: A population based study. Neurology 2006;67:1809–12.

13 Miley M, Wellik K, Wingerchuk D, et al. Does cervical manipulative therapy cause vertebral artery dissection and stroke? Neurologist 2008;14(1):66–73.

14 Boyle E, Cote P, Grier AR, et al. Examining vertebrobasilar artery stroke in two Canadian provinces. Spine 2008;33(4S):S170–5.

15 Coulter ID, Hurwitz EL, Adams AH, et al. The Appropriateness of Manipulation and Mobilization of the Cervical Spine. Santa Monica, CA: RAND; 1996.

16 Reid D, Hing W. AJP Forum: Pre-manipulative testing of the cervical spine. Aust J Physiother 2001;47:164.

17 Powell FC, Hanigan WC, Olivero WC. A risk/benefit analysis of spinal manipulation therapy for relief of lumbar or cervical pain. Neurosurgery 1993;33:73–9.

18 Ernst E. Manipulation of the cervical spine: A systematic review of case reports of serious adverse events, 1995–2001. Med J Aust 2002;176(8):376–80.

19 Ernst E. Adverse effects of spinal manipulation: A systematic review. J R Soc Med 2007;100(7): 330–8.

20 Di Fabio RP. Manipulation of the cervical spine: Risks and benefits. Phys Ther 1999;79(1):51–65.

21 Haldeman S, Kohlbeck F, McGregor M. Risk factors and precipitating neck movements causing vertebrobasilar artery dissection after cervical trauma and spinal manipulation. Spine 1999;24(8):785–94.

22 Endo K, Ichimaru K, Shimura H, et al. Cervical vertigo after hair shampoo treatment at a hairdressing salon: A case report. Spine 2000;25(5):632–4.

23 Haneline M, Lewkovich G. An analysis of the etiology of cervical artery dissections: 1994 to 2003. J Manipulative Physiol Ther 2005;28(8):617–22.

24 Taylor A, Kerry R. Neck pain and headache as a result of internal carotid artery dissection: Implications for manual therapists. Man Ther 2005;10(1):73–7.

25 Rubinstein S, Haldeman S, van Tulder M. An etiologic model to help explain the pathogenesis of cervical artery dissection: Implications for cervical manipulation. J Manipulative Physiol Ther 2006;29(4):336–8.

26 Maroon J, Gardner P, Abla A, et al. Golfer's stroke: Golf-induced stroke from vertebral artery dissection. Surg Neurol 2007;67(2):163–8.

27 Yamada SM, Goto Y, Murakami M, et al. Vertebral artery dissection caused by swinging a golf club: Case report and literature review. Clin J Sport Med 2014;24(2):155–7.

28 Schneck M, Simionescu M, Bijari A. Bilateral vertebral artery dissection possibly precipitated in delayed fashion as a result of roller coaster rides. J Stroke Cerebrovasc Dis 2008;17(1):39–41.

29 Cassidy J, Boyle E, Cote P, et al. Risk of Vertebrobasilar stroke and chiropractic care. Results of a population-based case-control and case-crossover study. Spine 2008;33(4S):176–83.

30 Smith W, Johnston S, Skalabrin E, et al. Spinal manipulative therapy is an independent risk factor for vertebral artery dissection. Neurology 2003;60(9):1424–8.

31 Williams L, Biller J. Vertebrobasilar dissection and cervical spine manipulation: A complex pain in the neck. Neurology 2003;60(9):1408–9.

32 Haldeman S, Carey P, Townsend M, et al. Clinical perceptions of the risk of vertebral artery dissection after cervical manipulation: The effect of referral bias. Spine J 2002;2(5):334–42.

33 Dittrich R, Rohsbach D, Heidbreder A, et al. Mild mechanical traumas are possible risk factors for cervical artery dissection. Cerebrovasc Dis 2007;23:275–81.

34 Thomas LC, Rivett DA, Attia JR, et al. Risk factors and clinical features of craniocervical arterial dissection. Man Ther 2011;16:351–6.

35 Engelter ST, Grond-Ginsbach C, Metso TM, et al. Cervical artery dissection and ischaemic stroke patients study group. Cervical artery dissection: Trauma and other potential mechanical trigger events. Neurology 2013;80:1950–7.

36 Haynes MJ, Vincent K, Fischhoff C, et al. Assessing the risk of stroke from neck manipulation: A systematic review. Int J Clin Pract 2012;66(10):940–7.

37 Marx P, Puschmann H, Haferkam PG, et al. Manipulative treatment of the cervical spine and stroke. Fortschr Neurol Psychiatr 2009;77(2):83–90.

38 Rushton A, Rivett D, Carlesso L, et al. International framework for examination of the cervical region for potential of cervical arterial dysfunction prior to orthopaedic manual therapy intervention, <www.ifompt.com>; 2012.

39 Biller J, Sacco RL, Albuquerque FC, et al. Cervical arterial dissections and association with cervical manipulative therapy: A statement for healthcare professionals from the American Heart Association / American Stroke Association. Stroke 2014;45(10):3155–74.

40 Oppenheim J, Spitzer D, Segal D. Nonvascular complications following spinal manipulation. Spine J 2005;5(6):660–7.

41 Chakraverty J, Curtis O, Hughes T, et al. Spinal cord injury following chiropractic manipulation to the neck. Acta Radiol 2011;52(10):1125–7.

42 Epstein NE, Forte CL. Medicolegal corner: Quadriplegia following chiropractic manipulation. Surg Neurol Int 2013;4(S5):S327–9.

43 Carnes D, Mars TS, Mullinger B, et al. Adverse events and manual therapy: A systematic review. Man Ther 2010;15:355–63.

44 Puentedura EJ, Landers MR, Cleland JA, et al. Thoracic spine thrust manipulation versus cervical spine thrust manipulation in patients with acute neck pain: A randomized clinical trial. J Orthop Sports Phys Ther 2011;41(4):208–20.

45 Chou R, Huffman L. Nonpharmacologic therapies for acute and chronic low back pain: A review of the evidence for an American Pain Society/American College of Physicians clinical practice guideline. Ann Intern Med 2007;147(7):492–504.

46 Hebert JJ, Stomski NJ, French SD, et al. Serious adverse events and spinal manipulative therapy of the low back region: A systematic review of

cases. J Manipulative Physiol Ther 2013;pii:S0161–4754(13)00068–7.

47 Walker BF, French SD, Grant W, et al. A Cochrane review of combined chiropractic interventions for low back pain. Spine 2011;36:230–42.

48 Dagenais S, Gay RE, Tricco AC, et al. NASS contemporary concepts in spine care: Spinal manipulation therapy for acute low back pain. Spine J 2010;10:918–40.

49 Rubinstein SM, Van Middelkoop M, Assendelft WJ, et al. Spinal manipulative therapy for chronic low back pain. Cochrane Database Syst Rev 2011;(2):CD008112.

50 Oliphant D. Safety of spinal manipulation in the treatment of lumbar disk herniations: A systematic review and risk assessment. J Manipulative Physiol Ther 2004;27(3): 197–210.

51 Haldeman S. Authors reply to Dr. Oppenheim et al. Nonvascular complications following spinal manipulation. Spine J 2006;6(4):474–5.

52 Thiel H, Bolton J, Docherty S, et al. Safety of chiropractic manipulation of the cervical spine. A prospective national survey. Spine 2007;32(21):2375–8.

53 Hurwitz E, Morgenstern H, Vassilaki M, et al. Frequency and clinical predictors of adverse reactions to chiropractic care in the UCLA neck pain study. Spine 2005;30(13):1477–84.

54 Senstad O, Leboeuf-Yde C, Borchgrevink C. Frequency and characteristics of side effects of spinal manipulative therapy. Spine 1997;22(4):435–40.

55 Leboeuf-Yde C, Hennius B, Rudberg E, et al. Side effects of chiropractic treatment: A prospective study. J Manipulative Physiol Ther 1997;20(8):511–15.

56 Cagnie B, Vinck E, Beernaert A, et al. How common are side effects of spinal manipulation and can these side effects be predicted? Man Ther 2004;9(3):151–6.

57 Rubinstein S, Leboeuf-Yde C, Knol D, et al. The benefits outweigh the risks for patients undergoing chiropractic care for neck pain: A prospective, multicenter, cohort study. J Manipulative Physiol Ther 2007;30(6):408–18.

58 Rubinstein S, Leboeuf-Yde C, Knol D, et al. Predictors of adverse events following chiropractic care for patients with neck pain. J Manipulative Physiol Ther 2008;31(2):93–103.

59 Donovan J, Kerber C, Donovan W, et al. Development of spontaneous intracranial hypotension concurrent with grade IV mobilization of the cervical and thoracic spine: A case report. Arch Phys Med Rehabil 2007;88(11):1472–3.

60 Michaeli A. Reported occurrence and nature of complications following manipulative physiotherapy in South Africa. Aust J Physiother 1993;39(4):309–15.

61 Jumper J, Horton J. Central retinal artery occlusion after manipulation of the neck by a chiropractor. Am J Opthalmol 1996;121(3): 321–2.

62 Tsuboi K. Retinal and cerebral artery embolism after 'shiatsu' on the neck. Stroke 2001;32(10): 2441.

63 Grant A, Wang N. Carotid dissection associated with a handheld electric massager. South Med J 2004;97(12):1262–3.

64 Magarey M, Rebbeck T, Coughlan B, et al. Pre-manipulative testing of the cervical spine: Review, revision and new clinical guidelines. Man Ther 2004;9(2):95–108.

65 Sweeney A, Doody C. Manual therapy for the cervical spine and reported adverse events: A survey of Irish Manipulative Physiotherapists. Man Ther 2010;15(1):32–6.

66 Posadzki P, Ernst E. The safety of massage therapy: An update of a systematic review. Focus Alternat Complement Ther 2013;18(1): 27–32.

67 Yin P, Gao N, Wu J, et al. Adverse events of massage therapy in pain-related conditions: A systematic review. Evid Based Complement Alternat Med 2014;480956.

68 Dabbs V, Lauretti W. A risk assessment of cervical manipulation vs. NSAIDs for the treatment of neck pain. J Manipulative Physiol Ther 1995;18(8):530–6.

69 Tramer MR, Moore RA, Reynolds DJ, et al. Quantitative estimation of rare adverse events which follow a biological progression: A new model applied to chronic NSAID use. Pain 2000;85:169–82.

70 Vincent C. The safety of acupuncture. BMJ 2001;323(7311):467–8.

71 Rickards LD. Therapeutic needling in osteopathic practice: An evidence–informed perspective. Int J Osteopath Med 2009;12(1): 2–13.

72 Zhang J, Shang H, Gao X, et al. Acupuncture related adverse events: A systematic review of the Chinese literature. Bull WHO 2010;88: 915C–921C.

73 Yamashita H, Tsukayama H, White AR, et al. Systematic review of adverse events following

acupuncture: The Japanese literature. Complement Ther Med 2001;9:98–104.

74 Ernst E, Sherman KJ. Is acupuncture a risk factor for hepatitis? Systematic Review of epidemiological studies. J Gastroenterol Hepatol 2003;18:1231–6.

75 Endres HG, Molsberger A, Lungenhausen M, et al. An internal standard for verifying the accuracy of serious adverse event reporting: The example of an acupuncture study of 190,924 patients. Eur J Med Res 2004;9:545–51.

76 Wheway J, Agbabiaka TB, Ernst E. Patient safety incidents from acupuncture treatments: A review of reports to the National Patient Safety Agency. Int J Risk Saf Med 2012;24(3):163–9.

77 Australian Acute Musculoskeletal Pain Guidelines Group. Evidence-based management of acute musculoskeletal pain. A guide for clinicians. Brisbane, Australia: Australian Academic Press Pty Ltd.; 2004.

78 Downie A, Williams C, Henschke N, et al. Red flags to screen for malignancy and fracture in patients with low back pain: A systematic review. BMJ 2013;347:f7095.

79 Drake R, Vogl W, Mitchell AW. Gray's Anatomy for Students, 2nd edn. St. Louis, MO: Elsevier; 2010.

80 Zweibel WJ. Introduction to Vascular Ultrasonography, 2nd edn. New York, NY: Harcourt Brace; 1986.

81 Barker S, Kesson M, Ashmore J, et al. Guidance for pre-manipulative testing of the cervical spine. Man Ther 2000;5(1):37–40.

82 Maigne R. Orthopaedic Medicine: A New Approach to Vertebral Manipulation. Springfield, IL: Charles C Thomas; 1972.

83 Maitland G. Vertebral Manipulation, 3rd edn. London, UK: Butterworth; 1973.

84 Oostendorp R. Vertebrobasilar insufficiency. Proceedings of the International Federation of Orthopaedic Manipulative Therapists Congress. Cambridge, UK: International Federation of Orthopaedic Manipulative Therapists; 1988.

85 Terret A. Vascular accidents from cervical spine manipulation: The mechanisms. Australian Chiropractors Association. J Chiropractic 1988;22(5):59–74.

86 Grant R. Vertebral artery insufficiency: A clinical protocol for pre-manipulative testing of the cervical spine. In: Boyling J, Palastanga N eds. Grieve's Modern Manual Therapy, 2nd edn. Edinburgh, UK: Churchill Livingstone; 1994: 371–80.

87 Chapman-Smith D. Cervical adjustment. Chiropractic Rep 1999;13(4):1–7.

88 Refshauge K. Rotation: A valid premanipulative dizziness test? Does it predict safe manipulation? J Manipulative Physiol Ther 1994;17(1):15–19.

89 Rivett D, Sharples K, Milburn PD. Effect of pre-manipulative test on vertebral artery and internal carotid artery blood flow: A pilot study. J Manipulative Physiol Ther 1999;22: 368–75.

90 Zaina C, Grant R, Johnson C, et al. The effect of cervical rotation on blood flow in the contralateral vertebral artery. Man Ther 2003;8(2):103–9.

91 Arnold C, Bourassa R, Langer T, et al. Doppler studies evaluating the effect of a physical therapy screening protocol on vertebral artery blood flow. Man Ther 2004;9(1):13–21.

92 Schmitt H. Anatomical structure of the cervical spine with reference to pathology of manipulation complications. J Man Med 1991;6:93–101.

93 Stevens A. Functional Doppler sonography of the vertebral artery and some considerations about manual techniques. J Man Med 1991;6: 102–5.

94 Haynes M. Doppler studies comparing the effects of cervical rotation and lateral flexion on vertebral artery blood flow. J Manipulative Physiol Ther 1996;19:378–84.

95 Mitchell J. Changes in vertebral artery blood flow following normal rotation of the cervical spine. J Manipulative Physiol Ther 2003;26(6): 347–51.

96 Mitchell J, Keene D, Dyson C, et al. Is cervical spine rotation, as used in the standard vertebrobasilar insufficiency test, associated with a measurable change in intracranial vertebral artery blood flow? Man Ther 2004;9(4):220–7.

97 Licht P, Christensen H, Hojgaard P, et al. Triplex ultrasound of vertebral artery flow during cervical rotation. J Manipulative Physiol Ther 1998;21:27–31.

98 Licht P, Christensen H, Hoilund-Carlsen P. Vertebral artery volume flow in human beings. J Manipulative Physiol Ther 1999;22: 363–7.

99 Licht P, Christensen H, Hoilund-Carlsen P. Is there a role for pre-manipulative testing before cervical manipulation? J Manipulative Physiol Ther 2000;23:175–9.

100 Haynes M, Milne N. Color duplex sonographic findings in human vertebral arteries during cervical rotation. J Clin Ultrasound 2000;29: 14–24.

101 Haynes M, Cala L, Melsom A, et al. Vertebral arteries and cervical rotation: Modeling and magnetic resonance angiography studies. J Manipulative Physiol Ther 2002;25(6):370–83.

102 Bowler N, Shamley D, Davies R. The effect of a simulated manipulation position on internal carotid and vertebral artery blood flow in healthy individuals. Man Ther 2011;16:87–93.

103 Thomas LC, Rivett DA, Bateman G, et al. Effect of selected manual therapy interventions for mechanical neck pain on vertebral and internal carotid arterial blood flow and cerebral inflow. Phys Ther 2013;93(11):1563–74.

104 Quesnele JJ, Triano JJ, Noseworthy MD, et al. Changes in vertebral artery blood flow following various head positions and cervical spine manipulation. J Manipulative Physiol Ther 2014;37(1):22–31.

105 Malo-Urries M, Tricas-Moreno JM, Lucha-Lopez O, et al. Vertebral and internal carotid artery flow during vascular premanipulative testing using duplex Doppler ultrasound measurements: A systematic review. Int J Osteopath Med 2012;15:103–10.

106 Gross A, Chesworth B, Binkley J. A case for evidence based practice in manual therapy. In: Boyling J, Jull G eds. Grieve's Modern Manual Therapy–The Vertebral Column, 3rd edn. Edinburgh, UK: Churchill Livingstone; 2005: Ch. 39.

107 Richter R, Reinking M. Evidence in practice. How does evidence on the diagnostic accuracy of the vertebral artery test influence teaching of the test in a professional physical therapist education program? Phys Ther 2005;85(6): 589–99.

108 Thiel H, Wallace K, Donat J, et al. Effect of various head and neck positions on vertebral artery flow. Clin Biomech 1994;9:105–10.

109 Cote P, Kreitz B, Cassidy J, et al. The validity of the extension-rotation test as a clinical screening procedure before neck manipulation: A secondary analysis. J Manipulative Physiol Ther 1996;19(3):159–64.

110 Rivett D, Milburn P, Chapple C. Negative pre- manipulative vertebral artery testing despite complete occlusion: A case of false negativity. Man Ther 1998;3(2):102–7.

111 Licht P, Christensen H, Hoilund-Carlsen P. Carotid artery blood flow during premanipulative testing. J Manipulative Physiol Ther 2002;25(9):568–72.

112 Westaway M, Stratford P, Symons B. False-negative extension/rotation pre-manipulative screening test on a patient with an atretic and hypoplastic vertebral artery. Man Ther 2003;8(2):120–7.

113 Hutting N, Verhagen A, Vijverman V, et al. Diagnostic accuracy of premanipulative vertebrobasilar insufficiency tests: A systematic review. Man Ther 2013;18:177–82.

114 Grant R. Vertebral artery testing–the Australian Physiotherapy Association Protocol after 6 years. Man Ther 1996;1(3):149–53.

115 Terrett A. Did the SMT practitioner cause the arterial injury? Chiropractic J Aust 2002;32(3): 99–119.

116 Thiel H, Rix G. Is it time to stop functional pre-manipulation testing of the cervical spine? Man Ther 2005;10(2):154–8.

117 Kerry R, Taylor A, Mitchell J, et al. Cervical arterial dysfunction and manual therapy: A critical literature review to inform professional practice. Man Ther 2008;13(4):278–88.

118 Symons B, Leonard T, Herzog W. Internal forces sustained by the vertebral artery during spinal manipulative therapy. J Manipulative Physiol Ther 2002;25(8):504–10.

119 Herzog W, Leonard TR, Symons B, et al. Vertebral artery strains during high-speed, low amplitude cervical spinal manipulation. J Electromyogr Kinesiol 2012;22(5):740–6.

120 Piper SL, Howarth SJ, Triano J, et al. Quantifying strain in the vertebral artery with simultaneous motion analysis of the head and neck: A preliminary investigation. Clin Biomech 2014;29(10):1099–107.

121 Biller J, Sacco RL, Albuquerque FC, et al. Cervical Arterial Dissections and Association with Cervical Manipulative Therapy. Stroke 2014;45:3155–74.

122 Micheli S, Paciaroni M, Corea F, et al. Cervical artery dissection: Emerging risk factors. Open Neurol J 2010;4:50–5.

123 Tehan P, Vaughan B, Gibbons P. Cervical Spine Manipulation Revisited. In-Touch Musculoskeletal Physiotherapy. Aust Physiother Assoc 2015;(1):15–18.

124 Silbert P, Mokri B, Schievink W. Headache and neck pain in spontaneous internal carotid and vertebral artery dissections. Neurology 1995;45:1517–22.

125 Taylor AJ, Kerry R. A 'system based' approach to risk assessment of the cervical spine prior to manual therapy. Int J Osteopath Med 2010;13(3):85–93.

126 Penning L, Wilmink J. Rotation of the cervical spine: A CT study in normals. Spine 1987;12(8):732–8.

127 Louri H, Stewart W. Spontaneous atlantoaxial dislocation. N Engl J Med 1961;265(14): 677–81.

128 Swinkels R, Beeton K, Alltree J. Pathogenesis of upper cervical instability. Man Ther 1996;1(3): 127–32.

129 Swinkels R, Oostendorp R. Upper cervical instability: Fact or fiction? J Manipulative Physiol Ther 1996;19(3):185–94.

130 Adams JC, Hamblen DL. Outline of Orthopaedics. Edinburgh, UK: Churchill Livingstone; 2001: Ch. 9.

131 Krauss WE, Bledsoe JM, Clarke MJ, et al. Rheumatoid arthritis of the craniovertebral junction. Neurosurgery 2010;66(Suppl. 3): 83–95.

132 Tredwell S, Newman D, Lockitch G. Instability of the upper cervical spine in Down syndrome. J Pediatr Orthop 1990;10:602–6.

133 Gabriel K, Mason D, Carango P. Occipito-atlantal translation in Down's syndrome. Spine 1990;15:997–1002.

134 Parfenchuck T, Bertrand S, Powers M, et al. Posterior occipitoatlantal hypermobility in Down syndrome: An analysis of 199 patients. J Pediatr Orthop 1994;14:304–8.

135 Matsuda Y, Sano N, Watanabe S, et al. Atlanto-occipital hypermobility in subjects with Down's syndrome. Spine 1995;20(21):2283–6.

136 Ugur H, Caglar S, Unlu A, et al. Infection-related atlantoaxial subluxation in two adults: Grisel syndrome or not? Acta Neurochir 2003;145:69–72.

137 Cattrysse E, Swinkels R, Oostendorp R, et al. Upper cervical instability: Are clinical tests reliable? Man Ther 1997;2(2):91–7.

138 Chiu W, Haan J, Cushing B, et al. Ligamentous injuries of the cervical spine in unreliable blunt trauma patients: Incidence, evaluation and outcome. J Trauma Inj Infect Crit Care 2001;50(3):457–64.

139 Dickman C, Greene K, Sonntag V. Injuries involving the transverse atlantal ligament: Classification and treatment guidelines based upon experience with 39 injuries. Neurosurgery 1996;38(1):44–50.

140 Pettman E. Stress tests of the craniovertebral joints. In: Boyling J, Palastanga N, editors. Grieve's Modern Manual Therapy. Edinburgh, UK: Churchill Livingstone; 1994: Ch. 38.

141 Hino H, Abumi K, Kanayama M, et al. Dynamic motion analysis of normal and unstable cervical spines using cineradiography. Spine 1999;24(2):163–8.

142 Soderman T, Olerud C, Shalabi A, et al. Static and dynamic CT imaging of the cervical spine in patients with rheumatoid arthritis. Skeletal Radiol 2015;44(2):241–8.

143 Sharp J, Purser D. Spontaneous atlantoaxial dislocation in ankylosing spondylitis and rheumatoid arthritis. Ann Rheum Dis 1961;20:47–77.

144 Uitvlught G, Indenbaum S. Clinical assessment of atlantoaxial instability using the Sharp–Purser test. Arthritis Rheum 1988;31(7): 370–4.

145 Meadows J. The Sharp-Purser test: A useful clinical tool or an exercise in futility and risk? J Man Manip Ther 1998;6(2):97–100.

146 Kaale B, Krakenes J, Albrektsen G, et al. Clinical assessment techniques for detecting ligament and membrane injuries in the upper cervical spine region–a comparison with MRI results. Man Ther 2008;13(5): 397–403.

147 Osmotherly PG, Rivett DA, Rowe LJ. The anterior shear and distraction tests for craniocervical instability. An evaluation using magnetic resonance imaging. Man Ther 2012;17(5):416–21.

148 Osmotherly PG, Rivett DA, Rowe LJ. Construct validity of clinical tests for alar ligament integrity: An evaluation using magnetic resonance imaging. Phys Ther 2012;92(5): 718–25.

149 Vick D, McKay C, Zengerle C. The safety of manipulative treatment: Review of the literature from 1925 to 1993. J Am Osteopath Assoc 1996;96(2):113–15.

6

Evidence-informed practice

High-velocity low-amplitude (HVLA) thrust techniques are widely used in patient care with increasing evidence of their effectiveness. However, the use of HVLA thrust techniques must be considered within the context of a comprehensive patient management plan, which may include the application of other osteopathic manipulative techniques and adjunctive therapies.

Various authors have described specific indications for the use of HVLA thrust techniques (Box 6.1).[1-30]

CAVITATION ASSOCIATED WITH HVLA THRUST TECHNIQUES

The aim of HVLA thrust techniques is to achieve joint cavitation that is accompanied by a 'popping' or 'cracking' sound. This audible release distinguishes HVLA procedures from other osteopathic manipulative techniques.

Research involving the metacarpophalangeal joint indicates that the audible release is generated by a cavitation mechanism resulting from a drop in the internal joint pressure.[31-34] Following cavitation, there is an increase in the size of the joint space and gas is found within that space.[31-35] Kawchuk et al, using real-time magnetic resonance imaging (MRI), reported that the mechanism of joint cracking is related to cavity formation rather than bubble collapse.[36] The gas bubble has been described as 80% carbon dioxide[32] or having the density of nitrogen.[14] The gas bubble remains within the joint for between 15 and 30 minutes,[31-33,35] which is consistent with the time taken for the gas to be reabsorbed into the synovial fluid.[32] An increased range of joint motion immediately following cavitation has been demonstrated.[35] Ultrasound imaging studies of the trapeziometacarpal articular cavity identified minute gas bubbles, also known as 'microcavities,' in 27.8% of pre manipulated joints. All post manipulative sonograms revealed numerous large conspicuous gas bubbles within the synovial fluid.[37]

The audible release in the lumbar spine is believed to originate from the apophysial joints.[38] Widening of lumbar zygapophysial joints after manipulation has been demonstrated by MRI following lumbar spine manipulation in asymptomatic subjects[39, 40] and low back pain subjects.[41] The situation in the cervical spine is less clear as neck manipulation did not demonstrate similar post manipulation apophysial joint space widening when assessed using computed tomography (CT).[42]

A number of studies have reported that thrust techniques are associated with a temporary increase in the range of spinal motion.[43-53] Longer-term effects of HVLA thrust techniques have also been reported,[54,55] and it is postulated that these

67

Box 6.1 Specific indications for HVLA thrust techniques as listed by various authors

- Hypomobility[1,2]
- Motion restriction[3–5]
- Joint fixation[6,7]
- Acute joint locking[2,8,9]
- Motion loss with somatic dysfunction[10,11]
- Somatic dysfunction[12–14]
- Restore bony alignment[4,15]
- Meniscoid entrapment[1,3,4,7,16]
- Adhesions[17]
- Displaced disc fragment[18]
- Pain modulation[1,5,9,19,20]
- Reflex relaxation of muscles[1,5,21–23]
- Reprogramming of the central nervous system[12]
- Release of endorphins[24]
- Clinical prediction rule[25–30]

may be due to reflex mechanisms that either directly cause muscle relaxation or inhibit pain.[5] Spinal manipulation applied to dysfunctional lumbar segments in patients with chronic low back pain demonstrated attenuation of the stretch reflex (erector spinae muscles) where an audible response was exhibited.[56] Lumbosacral spinal manipulation was found to produce a significant decrease in corticospinal and spinal reflex excitability compared with controls.[57] Studies of pain pressure threshold before and following spinal manipulation have been undertaken[58–60] with some demonstrating a positive effect.[58,60]

Some authors have reported benefits from HVLA thrust techniques without the accompanying audible release.[61,62] There continues to be speculation as to the level and side of apophysial joint cavitation when HVLA thrust techniques are applied to the spine.[63–66] It is likely that the level and side of cavitation will be dependent on a range of factors that might include spinal positioning and locking, the specific technique applied, operator skill and patient compliance and whether the patient is symptomatic or asymptomatic. MRI studies before and after sidelying lumbar manipulation identified that 93.5% of cavitations occurred in the upper apophyseal joints.[67] The authors also reported that 71% of cavitations occurred within the target area, which would indicate that there is a potential for some specificity when applying thrust techniques to the lumbosacral spine. A study on manipulation of the upper cervical spine recorded bilateral cavitation occurring in 91.9% of subjects when a single rotary thrust manipulation was applied to the C1–2 articulation.[68]

The aim of HVLA thrust techniques is to achieve cavitation within the normal range of zygapophysial joint motion and not at the anatomical end range.

Repeated 'cracking' or 'popping' of the joints of the hand, associated with cavitation, has not been shown to be linked with an increased incidence of degenerative change.[69–71]

EVIDENCE SUMMARY

Best practice requires practitioners to embrace the principles of evidence-based medicine (EBM). EBM incorporates the best results from clinical and epidemiological research with individual clinical experience and expertise whilst taking account of patient preferences.[72,73]

In manual medicine the focus of critical review or assessment of the efficacy of treatment is often based solely upon research evidence. However, clinical experience and patient preferences should also play an important role in deciding the best treatment approach.

Practice-based evidence (PBE) is evidence that individual clinicians acquire through their training, clinical experience and practice, which also takes account of patient preferences (Fig. 6.1). Evidence-rich areas are in the minority in musculoskeletal medicine practice, requiring practitioners to rely more heavily upon their PBE. This,

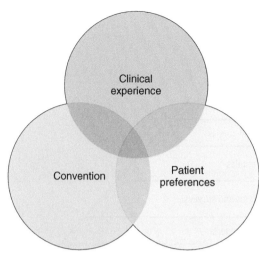

Figure 6.1 Practice-based evidence.

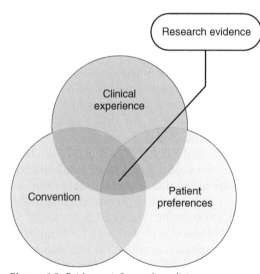

Figure 6.2 Evidence-informed medicine.

however, should be informed by the best available research. Best practice should take account of training, clinical experience, patient preference and research evidence (Fig. 6.2).

Evidence for efficacy of interventions such as spinal manipulation can be assessed according to a hierarchy of evidence that exists in the literature for that intervention (Fig. 6.3).

Recommendations arising from a review of the research reflect the strength of evidence and methodological quality, but not necessarily the clinical importance.

Research evidence can be synthesized in a number of different ways. A systematic review, which is the systematic synthesis of evidence across all trials for a given intervention, can be undertaken.

SYNTHESES

- Systematic reviews including meta-analyses
- Decision and economic analyses
- Guidelines

Meta-analysis is a systematic review that uses special statistical methods for combining the results of several studies. Recommendations based on research evidence can be used to develop clinical practice guidelines and standards for third-party payers and policy makers.

Bronfort et al[74] reported that between 1979 and 2002 there have been in excess of 50 mostly qualitative, nonsystematic reviews published relating to manipulation and mobilization treatment for back and neck pain. A number of systematic reviews and meta-analyses have also been undertaken to attempt to determine the efficacy of spinal manipulation on low back pain,[75–91] back and neck pain,[92] neck pain[93–100] and headache.[101–103]

Bronfort et al[74] undertook an extensive search of computerized and bibliographic literature databases up to the end of 2002 relating to the efficacy of spinal manipulation and mobilization for low back and neck pain and concluded that the use of spinal manipulative therapy and/or mobilization is a viable option for the treatment of both low back pain and neck pain. This systematic review identified the paucity of high-quality trials distinguishing between acute and chronic presentations and recommended that further research should examine the value of spinal manipulation and mobilization for well-defined subgroups of patients and

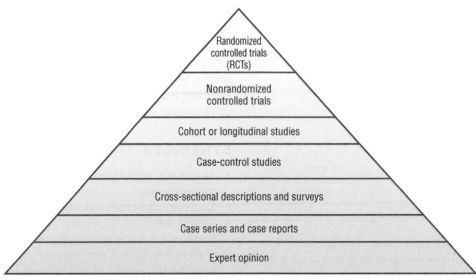

Figure 6.3 Hierarchy of evidence.

determine the cost-effectiveness of different treatment approaches.

A Cochrane database systematic review on spinal manipulative therapy for low back pain concluded that there is no evidence that spinal manipulation is superior to other standard treatments for patients suffering acute or chronic low back pain.[83] An update of a Cochrane review identified that there is no clinically relevant difference between spinal manipulative therapy and other interventions for reducing pain and improving function in patients with chronic low back pain.[86] However, the decision to refer patients for spinal manipulative therapy should also be based upon consideration of costs, patient preferences and the relative safety of interventions.[87] A systematic review of randomized controlled trials (RCTs) relating to a range of complementary therapies for nonspecific back pain, concluded that spinal manipulation has real but modest benefits for acute and chronic low back pain and that the risks of lumbar manipulation are low.[80] A systematic review relating to chronic low back pain concluded that both

spinal manipulation and mobilization are viable treatment options and are at least as effective as other commonly used interventions with a low risk of serious adverse events.[85]

The United Kingdom Back Pain Exercise and Manipulation (UK BEAM) randomized trial concluded that spinal manipulation over a 12-week period produced statistically significant benefits relative to best care in general practice at both 3 and 12 months[104] and that spinal manipulation was also a cost-effective addition to general practice best care.[105] The joint clinical practice guideline from the American College of Physicians and the American Pain Society states that practitioners should consider using spinal manipulation for acute, subacute or chronic low back pain in those patients who do not improve with self-care options.[106] A prospective single-blinded, placebo-controlled study assessing the effectiveness of spinal manipulation for chronic nonspecific low back pain found spinal manipulation to be effective. The authors suggested that to obtain longer-term benefit, patients should receive maintenance spinal manipulation after an initial period of more intense manipulative therapy.[107]

A Cochrane review of manipulation and mobilization for mechanical neck pain concluded that manipulation when combined with exercise and/or mobilization is beneficial for persistent mechanical neck disorders with or without headache, providing strong evidence for using a multimodal treatment approach.[95] Vernon et al[96] carried out a systematic analysis of group change scores in RCTs of patients treated with manual therapy who were suffering from chronic neck pain not due to whiplash and excluding headache or arm pain. They concluded that patients randomized to receive spinal manipulation or mobilization showed clinically important improvements at 6, 12 and up to 104 weeks after treatment. The Bone and Joint Decade 2000–2010 task force on neck pain and its associated disorders reported that the evidence favours supervised exercise sessions with or without manual therapy over usual or no care for both whiplash-associated disorders and neck disorders without trauma.[97] The task force reported that manipulation and mobilization yielded comparable clinical outcomes. A systematic review of controlled clinical trials relevant to chiropractic practice concluded that interventions commonly used in chiropractic care (including spinal manipulation) improve outcomes for acute and chronic neck pain.[100]

A systematic review of the efficacy of spinal manipulation for chronic headache concluded that spinal manipulative therapy has an effect comparable with commonly prescribed prophylactic tension headache and migraine medications.[101] Bryans et al undertook a systematic review of controlled clinical trials relevant to chiropractic practice and concluded that chiropractic care (including spinal manipulation) improves migraine and cervicogenic headaches with the type, frequency, dosage and duration of

treatment based on guideline recommendations, clinical experience and clinical findings.[102]

A comprehensive summary of the scientific evidence (systematic reviews, randomized clinical trials, evidence-based guidelines) relating to the effectiveness of manual therapies concluded that spinal manipulation/mobilization is effective in adults for acute, subacute and chronic low back pain; acute and subacute neck pain; cervicogenic headache and cervicogenic dizziness.[108]

In an effort to increase consistency in the management of spinal disorders, available evidence is reviewed by expert committees to establish clinical guidelines. Clinical guidelines for the management of low back pain have been developed in at least 13 different countries. Since the available evidence is international, there would be an expectation that all the guidelines regarding diagnosis and treatment would offer broadly similar recommendations.[106] Willem et al[82] noted that all national guidelines on the management of low back pain included the use of spinal manipulation. However, the data upon which national recommendations are based have been interpreted differently, leading to conflicting guidelines between countries for the use of spinal manipulation in the management of both acute and chronic back pain. Following an overview of clinical guidelines for the management of nonspecific low back pain in primary care, Koes et al[109] noted similar recommendations for diagnostic classification and the use of diagnostic and therapeutic interventions but discrepancies in recommendations regarding spinal manipulation and drug treatment for acute and chronic low back pain. The National Institute for Health and Clinical Excellence published guidelines for the management of nonspecific low back pain lasting for more than 6 weeks but less than 12 months.[110] Taking into account patient preferences, one of three treatment options was proposed—an exercise program, a course of manual therapy or a course of acupuncture. A practitioner should consider offering another of these options if the chosen treatment does not result in satisfactory improvement. The manual therapy treatment option comprised a course of manual therapy, including spinal manipulation, to a maximum of nine sessions over a period of up to 12 weeks.

Manual therapy approaches, including HVLA thrust techniques, have been negatively impacted by poorly designed and implemented research studies.[111] Practitioners of manipulative therapy are not a homogeneous group and have differing levels of training and skill in the application of manipulative techniques. Patients with spinal pain are also not a homogeneous group, which makes comparison of like with like extremely difficult. However, practitioners have demonstrated an ability, using signs and symptoms, to identify subgroups of patients with low back pain and then match them to specific treatment approaches. Those patients matched by the practitioner to specific interventions showed statistically significant improvement compared with nonmatched controls.[112] Several classification systems for spinal and pelvic girdle pain have been proposed in an attempt to address this problem and identify the subgroups of patients who are likely to respond positively to specific interventions.[113-122]

Research into the predictive value of specific clinical findings to identify patients with spinal pain who are likely to benefit from spinal manipulation has led to the development of clinical prediction rules. Clinical prediction rules consist of combinations of variables obtained from self-report measures, patient history and examination that assist in identifying those patients with spinal pain most likely to respond to spinal manipulation.[25-28,30,123]

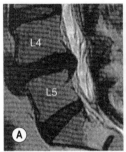 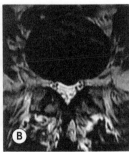

Figure 6.4 L4–5 disc protrusion. **A,** Sagittal view. **B,** Axial view. (From Edelman RR, Hesselink JD, Zlatkin MB, Crues JV. Clinical Magnetic Resonance Imaging, 3rd edn, St. Louis, MO: Elsevier; 2009.)

HVLA THRUST TECHNIQUES AND DISC LESIONS

The diagnosis of disc pathology is achieved by clinical examination and imaging modalities, including CT and MRI (Fig. 6.4).[124] A number of studies have reported imaging evidence of a disc abnormality in asymptomatic individuals.[125-132] Another study has reported patients with low back pain and imaging evidence of disc abnormality responding favourably to manipulative treatment without any alteration in the MRI findings.[133] Abnormal disc imaging findings may frequently be coincidental to a patient's symptoms and are not reliable predictors for the presence, development or duration of spinal pain. It has been reported that a high rate of asymptomatic subjects have disc herniation on MRI imaging and that clinicians need to be aware that MRI images are not necessarily a causal explanation of a patient's pain.[131] The diagnosis of discogenic pain should not be made from imaging findings alone but must also take into account a patient's age, clinical signs and symptoms.

The use of HVLA thrust techniques for patients with disc bulging or herniation is often cited as being controversial, but there are authors who support the use of manipulation and research evidence indicating positive outcomes in the treatment of patients with MRI documented disc herniations[133-141] and in patients with radiculopathy.[139,142-145] The North American Spine Society has published *Evidence–Based Clinical Guidelines for Diagnosis and Treatment of Lumbar Disc Herniation with Radiculopathy*, stating that spinal manipulation is an option for symptomatic relief in patients with lumbar disc herniation with radiculopathy.[146] A prospective randomized clinical study of 40 patients with unilateral lumbar radiculopathy secondary to lumbar disc herniation, who failed at least 3 months of nonoperative management, were randomized to either surgical microdiscectomy or standardized chiropractic spinal manipulation.[139] Significant improvement in both treatment groups compared with baseline scores over time was observed in all outcome measures. After 1 year, follow-up intent-to-treat analysis did not reveal a difference in outcome based on the original treatment received. Sixty percent of patients with sciatica who had failed other medical management benefited from spinal manipulation to the same degree as if they underwent surgical intervention. The 40% of patients that did not improve with spinal manipulation crossed from spinal manipulation to surgery and improved to the same degree as their primary surgical counterparts. The authors concluded that patients with symptomatic lumbar disc herniation failing medical management should consider spinal manipulation followed by surgery, if warranted.

A review of the published data on the efficacy of spinal manipulation in the management of disc herniation, including published data on harms, reported that adverse events appear to be rare and manipulation is likely to be safe when used by appropriately trained practitioners.[147] However, there have been case reports of ruptured cervical disc[148] and lumbar disc herniation progressing to cauda equina syndrome following manipulative procedures.[149,150] What is not known is whether the disc herniation would have progressed without manipulation or whether the force and torque of the manipulation was a factor. A systematic review of the safety of spinal manipulation in the treatment of lumbar disc herniations reported the risk of a patient suffering a clinically worsened disc herniation or cauda equina syndrome following spinal manipulation to be less than 1 in 3.7 million.[151] A systematic review of HVLA thrust techniques concluded that the evidence does not support the hypothesis that spinal manipulation is inherently unsafe in cases of symptomatic lumbar disc disease.[152]

HVLA THRUST TECHNIQUES IN THE PREGNANT AND POSTPARTUM POPULATION

Musculoskeletal pain, especially lumbopelvic pain, is a common occurrence during pregnancy and the postpartum period. Low back pain has been reported to occur as frequently as in 35% to 45% of pregnant women.[153-155] Skaggs et al[156] identified pregnancy-related pain at three major sites: low back, pelvic girdle and mid-back. It has been postulated that spinal pain experienced during pregnancy is multifactorial, but some of the proposed mechanisms include influence of relaxin levels producing ligamentous laxity, maternal weight gain and biomechanical changes due to altered posture.

Many pregnant women express a preference to avoid using medicines in the management of spinal pain and seek nonpharmacological treatment options. In a population-based survey of South Australian women, Stapleton et al[153] reported that 11% of women with low back pain in pregnancy underwent chiropractic treatment. There is a paucity of published studies investigating the clinical effectiveness of HVLA thrust techniques in the management of pregnancy-related and postpartum spinal and pelvic girdle pain. A retrospective case series described the results of chiropractic treatment, including spinal manipulation, for 17 women with low back pain when pregnant.[157] Of the 17 cases, 16 demonstrated clinical improvement in pain intensity throughout the course of treatment, but no conclusions on effectiveness can be drawn from any case series. A systematic review reported that six studies demonstrated that chiropractic care is associated with improved outcomes in pregnancy-related low back pain.[158] However, the authors stated that the lack of randomized trials and control groups preclude any definitive statement as to the efficacy of chiropractic care for pregnancy-related low back pain. In another systematic review of manipulative therapy for pregnancy and related conditions, Khorsan et al[155] concluded that definitive evidence that establishes clinical effectiveness has not yet been presented. A prospective cohort outcomes study with short-term, medium-term and 1-year follow-up found that a large proportion of pregnant patients with low back or pelvic pain undergoing chiropractic treatment reported improvement in their symptoms at all time points up to 1 year.[159] However, because there was no control group or other treatment group for comparison, the outcomes reported cannot necessarily be assumed to arise from the treatment.

The safety of spinal manipulation during pregnancy and the postpartum period has been a matter of debate. Spontaneous abortion is a common complication of early pregnancy. The overall risk of spontaneous abortion after 15 weeks is low for chromosomally and structurally normal foetuses.[160] If a woman has had manipulation applied to the spine or pelvis, especially in the first trimester of pregnancy, and suffers a spontaneous abortion, she may associate the two events even though

there is no published evidence there is any causal connection between HVLA thrust techniques and spontaneous abortion. Serious adverse events from spinal manipulation to pregnant women or those in the early postpartum period are very rare with only 7 cases reported in the literature, and all these serious adverse events were related to treating the cervical spine.[161] Further research is necessary to establish both the clinical effectiveness and the risks associated with using HVLA thrust techniques in the pregnant and postpartum populations. Because safe and effective treatments for pregnancy-related spinal and pelvic girdle pain are limited, practitioners may consider HVLA thrust techniques as a treatment option, in a multimodal approach, for patients who have a preference for this approach if no contraindications are present. As the pregnancy develops, modifications in technique delivery often have to be made to ensure patient comfort and avoid abdominal compression.

HVLA THRUST TECHNIQUES IN THE PAEDIATRIC POPULATION

A systematic literature review reported that idiopathic adolescent spinal pain is a significant problem and that prevalence figures approach those of adults.[162] Is it appropriate to use HVLA thrust techniques in the treatment of paediatric conditions?

A number of studies have shown that chiropractors and osteopaths do treat children and adolescents and that treatment does include the use of spinal manipulation.[163–166] With increasing age, children are more likely to present with musculoskeletal conditions, whereas younger children commonly present with nonmusculoskeletal conditions.[163–165] Some examples of nonmusculoskeletal conditions that chiropractors report treating are infantile colic, enuresis, asthma and otitis media.[167] A number of reviews of the literature have investigated the effectiveness of spinal manipulative therapy for paediatric conditions,[168-173] but there does not appear to have been even one RCT that has investigated the effectiveness of spinal manipulative therapy for spinal pain in children and adolescents. There is currently a paucity of high-quality research evidence to support or refute the effectiveness of using HVLA thrust techniques when treating paediatric conditions.

Although spinal manipulation is used in children and adolescents, there is limited understanding of paediatric risk estimates. A systematic review by Vohra et al[174] identified a total of 34 adverse incidents reported in the published literature. Fourteen cases of direct adverse events were identified, 9 of which were classified as serious and resulted in hospitalization, permanent disability or death. Twenty cases of delayed diagnosis and/or inappropriate provision of chiropractic care that resulted in indirect adverse events were also identified. The type of spinal manipulation associated with the adverse incidents was unspecified in all cases. The review authors noted that case reports and case series are only a type of passive surveillance and as such do not provide high-quality information regarding the true incidence of adverse events. A 2010 update of the review by Vohra et al on possible adverse events in children treated by spinal manipulation concluded that there was still insufficient evidence related to adverse events and manual therapy to accurately estimate risk.[175] In a literature review of cases of adverse events in infants and children treated by chiropractors or other manual therapists, Todd et al[176] identified 15 serious adverse events and reported that underlying pre-existing pathology was present in a majority of the cases. Before applying HVLA thrust techniques to children, practitioners should reflect on their training and clinical experience and decide whether they are able to adequately assess their paediatric patients

and make a diagnosis. The view has also been expressed that manipulation is contraindicated for children whose epiphyseal plates have not closed,[2] but there is no research evidence available to support this opinion.

From the limited data available, there appears to be a low incidence of serious adverse events associated with spinal HVLA thrust techniques applied to children and adolescents but further research is needed to establish an accurate risk profile.

When treating children, especially young children, consideration should be given to their ability to provide an adequate history and give appropriate feedback on any treatment intervention that is used. Some practitioners choose not to use HVLA thrust techniques in the paediatric population until they judge that a child is capable of providing an adequate history and is able to give appropriate feedback.

Given the limited evidence as to the clinical effectiveness and risk profile of using HVLA thrust techniques in the treatment of children and adolescents, a practitioner can only be guided by clinical experience and patient preference in deciding whether to use these techniques in the management of paediatric conditions. When HVLA thrust techniques are applied to adolescents and children, a minimal leverage, not end range, approach is recommended with the intervention applying the lowest force necessary to achieve cavitation.

CLINICAL DECISION MAKING

Clinical decision making is the ability to collate and synthesize information, make decisions and appropriately implement these decisions in the clinical environment. At our present state of knowledge, what should guide our clinical decision making to incorporate HVLA thrust techniques within a treatment regimen? All healthcare practitioners utilize a clinical

Box 6.2 Clinical decision making

- Exclude contraindications
- Determine influence of psychosocial factors
- Identify presence of a treatable lesion–somatic dysfunction
- Perform risk–benefit analysis
- Identify patient preference for treatment approach
- Refer for further assessment, if indicated, or decide upon appropriate treatment which may include co-management

Box 6.3 Failure of therapy

- Therapy effective/ineffective?
- Therapist efficient/inefficient?
- Unidentified psychosocial risk factors?
- Clinical decision making–right/wrong?

decision-making process before the application of a therapeutic intervention, such as HVLA thrust technique (Box 6.2).

If a patient fails to respond to spinal manipulation, the practitioner must reflect upon a number of potential reasons why this might be the case (Box 6.3). Failure of a patient to respond positively may not be a failure due to the technique per se but can result from factors such as initial incorrect choice of technique, inadequate training and poor technical delivery of the technique, inappropriate patient positioning, patient inability to relax and unidentified psychosocial and chronic pain risk factors.

Exclude Contraindications

Although the majority of patients who present with spinal pain will not have serious pathology, it is imperative that practitioners maintain vigilance in identifying red flags. The term 'red flags' refers to clinical features that may indicate a serious condition requiring urgent

evaluation. The following may indicate the presence of red flags:
- Patient younger than 20 years or older than 50 years with first onset of spinal pain
- Pain following trauma
- Constant and worsening pain
- Past or present history of malignancy
- Long-term corticosteroid use
- General malaise
- Night sweats / pyrexia
- Weight loss
- Neurological symptoms and signs.

Determine Influence of Psychosocial Risk Factors

There are psychosocial risk factors associated with chronic pain, disability and failure to return to work.[177-186] They are subjective and include negative coping strategies, fear avoidance behaviour, anxiety, depression and distress. Practitioners should screen for adverse prognostic factors, and, if identified, treatment should aim to reduce dependency on medication and other passive forms of treatment, including manipulative therapy, and encourage the development of self-management skills. Despite widespread study, uncertainty remains regarding which risk factors for poor recovery are associated with particular outcomes and the strength of those associations.[187,188]

Identify the Presence of a Treatable Lesion–Somatic Dysfunction

A number of treatment models use elements of T-A-R-T as the basis for the selection of manipulative techniques, including HVLA thrust techniques.[11,12,14,21,189,190] The authors advocate that the current convention for the diagnosis of somatic dysfunction T-A-R-T should be expanded to include patient feedback relating to pain provocation and the reproduction of familiar symptoms. We recommend that somatic dysfunction is identified by the S-T-A-R-T of diagnosis and is made on the basis of a number of

> **Box 6.4** Diagnosis of somatic dysfunction
>
> - **S** relates to symptom reproduction
> - **T** relates to tissue tenderness
> - **A** relates to asymmetry
> - **R** relates to range of motion
> - **T** relates to tissue texture changes

positive findings relating to symptom reproduction, tissue tenderness, asymmetry, range of motion and tissue texture changes (Box 6.4).

Decide upon Appropriate Intervention

There is research evidence demonstrating the effects of HVLA thrust techniques in increasing range of motion,[43–51] altering pain perception,[58–60,191] reducing pain[192] and altering autonomic reflex activity.[193] However, the rationale for the use of these techniques should also be informed by research showing evidence of efficacy.

Broadly speaking, manipulative techniques should be selected based upon research evidence, PBE, patient preference and the practitioner's training and experience in the delivery of HVLA thrust techniques.

Research evidence

Research evidence supports the use of spinal manipulation in cervicogenic headache, in mechanical neck pain, and in patients suffering with acute and chronic mechanical low back pain. Clinical prediction rules allow practitioners to identify subgroups of patients who are likely to positively respond to spinal manipulation.

Practice-based evidence

Spinal manipulation is a therapeutic intervention that has been used by various cultures and whose use has been documented over time dating from Hippocrates. Spinal manipulation remains one of the most commonly used osteopathic manipulative treatment techniques.

Patient preference

Although research and practice-based evidence support the use of spinal manipulation in the hands of appropriately trained and experienced practitioners, some patients will express a preference for alternative treatment techniques. Conversely other patients who have had a positive response to spinal manipulation will commonly express a preference for HVLA thrust techniques to be used in treatment.

Practitioner training and experience

The key to safety is dependent on appropriate training, a thorough patient history and physical assessment before the application of any manipulative procedure. Appropriate training in the use of HVLA thrust techniques and subsequent skill refinement through regular practice are key elements for safe practice and professional competence.[194,195]

In clinical practice, the treatment of spinal pain and dysfunction commonly combines several interventions such as manipulation, mobilization and exercise with evidence supporting a multimodal approach.[143,196–202] There is currently no evidence to guide the clinician with regard to the following aspects of manipulative treatment interventions:

1. Which HVLA thrust technique to use
2. How specific we need to be
3. Direction of thrust needed
4. The combination of manual therapy techniques that will be most effective
5. The most effective sequencing of technique within a multimodal approach.

In the absence of research evidence, the decision regarding these aspects of treatment can only be made upon the basis of practitioner training and experience.

CONCLUSION

Practitioners rely upon theoretical and clinical models to justify the use of HVLA thrust techniques in clinical practice. Best practice also requires incorporating the results from clinical and epidemiological research with the individual clinical experience and expertise of the practitioner while taking account of patient preferences. Osteopaths have used HVLA thrust techniques for the treatment of somatic dysfunction for many years with increasing research evidence to support the use of these techniques in clinical practice. Clinical decision making relating to the use of these techniques requires the identification and exclusion of contraindications, recognition of the impact of psychosocial issues upon patient presentation and prognosis, the identification of a treatable lesion, patient preference and analysis of benefits versus risks. The treatment of spinal pain and dysfunction commonly combines several interventions e.g. manipulation, mobilization and exercise, with evidence supporting a multimodal approach.

References

1 Kenna C, Murtagh J. Back Pain and Spinal Manipulation, 2nd edn. Oxford, UK: Butterworth-Heinemann; 1989.

2 Bruckner P, Khan K. Clinical Sports Medicine, 4th edn. New York, NY: McGraw-Hill; 2012: Ch. 13.

3 Lewit K. Manipulative Therapy in Rehabilitation of the Locomotor System, 2nd edn. Oxford, UK: Butterworth-Heinemann; 1991.

4 Maigne R. Diagnosis and Treatment of Pain of Vertebral Origin. Baltimore, MD: Williams & Wilkins; 1996.

5 Brodeur R. The audible release associated with joint manipulation. J Manipulative Physiol Ther 1995;18(3):155–64.

6 Eder M, Tilscher H. Chiropractic Therapy. Diagnosis and Treatment. Gaithersburg, MD: Aspen; 1990.

7 Sammut E, Searle-Barnes P. Osteopathic Diagnosis. Cheltenham, UK: Stanley Thornes; 1998.

8 Gainsbury J. High-velocity thrust and pathophysiology of segmental dysfunction. In: Glasgow E, Twomey L, Sculle E, et al. eds. Aspects of Manipulative Therapy, 2nd edn. Melbourne, Australia: Churchill Livingstone; 1985: Ch. 13.

9 Zusman M. What does manipulation do? The need for basic research. In: Boyling J, Palastanga M eds. Grieve's Modern Manual Therapy, 2nd edn. New York, NY: Churchill Livingstone; 1994: Ch. 47.

10 Kuchera W, Kuchera M. Osteopathic Principles in Practice. Kirksville, MO: KCOM; 1992.

11 Kappler R, Jones J. Thrust (high-velocity/low-amplitude) techniques. In: Ward R ed. Foundations for Osteopathic Medicine. Philadelphia, PA: Lippincott Williams & Wilkins; 2003: Ch. 56.

12 Bourdillon J, Day E, Bookhout M. Spinal Manipulation, 5th edn. Oxford, UK: Butterworth-Heinemann; 1992.

13 Kimberly P. Formulating a prescription for osteopathic manipulative treatment. In: Beal M ed. The Principles of Palpatory Diagnosis and Manipulative Technique. Newark, NJ: American Academy of Osteopathy; 1992: 146–52.

14 DeStefano L. Greenman's principles of manual medicine, 4th edn. Philadelphia, PA: Wolters Kluwer / Lippincott Williams & Wilkins; 2010.

15 Nyberg R, Basmajian J. Rationale for the use of spinal manipulation. In: Basmajian J, Nyberg R eds. Rational Manual Therapies. Baltimore, MD: Williams & Wilkins; 1993: Ch. 17.

16 Bogduk N, Twomey L. Clinical Anatomy of the Lumbar Spine, 2nd edn. Melbourne, Australia: Churchill Livingstone; 1991.

17 Stoddard A. Manual of Osteopathic Practice. London, UK: Hutchinson; 1969.

18 Cyriax J. Textbook of Orthopaedic Medicine, vol. 1. London, UK: Baillière Tindall; 1975.

19 Terrett A, Vernon H. Manipulation and pain tolerance. A controlled study on the effect of spinal manipulation on paraspinal cutaneous pain tolerance levels. Am J Phys Med 1984;63:217–25.

20 Hoehler F, Tobis J, Buerger A. Spinal manipulation for low back pain. J Am Med Assoc 1981;245:1835–8.

21 Kuchera W, Kuchera M. Osteopathic Principles in Practice. Dayton, OH: Greyden Press; 1994: 292.

22 Neumann H. Introduction to Manual Medicine. Berlin, Germany: Springer; 1989.

23 Fisk J. A controlled trial of manipulation in a selected group of patients with low back pain favouring one side. N Z Med J 1979;90:288–91.

24 Vernon H, Dharmi I, Howley T, et al. Spinal manipulation and beta-endorphin: A controlled study of the effect of a spinal manipulation on plasma beta-endorphin levels in normal males. J Manipulative Physiol Ther 1986;9:115–23.

25 Flynn T, Fritz J, Whitman J, et al. A clinical prediction rule for classifying patients with low back pain who demonstrate short term improvement with spinal manipulation. Spine 2002;27(24):2835–43.

26 Childs J, Fritz J, Flynn T, et al. A clinical prediction rule to identify patients with low back pain most likely to benefit from spinal manipulation: A validation study. Ann Intern Med 2004;141(12):920–8.

27 Tseng Y, Wang W, Chen W, et al. Predictors for the immediate responders to cervical manipulation in patients with neck pain. Man Ther 2006;11(4):306–15.

28 Cleland J, Childs J, Fritz J, et al. Development of a clinical prediction rule for guiding treatment of a subgroup of patients with neck pain: Use of thoracic spine manipulation, exercise, and patient education. Phys Ther 2007;87(1):9–23.

29 Puentedura EJ, Landers MR, Cleland JA, et al. Thoracic spine thrust manipulation versus cervical spine thrust manipulation in patients with acute neck pain: A randomized clinical trial. Orthop Sports Phys Ther 2011;41(4):208–20.

30 Puentedura EJ, Cleland JA, Landers MR, et al. Development of a clinical prediction rule to identify patients with neck pain likely to benefit from thrust joint manipulation to the cervical spine. J Orthop Sports Phys Ther 2012;42(7):577–92.

31 Roston J, Haines R. Cracking in the metacarpophalangeal joint. J Anat 1947;81:165–73.

32 Unsworth A, Dowson D, Wright V. Cracking joints: A bioengineering study of cavitation in the metacarpophalangeal joint. Ann Rheum Dis 1972;30:348–58.

33 Meal G, Scott R. Analysis of the joint crack by simultaneous recording of sound and tension.

J Manipulative Physiol Ther 1986;9: 189–95.

34 Watson P, Mollan R. Cineradiography of a cracking joint. Br J Radiol 1990;63:145–7.

35 Mierau D, Cassidy J, Bowen V, et al. Manipulation and mobilization of the third metacarpophalangeal joint: A quantitative radiographic and range of motion study. Man Med 1988;3:135–40.

36 Kawchuk GN, Fryer J, Jaremko JL, et al. Real-time visualization of joint cavitation. PLoS ONE 2015;10(4):e0119470.

37 Jones AR, Yelverton CJ, Bester C. Ultrasound imaging of the trapeziometacarpal articular cavity to investigate the presence of intraarticular gas bubbles after chiropractic manipulation. J Manipulative Physiol Ther 2014;37(7):476–84.

38 Bereznick D, Pecora C, Ross J, et al. The refractory period of the audible 'crack' after lumbar manipulation: A preliminary study. J Manipulative Physiol Ther 2008;31(3):199–203.

39 Cramer G, Gregerson D, Knudsen J, et al. The effects of side-posture positioning and spinal adjusting on the lumbar Z joints. Spine 2002;27(22):2459–66.

40 Cramer GD, Ross K, Pocius J, et al. Evaluating the relationship among cavitation, zygapophyseal joint gapping and spinal manipulation: An exploratory case series. J Manipulative Physiol Ther 2011;34(1):2–14.

41 Cramer GD, Cambron J, Cantu J. Magnetic resonance imaging zygapophyseal joint space changes (gapping) in low back pain patients following spinal manipulation and side-posture positioning: A randomised controlled mechanisms trial with blinding. J Manipulative Physiol Ther 2013;36(4):203–17.

42 Cascioli V, Corr P, Till A. An investigation into the production of intra-articular gas bubbles and increase in joint space in the zygapophysial joints of the cervical spine in asymptomatic subjects after spinal manipulation. J Manipulative Physiol Ther 2003;26(6):356–64.

43 Howe DH, Newcombe RG, Wade MT. Manipulation of the cervical spine: A pilot study. J R Coll Gen Pract 1983;33(254):574–9.

44 Nansel D, Cremata E, Carlson J, et al. Effect of unilateral spinal adjustments on goniometrically assessed cervical lateral-flexion end-range asymmetries in otherwise asymptomatic subjects. J Manipulative Physiol Ther 1989;12(6):419–27.

45 Nansel D, Peneff A, Carlson J, et al. Time course considerations for the effects of unilateral lower cervical adjustments with respect to the amelioration of cervical lateral-flexion passive end-range asymmetry. J Manipulative Physiol Ther 1990;13(6):297–304.

46 Cassidy JD, Quon JA, Lafrance LJ, et al. The effect of manipulation on pain and range of motion in the cervical spine: A pilot study. J Manipulative Physiol Ther 1992;15(8):495–500.

47 Nansel D, Peneff A, Quitoriano D. Effectiveness of upper versus lower cervical adjustments with respect to the amelioration of passive rotational versus lateral-flexion end-range asymmetries in otherwise asymptomatic subjects. J Manipulative Physiol Ther 1992;15(2):99–105.

48 Nilsson N, Christenson HW, Hartrigson J. Lasting changes in passive range of motion after spinal manipulation: A randomised, blind, controlled trial. J Manipulative Physiol Ther 1996;19(3):165–8.

49 Surkitt D, Gibbons P, McLaughlin P. High velocity low amplitude manipulation of the atlanto-axial joint: Effect on atlanto-axial and cervical spine rotation asymmetry in asymptomatic subjects. J Osteopath Med 2000;3(1):13–19.

50 Clements B, Gibbons P, McLaughlin P. The amelioration of atlanto-axial asymmetry using high velocity low amplitude manipulation: Is the direction of thrust important? J Osteopath Med 2001;4(1):8–14.

51 Martinez-Segura R, Fernadez-de-la Penas C, et al. Immediate effects on neck pain and active range of motion after a single cervical high velocity low amplitude manipulation in subjects presenting with mechanical neck pain: A randomized controlled trial. J Manipulative Physiol Ther 2006;29(7):511–17.

52 Branney J, Breen AC. Does inter-vertebral range of motion increase after spinal manipulation? A prospective cohort study. Chiropr Man Therap 2014;22:24.

53 Snodgrass SJ, Cleland JA, Haskins R, et al. The clinical utility of cervical range of motion in diagnosis, prognosis and evaluating the effects of manipulation: A systematic review. Physiotherapy 2014;100(4):290–304.

54 Stodolny J, Chmielewski H. Manual therapy in the treatment of patients with cervical migraine. Man Med 1989;4:49–51.

55 Nordemar R, Thorner C. Treatment of acute cervical pain: A comparative group study. Pain 1981;10:93–101.

56 Clark BC, Goss DA, Walkowski S, et al. Neurophysiologic effects of spinal manipulation in patients with chronic low back pain. BMC Musculoskelet Disord 2011;12:170.

57 Fryer G, Pearce AJ. The effect of lumbosacral manipulation on corticospinal and spinal reflex excitability on asymptomatic participants. J Manipulative Physiol Ther 2012;35(2):86–93.

58 Coronado RA, Gay CW, Bialosky JE, et al. Changes in pain sensitivity following spinal manipulation: A systematic review and meta-analysis. J Electromyogr Kinesiol 2012;22(5):752–67.

59 Gazin M, Zegarra-Parodi R. Compression musculaire ischémique versus technique manipulative du rachis cervical: effets sur le seuil de douleur à la pression du trapèze supérieur. La Revue de l'Ostéopathie 2011;3:5–12.

60 De Oliveira RF, Liebano RE, Da Cunha Menezes Costa L, et al. Immediate effects of region-specific and non-region-specific spinal manipulative therapy in patients with chronic low back pain: A randomized controlled trial. Phys Ther 2013;93(6):748–56.

61 Flynn T, Fritz J, Wainner R, et al. The audible pop is not necessary for successful spinal high-velocity thrust manipulation in individuals with low back pain. Arch Phys Med Rehabil 2003;84:1057–60.

62 Flynn T, Childs J, Fritz J. The audible pop from high-velocity thrust manipulation and outcome in individuals with low back pain. J Manipulative Physiol Ther 2006;29(1):40–5.

63 Reggars J, Pollard H. Analysis of zygapophysial joint cracking during chiropractic manipulation. J Manipulative Physiol Ther 1995;18(2):65–71.

64 Beffa R, Mathews R. Does the adjustment cavitate the targeted joint? An investigation into the location of cavitation sounds. J Manipulative Physiol Ther 2004;27(2):e2.

65 Ross J, Bereznick D, McGill S. Determining cavitation location during lumbar and thoracic spinal manipulation. Is spinal manipulation accurate and specific? Spine 2004;29(13):1452–7.

66 Bolton A, Moran R, Standen C. An investigation into the side of joint cavitation associated with cervical spine manipulation. Int J Osteopath Med 2007;10(4):88–96.

67 Cramer GD, Ross JK, Raju PK, et al. Distribution of cavitations as identified with accelerometry during lumbar spinal manipulation. J Manipulative Physiol Ther 2011;34(9):572–83.

68 Dunning J, Mourad F, Barbero M, et al. Bilateral and multiple cavitation sounds during upper cervical thrust manipulation. BMC Musculoskelet Disord 2013;14(24):1–12.

69 Swezey R, Swezey S. The consequences of habitual knuckle cracking. West J Med 1975;122:377–9.

70 Castellanos J, Axelrod D. Effect of habitual knuckle cracking on hand function. Ann Rheum Dis 1990;49:308–9.

71 De Weber K, Olszewski M, Ortolano R. Knuckle cracking and hand osteoarthritis. J Am Board Fam Med 2011;24(2):169–74.

72 Sackett D, Richardson W, Rosenberg W, et al. Evidence Based Medicine. How to Practice & Teach EBM. New York, NY: Churchill Livingstone; 1997.

73 Pedersen T, Gluud C, Gotzsche P, et al. What is evidence-based medicine? Ugeskr Laeg 2001;163(27):3769–72.

74 Bronfort G, Hass M, Evans R, et al. Efficacy of spinal manipulation and mobilization for low back and neck pain: A systematic review and best evidence synthesis. Spine J 2004;4(3):335–56.

75 Koes B, Assendelft W, Heijden G, et al. Spinal manipulation for low back pain. An updated systematic review of randomized clinical trials. Spine 1996;21(24):2860–71.

76 van Tulder M, Koes B, Bouter L. Conservative treatment of acute and chronic nonspecific low back pain. A systematic review of randomized controlled trials of the most common interventions. Spine 1997;22(18):2128–56.

77 Bronfort G. Spinal manipulation: Current state of research and its indications. Neurol Clin 1999;17(1):91–111.

78 Ferreira M, Ferreira P, Latimer J, et al. Does spinal manipulative therapy help people with chronic low back pain? Aust J Physiother 2002;48(4):277–84.

79 Pengel H, Maher C, Refshauge K. Systematic review of conservative interventions for subacute low back pain. Clin Rehabil 2002;16(8):811–20.

80 Cherkin D, Sherman K, Deyo R, et al. A review of the evidence for the effectiveness, safety, and cost of acupuncture, massage therapy, and spinal manipulation for back pain. Ann Intern Med 2003;138(11):898–906.

81 Ferreira M, Ferreira P, Latimer J, et al. Efficacy of spinal manipulative therapy for low back pain of less than three months' duration. J Manipulative Physiol Ther 2003;26(9):593–601.

82 Willem J, Assendelft W, Morton S, et al. Spinal manipulative therapy for low back pain. A meta-analysis of effectiveness relative to other therapies. Ann Intern Med 2003;138(11):871–81.

83 Assendelft W, Morton S, Yu E, et al. Spinal manipulative therapy for low back pain. Cochrane Database Syst Rev 2004;(1):CD000447.

84 Van Tulder M, Koes B, Malmivaara A. Outcome of non-invasive treatment modalities on back pain: An evidence review. Eur Spine J 2006;15(Suppl. 1):S64–81.

85 Bronfort G, Haas M, Evans R, et al. Evidence-informed management of chronic low back pain with spinal manipulation and mobilization. Spine J 2008;8(1):213–25.

86 Rubinstein SM, Van Middelkoop M, Assendelft WJ, et al. Spinal manipulative therapy for chronic low back pain. An update of a Cochrane Review. Spine 2011;36(13):E825–46.

87 Rubinstein SM, Terwee CB, Assendelft WJ, et al. Spinal manipulative therapy for acute low back pain. Cochrane Database Syst Rev 2012;(9):CD008880.

88 Kuczynski JJ, Schwieterman B, Columber K, et al. Effectiveness of physical therapist administered spinal manipulation for the treatment of low back pain: A systematic review of the literature. Int J Sports Phys Ther 2012;7(6):647–62.

89 Rubinstein SM, Terwee CB, Assendelft WJ, et al. Spinal manipulative therapy for acute low back pain: An update of the Cochrane review. Spine 2013;38(3):E158–77.

90 Hidalgo B, Detrembleur C, Hall T, et al. The efficacy of manual therapy and exercise for different stages of non-specific low back pain: An update of systematic reviews. J Man Manip Ther 2014;22(2):59–74.

91 Menke JM. Do manual therapies help low back pain?: a comparative effectiveness meta-analysis. Spine 2014;39:E463–72.

92 Mior S. Manipulation and mobilization in the treatment of chronic pain. Clin J Pain 2001;17(4):S70–6.

93 Hurwitz E, Aker P, Adams A, et al. Manipulation and mobilization of the cervical spine. A systematic review of the literature. Spine 1996;21(15):1746–59.

94 Gross A, Kay T, Hondras M, et al. Manual therapy for mechanical neck disorders: A systematic review. Man Ther 2002;7(3):131–49.

95 Gross A, Hoving J, Haines T, et al. A Cochrane review of manipulation and mobilization for mechanical neck disorders. Spine 2004;29(14):1541–8.

96 Vernon H, Humphreys K, Hagino C. Chronic mechanical neck pain in adults treated by manual therapy: A systematic review of change scores in randomized clinical trials. J Manipulative Physiol Ther 2007;30(3):215–27.

97 Hurwitz E, Carragee E, van der Velde G, et al. Treatment of neck pain: Non-invasive interventions. Results of the bone and joint decade 2000-2010 task force on neck pain and its associated disorders. Eur Spine J 2008;17(Suppl1):123–52.

98 Gross A, Miller J, D'Sylva J, et al. Manipulation or mobilisation for neck pain: A Cochrane review. Man Ther 2010;15(4):315–33.

99 Miller J, Gross A, D'Sylva J, et al. Manual therapy and exercise for neck pain: A systematic review. Man Ther 2010;15(4):334–54.

100 Bryans R, Decina P, Descarreaux M, et al. Evidence-based guidelines for the chiropractic treatment of adults with neck pain. J Manipulative Physiol Ther 2014;37(1):42–63.

101 Bronfort G, Assendelft W, Evans R, et al. Efficacy of spinal manipulation for chronic headache: A systematic review. J Manipulative Physiol Ther 2001;24(7):457–66.

102 Bryans R, Descarreaux M, Duranleau M, et al. Evidence-based guidelines for the chiropractic treatment of adults with headache. J Manipulative Physiol Ther 2011;34(5):274–89.

103 Chaibi A, Russell MB. Manual therapies for cervicogenic headache: A systematic review. J Headache Pain 2012;13:351–9.

104 UK BEAM Trial Team. United Kingdom Back Pain Exercise and Manipulation (UK BEAM) randomised trial: Effectiveness of physical treatments for back pain in primary care. BMJ 2004;329(7479):1377.

105 UK BEAM Trial Team. United Kingdom back pain exercise and manipulation (UK BEAM) randomised trial: Cost effectiveness of physical treatments for back pain in primary care. BMJ 2004;329(7479):1381. Epub.

106 Chou R, Qaseem A, Snow V, et al. Diagnosis and treatment of low back pain: A joint clinical practice guideline from the American College of Physicians and the American Pain Society. Ann Intern Med 2007;147(7):478–91.

107 Senna MK, Machaly SA. Does maintained spinal manipulation therapy for chronic nonspecific low back pain result in better long term outcome? Spine 2011;36(18):1427–37.

108 Bronfort G, Haas M, Evans R, et al. Effectiveness of manual therapies: The UK evidence report. Chiropr Osteopat 2010;18:1–33.

109 Koes BW, Van Tulder M, Lin CW, et al. An updated overview of clinical guidelines for the management of non-specific low back pain in primary care. Eur Spine J 2010;19(12):2075–94.

110 National Institute for Health and Care Excellence Clinical Guideline 88. Low Back Pain. Early Management of Persistent Non-Specific Low Back Pain. <guidance.nice.org.uk/cg88>; 2009.

111 Rubinstein SM, Van Eekelen R, Oosterhuis T, et al. The risk of bias and sample size of trials of spinal manipulative therapy for low back and neck pain: Analysis and recommendations. J Manipulative Physiol Ther 2014;37(8):523–41.

112 Brennan G, Fritz J, Hunter S, et al. Identifying subgroups of patients with acute/subacute nonspecific low back pain. Spine 2006;31(6):623–31.

113 Fritz J, Delitto A, Erhard R. Comparison of classification-based physical therapy with therapy based on clinical practice guidelines for patients with acute low back pain: A randomized clinical trial. Spine 2003;28(13):1363–71.

114 Childs J, Fritz J, Piva S, et al. Proposal of a classification system for patients with neck pain. J Orthop Sports Phys Ther 2004;34(11):686–96.

115 O'Sullivan P. Diagnosis and classification of chronic low back pain disorders: Maladaptive movement and motor control impairments as underlying mechanism. Man Ther 2005;10(4):242–55.

116 Fritz J, Brennan G. Preliminary examination of a proposed treatment-based classification system for patients receiving physical therapy interventions for neck pain. Phys Ther 2007;87(5):513–24.

117 Billis E, McCarthy C, Oldham J. Subclassification of low back pain: A cross-country comparison. Eur Spine J 2007;16(7):865–79.

118 Fritz J, Cleland J, Childs J. Subgrouping patients with low back pain: Evolution of a classification approach to physical therapy. J Orthop Sports Phys Ther 2007;37(6):290–302.

119 Fritz J, Lindsay W, Matheson J, et al. Is there a subgroup of patients with low back pain likely to benefit from mechanical traction? Results of a randomized clinical trial and subgrouping analysis. Spine 2007;32(26):E793–800.

120 O'Sullivan P, Beals D. Diagnosis and classification of pelvic girdle pain disorders–Part 1: A mechanism based approach within a biopsychosocial framework. Man Ther 2007;12(2):86–97.

121 Burns SA, Foresman E, Kraycsir SJ, et al. A treatment-based classification approach to examination and intervention of lumbar disorders. Sports Health 2011;3(4):362–72.

122 Vining R, Potocki E, Seidman M, et al. An evidence-based diagnostic classification system for low back pain. J Can Chiropr Assoc 2013;57(3):189–204.

123 Cleland JA, Mintken PE, Carpenter K, et al. Examination of a clinical prediction rule to identify patients with neck pain likely to benefit from thoracic spine thrust manipulation and a general cervical range of motion exercise: Multi-center randomized clinical trial. Phys Ther 2010;90(9):1239–50.

124 Edelman RR, Hesselink JD, Zlatkin MB, et al. Clinical Magnetic Resonance Imaging, 3rd edn. Philadelphia, PA: Saunders; 2009.

125 Boden S, Davis D, Dina T, et al. Abnormal magnetic-resonance scans of the lumbar spine in asymptomatic subjects. J Bone Joint Surg Am 1990;72-A(3):403–8.

126 Jensen M, Brant-Zawadzki M, Obuchowski N, et al. Magnetic resonance imaging of the lumbar spine in people without back pain. N Engl J Med 1994;331(2):69–73.

127 Boos N, Rieder R, Schade V, et al. The diagnostic accuracy of magnetic resonance imaging, work perception, and psychosocial factors in identifying symptomatic disc herniations. Spine 1995;20(4):2613–25.

128 Brant-Zawadzki M, Jensen M, Obuchowski N, et al. Interobserver and intraobserver variability in interpretation of lumbar disc abnormalities. Spine 1995;20(11):1257–64.

129 Wood K, Blair J, Aepple D, et al. The natural history of asymptomatic thoracic disc herniations. Spine 1997;22(5):525–9.

130 Borenstein D, O' Mara J, Boden S, et al. The value of magnetic resonance imaging of the lumbar spine to predict low-back pain in asymptomatic subjects. J Bone Joint Surg Am 2001;83-A(9):1306–11.

131 Ernst C, Stadnik T, Peeters E, et al. Prevalence of annular tears and disc herniations on MR images of the cervical spine in symptom free volunteers. Eur J Radiol 2005;55(3):409–14.

132 Nakashima H, Yukawa Y, Suda K, et al. Abnormal findings on magnetic resonance images of the cervical spine in 1211 asymptomatic subjects. Spine 2015;40(6):392–8.

133 Santillia V, Beghi E, Finucci S. Chiropractic manipulation in the treatment of acute back pain and sciatica with disc protrusion: A randomized double-blind clinical trial of active and simulated spinal manipulations. Spine J 2006;6(2):131–7.

134 Cyriax R. Textbook of Orthopaedic Medicine, vol. 2. London, UK: Baillière Tindall; 1984.

135 Maigne R. Diagnosis and Treatment of Pain of Vertebral Origin: A Manual Medicine Approach. Baltimore, MD: Williams & Wilkins; 1996.

136 BenEliyahu D. Magnetic resonance imaging and clinical follow-up: Study of 27 patients receiving chiropractic care for cervical and lumbar disc herniations. J Manipulative Physiol Ther 1996;19(9):597–606.

137 Herzog W. Clinical Biomechanics of Spinal Manipulation. New York, NY: Churchill Livingstone; 2000.

138 Burton A, Tillotson K, Cleary J. Single-blind randomised controlled trial of chemonucleolysis and manipulation in the treatment of symptomatic lumbar disc herniation. Eur Spine J 2000;9(3):202–7.

139 McMorland G, Suter E, Casha S, et al. Manipulation or microdiskectomy for sciatica? A prospective randomized clinical study. J Manipulative Physiol Ther 2010;33(8):576–84.

140 Peterson CK, Schmid C, Leeman S, et al. Outcomes from magnetic resonance imaging–confirmed symptomatic cervical disk herniation patients treated with high-velocity, low-amplitude spinal manipulative therapy: A prospective cohort study with 3-month follow-up. J Manipulative Physiol Ther 2013;36(8):461–7.

141 Leeman S, Peterson CK, Schmid C, et al. Outcomes of acute and chronic patients with magnetic resonance imaging-confirmed symptomatic lumbar disc herniations receiving high-velocity, low-amplitude, spinal manipulative therapy: A prospective observational cohort study

with one year follow up. J Manipulative Physiol Ther 2014;37(3):155–63.

142 Hahne AJ, Ford JJ, McMeeken JM. Conservative management of lumbar disc herniation with associated radiculopathy: A systematic review. Spine 2010;35(11):E488–504.

143 Boyles R, Toy P, Mellon J, et al. Effectiveness of manual physical therapy in the treatment of cervical radiculopathy: A systematic review. J Man Manip Ther 2011;19(3):135–42.

144 Leininger B, Bronfort G, Evans R, et al. Spinal manipulation or mobilisation for radiculopathy: A systematic review. Phys Med Rehabil Clin N Am 2011;22(1):105–25.

145 Rodine RJ, Vernon H. Cervical radiculopathy: A systematic review on treatment by spinal manipulation and measurement with the neck disability index. J Can Chiropr Assoc 2012;56(1):18–28.

146 North American Spine Society. Evidence-Based Clinical Guidelines Committee. Clinical Guidelines for Diagnosis and Treatment of Lumbar Disc Herniation with Radiculopathy. Burr Ridge, IL: NASS; 2012.

147 Snelling N. Spinal manipulation in patients with disc herniation: A critical review of risk and benefit. Int J Osteopath Med 2006;9(3):77–84.

148 Tseng S, Lin S, Chen Y, et al. Ruptured cervical disc after spinal manipulation therapy. Spine 2002;27(3):E80–2.

149 Haldeman S, Rubinstein S. Cauda equina syndrome in patients undergoing manipulation of the lumbar spine. Spine 1992;17(12):1469–73.

150 Markowitz H, Dolce D. Cauda equina syndrome due to sequestrated recurrent disk herniation after chiropractic manipulation. Orthopedics 1997;20(7):652–3.

151 Oliphant D. Safety of spinal manipulation in the treatment of lumbar disk herniations: A systematic review and risk assessment. J Manipulative Physiol Ther 2004;27(3):197–210.

152 Lisi A, Holmes E, Ammendolia C. High-velocity low-amplitude spinal manipulation for symptomatic lumbar disk disease: A systematic review of the literature. J Manipulative Physiol Ther 2005;28(6):429–42.

153 Stapleton D, Maclennan A, Kristiansson P. The prevalence of recalled low back pain during and after pregnancy: A South Australian population survey. Aust NZ Obstet Gynaecol 2002;42(5):482–5.

154 Wu WH, Meijer OG, Uegaki K, et al. Pregnancy-related pelvic girdle pain (PPP), I: Terminology, clinical presentation and prevalence. Eur Spine J 2004;13(7):575–89.

155 Khorsan R, Hawk C, Lisi A, et al. Manipulative therapy for pregnancy and related conditions: A systematic review. Obstet Gynecol Survey 2009;64(6):416–27.

156 Skaggs CD, Prather H, Gross G, et al. Back and pelvic pain in an underserved United States pregnant population: A preliminary descriptive survey. J Manipulative Physiol Ther 2007;30(2):130–4.

157 Lisi A. Chiropractic spinal manipulation for low back pain of pregnancy: A retrospective case series. J Midwifery Women Health 2006;51(1):e7–10.

158 Stuber KJ, Smith DL. Chiropractic treatment of pregnancy-related low back pain: A systematic review of the evidence. J Manipulative Physiol Ther 2008;31(6):447–54.

159 Peterson CK, Muhlemann D, Humphreys BK. Outcomes of pregnant patients with low back pain undergoing chiropractic treatment: A prospective cohort study with short term, medium term and 1 year follow up. Chiropr Man Therap 2014;22(15):1–7.

160 Wyatt PR, Owolabi T, Meier C, et al. Age-specific risk of fetal loss observed in a second trimester serum screening population. Am J Obstet Gynecol 2005;192:240–6.

161 Stuber KJ, Wynd S, Weis CA. Adverse events from spinal manipulation in the pregnant and postpartum periods: A critical review of the literature. Chiropr Man Therap 2012;20:8.

162 Jeffries LJ, Milanese SF, Grimmer-Somers KA. Epidemiology of adolescent spinal pain: A systematic overview of the research literature. Spine 2007;32(23):2630–7.

163 Verhoef M. Survey of Canadian chiropractors' involvement in the treatment of patients under the age of 18. J Can Chiro Assoc 1999;43(1):50–7.

164 Durant CL, Verhoef MJ, Conway PJ, et al. Chiropractic treatment of patients younger than 18 years of age: Frequency, patterns and chiropractors' beliefs. Paediatr Child Health 2001;6(7):433–8.

165 Hestbaek L, Jorgensen A, Hartvigsen J. A description of children and adolescents in Danish chiropractic practice: Results from a nationwide study. J Manipulative Physiol Ther 2009;32(8):607–15.

166 Fawkes C, Leach J, Mathias S, et al. The Standardised Data Collection

Project–Standardised Data Collection Within Osteopathic Practice in the UK: Development and First Use of a Tool to Profile Osteopathic Care in 2009. London, UK: National Council for Osteopathic Research; 2010.

167 Ferrance RJ, Miller J. Chiropractic diagnosis and management of non-musculoskeletal conditions in children and adolescents. Chiropr Osteopat 2010;18(14):1–8.

168 Gotlib A, Rupert R. Assessing the evidence for the use of chiropractic manipulation in paediatric health conditions: A systematic review. Paediatr Child Health 2005;10(3):157–61.

169 Gotlib A, Rupert R. Chiropractic manipulation in pediatric health conditions–an updated systematic review. Chiropr Osteopat 2008;16(11):1–6.

170 Hestbaek L, Stochkendahl MJ. The evidence base for chiropractic treatment of musculoskeletal conditions in children and adolescents: The emperor's new suit? Chiropr Osteopat 2010;18(15):1–4.

171 Posadzki P, Lee MS, Ernst E. Osteopathic manipulative treatment for pediatric conditions: a systematic review. Pediatrics 2013;132(1):140–52.

172 Posadzki P, Ernst E. Is spinal manipulation effective for paediatric conditions? An overview of systematic reviews. Focus Altern Complement Ther 2012;17(1):22–6.

173 Gleberzon BJ, Arts J, Mei A, et al. The use of spinal manipulative therapy for pediatric health conditions: A systematic review of the literature. J Can Chiropr Assoc 2012;56(2):128–41.

174 Vohra S, Johnson B, Cramer K, et al. Adverse events associated with pediatric spinal manipulation: A systematic review. Pediatrics 2007;119(1):e275–83.

175 Humphreys BK. Possible adverse events in children treated by manual therapy: A review. Chiropr Osteopat 2010;18(12):1–7.

176 Todd AJ, Carroll MT, Robinson A, et al. Adverse events due to chiropractic and other manual therapies for infants and children: A review of the literature. J Manipulative Physiol Ther 2014;pii:S0161-4754(14)00178-X.

177 Grotle M, Vollestad N, Veierod M, et al. Fear-avoidance beliefs and distress in relation to disability in acute and chronic low back pain. Pain 2004;112(3):343–52.

178 Steenstra I, Verbeek J, Heymans M, et al. Prognostic factors for duration of sick leave in patients sick listed with acute low back pain: A systematic review of the literature. Occup Environ Med 2005;62(12):851–60.

179 Grotle M, Vollestad N, Brox J. Clinical course and impact of fear-avoidance beliefs in low back pain: Prospective cohort study of acute and chronic low back pain. Spine 2006;31(9):1038–46.

180 Iles R, Davidson M, Taylor N. A systematic review of psychosocial predictors of failure to return to work in non-chronic non-specific low back pain. Occup Environ Med 2008;65(8):507–17. Epub.

181 Grotle M, Brox J, Glomsrod B, et al. Prognostic factors in first-time care seekers due to acute low back pain. Eur J Pain 2007;11(3):290–8.

182 Keeley P, Creed F, Tomenson B, et al. Psychosocial predictors of health-related quality of life and health service utilisation in people with chronic low back pain. Pain 2008;135(1–2):142–50. Epub.

183 Henschke N, Maher C, Refshauge K, et al. Prognosis in patients with recent onset low back pain in Australian primary care: Inception cohort study. BMJ 2008;337:a171.

184 Carroll L, Hogg-Johnson S, van der Velde G, et al. Course and prognostic factors for neck pain in the general population. Results of the bone and joint decade 2000-2010 Task Force on neck pain and its associated disorders. Spine 2008;33(4S):S75–82.

185 Landers M, Creger R, Baker C, et al. The use of fear-avoidance beliefs and nonorganic signs in predicting prolonged disability in patients with neck pain. Man Ther 2008;13(3):239–48.

186 Nicholas MK, Linton SJ, Watson PJ, et al. Early identification and management of psychological risk factors ("Yellow Flags") in patients with low back pain: A reappraisal. Phys Ther 2011;91(5):737–53.

187 Kent P, Keating J. Can we predict poor recovery from recent-onset nonspecific low back pain? A systematic review. Man Ther 2008;13(1):12–28.

188 Ramond A, Bouton C, Richard I, et al. Psychosocial risk factors for chronic low back pain in primary care: A systematic review. Fam Pract 2011;28(1):12–21.

189 DiGiovanna EL, Schiowitz S, Dowling DJ. An Osteopathic Approach to Diagnosis and Treatment, 3rd edn. Philadelphia, PA: Lippincott Williams & Wilkins; 2005.

190 Mitchell F. The Muscle Energy Manual. East Lansing, MI: MET; 1995.

191 Cleland J, Childs J, McRae M, et al. Immediate effects of thoracic manipulation in patients

with neck pain: A randomized clinical trial. Man Ther 2005;10(2):127–35.

192 Fernadez-de-la Penas C, Palomeque-del-Cerro L, Rodriguez-Blanco C, et al. Changes in neck pain and active range of motion after a single thoracic spine manipulation in subjects presenting with mechanical neck pain: A case series. J Manipulative Physiol Ther 2007;30(4):312–20.

193 Gibbons P, Gosling C, Holmes M. The short term effects of cervical manipulation on edge light pupil cycle time: A pilot study. J Manipulative Physiol Ther 2000;23(7):465–9.

194 Chou R, Huffman L. Non pharmacologic therapies for acute and chronic low back pain: A review of the evidence for an American Pain Society / American College of Physicians clinical practice guideline. Ann Intern Med 2007;147(7):492–504.

195 Carnes D, Mars TS, Mullinger B, et al. Adverse events and manual therapy: A systematic review. Man Ther 2010;15(4):355–63.

196 Jull G, Trott P, Potter H, et al. A randomized controlled trial of exercise and manipulative therapy for cervicogenic headache. Spine 2002;27(17):1835–43.

197 Gross A, Kay T, Kennedy C, et al. Clinical practice guideline on the use of manipulation or mobilization in the treatment of adults with mechanical neck disorders. Man Ther 2002;7(4):193–205.

198 Grunnesjo M, Bogefeldt B, Svardsudd K, et al. A randomized controlled clinical trial of stay-active care versus manual therapy in addition to stay-active care: Functional variables and pain. J Manipulative Physiol Ther 2004;27(7):431–41.

199 Gross A, Goldsmith A, Hoving J, et al. Conservative management of mechanical neck disorders: A systematic review. J Rheumatol 2007;34(5):1083–102.

200 Walker M, Boyles R, Young B, et al. The effectiveness of manual physical therapy and exercise for mechanical neck pain. A randomized clinical trial. Spine 2008;33(22):2371–8.

201 Leaver AM, Refshauge KM, Maher CG, et al. Conservative interventions provide short-term relief for non-specific neck pain: A systematic review. J Physiother 2010;56(2):73–85.

202 Forbush SW, Cox T, Wilson E. Treatment of patients with degenerative cervical radiculopathy using a multi-modal conservative approach in a geriatric population: A case series. J Orthop Sports Phys Ther 2011;41(10):723–33.

7

Consent

Practitioners should incorporate all proposed treatment techniques, modalities and advice for an individual patient's management into the informed consent process, and a patient's consent should not just be limited to the use of high-velocity low-amplitude (HVLA) thrust techniques.

So that patients have an informed choice about their healthcare, it is important to couple information with high-quality advice about the potential risks, benefits, and uncertainties of clinical options when assisting them in selecting the treatment that best accommodates their personal preferences.[1] For consent to be valid, it must be informed. This can only be achieved if a patient understands the nature of any proposed treatment, the associated risks and benefits, alternative treatment options and the rationale for the proposed treatment. Shared decision making is regarded as the optimal approach to obtaining informed consent for treatment, and patients need to be competent to make decisions and to understand the information given to them. The specific requirements of informed consent will vary from country to country according to the local laws, customs and norms.[2]

Informed consent may be defined as 'the voluntary and revocable agreement of a competent individual to participate in a therapeutic or research procedure, based on an adequate understanding of its nature, purpose and implications'.[3] Informed consent comprises four elements, each of which should be present to a satisfactory degree if consent is to be valid (Fig. 7.1).[4]

When a health practitioner provides information to a patient, it should be free of any controlling or coercive influences. The information should also be presented in a relevant and meaningful manner that is both intellectually and emotionally comprehensible to the patient.[5]

The Osteopathy Board of Australia[6] recommends that in order for patients to provide informed consent, they have a right to sufficient information for their understanding of the following:

1. The diagnosis and likely outcome of the condition
2. An explanation of the recommended treatment
3. The risks of the procedure and common side effects
4. Possible complications
5. Specific details of the treatment
6. Any other options for treatment and their probability of success
7. Cost of treatment
8. Option to defer treatment
9. Right to withdraw consent to treatment at any time.

Gaining a patient's consent to treatment is not a one-off activity either when a form is signed or when the patient first attends for treatment. Practitioners have an ongoing

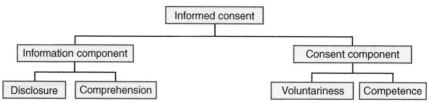

Figure 7.1 The elements of informed consent. (From Sim, 1996.[4])

responsibility to ensure that the consent process is repeated when patients return after a period of absence or when their condition or treatment plan changes.[6]

INFORMATION EXCHANGE

The traditional method of communication in the clinical encounter is verbal, but this form of communication can be enhanced by written information. To be effective, the written information should be both legible and readable.[7] Videotaped material has also been shown to be effective in patient education, particularly with regard to short-term knowledge.[8] Delany[9] advocates that a combination of verbal, written and audiovisual information be provided to patients. Use of written or electronic tools can help to clarify choices for patients, but these communication aids cannot replace the human element in facilitating informed choice.[1]

How to Explain the Risks of Treatment Involving Spinal and Sacroiliac HVLA Thrust Techniques

A survey of a sample of UK osteopathic patients revealed that 98% of 124 respondents thought that having information about rare yet potentially severe risks of treatment was important.[10] Risks and possible harms should be discussed with patients both when they are rare but carry a significant risk of detriment and also when an adverse outcome is common, regardless of whether the detriment to the patient is slight or severe. The following

potential complications need to be discussed when treating specific regions of the spine and pelvis with HVLA thrust techniques:

Transient complications

Cervical spine/thoracic spine/lumbar spine/pelvis

Substantive complications

Cervical spine

- Disc herniation/prolapse
- Nerve root compression
- Cervical and upper thoracic spine strain.

Thoracic spine and rib cage

- Rib/vertebrae fracture
- Shoulder girdle, thoracic spine and rib cage strain.

Lumbar spine and pelvis

- Vertebra fracture
- Disc herniation/prolapse
- Nerve root compression
- Shoulder girdle, thoracic spine/rib cage and lumbopelvic region strain.

Rare and very serious complications

Cervical spine

- Stroke
- Spinal cord compression.

Thoracic spine and rib cage

- Spinal cord compression.

Lumbar spine and pelvis

- Cauda equina syndrome.

Practitioners have a responsibility to inform patients of the very rare but potentially serious complications when treating the thoracic and lumbar spinal regions as well as when treatment is directed at the cervical spine.

More detailed information about the potential complications of treatment involving HVLA thrust techniques can be found in Chapter 5.

When explaining possible complications associated with any proposed treatment, they need to be discussed in language that the lay person can understand and in a manner that explains the risks sensitively and in context. A patient can generally understand that there is a very low risk of serious injury or death associated with travelling in a motor vehicle or taking commonly prescribed medicines, e.g. nonsteroidal antiinflammatory drugs. Patients can generally comprehend that risk can be mitigated to some extent but cannot be totally removed from everyday life. The very rare and serious complications that have been associated with the use of HVLA thrust techniques can be explained and discussed in this context and some possible approaches are given below:

Cervical and cervicothoracic spine

The treatment I am recommending is to use some hands-on treatment in conjunction with an exercise program. The hands-on treatment will involve a combination of massage, stretching, rhythmic movement and impulse techniques where you may hear a popping or cracking sound. This treatment approach can be associated with some short-term increase of symptoms, most commonly a short-term increase of the pain you have come to see me about. This is nothing to be concerned about, and the increase of symptoms usually settles in 24 to 72 hours. If the increase in pain or discomfort persists for longer than this, I would like you to contact me.

There have been some reports that this treatment approach has caused or aggravated a disc injury or a pinched nerve and in some instances strained the neck or upper back. It is very important that you let me know if anything I am doing is painful or uncomfortable so I can adjust the treatment to minimize the risk of any of these possible reactions.

Do you ever travel in a motor car? Each time you do this, you know there is a very small risk of being injured or killed, but you accept that the benefits of being able to travel in your car outweigh the risk of being seriously injured or killed, even though you might drive very carefully and keep your car well maintained. It is the same situation with the treatment I am recommending. A few cases of damage to the spinal cord and a rare form of stroke have been associated with this treatment approach, but a number of these rare incidents were due to the patient not being properly assessed. I have listened to your history and examined you, and I cannot find any reason to think you would be at an increased risk of any of these rare reactions as a result of the proposed treatment. Do you have any questions?

Thoracic spine and rib cage

The treatment I am recommending is to use some hands-on treatment in conjunction with an exercise program. The hands-on treatment will involve a combination of massage, stretching, rhythmic movement and impulse techniques where you may hear a popping or cracking sound. This treatment approach can be associated with some short-term increase of symptoms, most commonly a short-term increase of the pain you have come to see me about. This is nothing to be concerned about, and the increase of symptoms usually settles in 24 to 72 hours. If the increase in pain or discomfort persists for longer than this, I would like you to contact me.

There have been some reports that this treatment approach has caused rib or vertebrae fractures and in some instances strained the shoulder region, mid-back or rib cage. It is very important that you let me know if anything that I am doing is painful or uncomfortable so I can adjust the treatment to minimize the risk of any of these possible reactions.

From your history, I am aware that you are taking some antiinflammatory medication that your doctor has prescribed for you. When someone regularly takes these medications, there is a very small risk of getting seriously ill or even dying. Because the doctor has assessed you and judged that you are not at risk because of any medical reason of these very serious complications, you have agreed to take the medicine on the basis that the benefit outweighs the very small risk of these serious complications. It is the same situation with the treatment I am recommending. A few cases of damage to the spinal cord have been associated with this treatment approach, but a number of these rare incidents were due to the patient not being properly assessed. I have listened to your history and examined you, and I cannot find any reason to think you would be at an increased risk of any of these rare reactions as a result of the proposed treatment. Do you have any questions?

Lumbar spine, thoracolumbar spine and pelvis

The treatment I am recommending is to use some hands-on treatment in conjunction with an exercise program. The hands-on treatment will involve a combination of massage, stretching, rhythmic movement and impulse techniques where you may hear a popping or cracking sound. This treatment approach can be associated with some short-term increase of symptoms, most commonly a short-term increase of the pain you have come to see me about. This is nothing to be concerned about, and the increase of symptoms usually settles in 24 to 72 hours. If the increase in pain

or discomfort persists for longer than this, I would like you to contact me.

There have been some reports that this treatment approach has caused a vertebral fracture, caused or aggravated a disc injury or a pinched nerve and in some instances strained the shoulder region, mid-, lower back or rib cage. It is very important that you let me know if anything that I am doing is painful or uncomfortable so I can adjust the treatment to minimize the risk of any of these possible reactions.

Do you ever travel in a motor car? Each time you do this, you know there is a very small risk of being injured or killed, but you accept that the benefits of being able to travel in your car outweigh the risk of being seriously injured or killed, even though you might drive very carefully and keep your car well maintained. It is the same situation with the treatment I am recommending. A few cases of damage to the nerves in the spinal canal of the lower back, which can lead to permanent bladder or bowel problems, have been associated with this treatment approach, but a number of these rare incidents were due to the patient not being properly assessed. I have listened to your history and examined you, and I cannot find any reason to think you would be at an increased risk of any of these rare reactions as a result of the proposed treatment. Do you have any questions?

The above examples constitute only part of the informed consent process and are related just to the explanation of risks. There are a number of other key elements that are necessary for obtaining informed consent in clinical practice:[11]

- Discussion of the clinical issue and the nature of the decision to be made
- Discussion of the alternatives
- Discussion of the benefits and risks
- Discussion of uncertainties associated with the decision
- Assessment of the patient's understanding
- Asking patients to express their preference.

Box 7.1 Consent/Complications

Transient	☐
Strain	☐
Disc	☐
Radiculopathy	☐
Fracture	☐
Spinal cord compression	☐
Stroke	☐
Cauda equina	☐

DOCUMENTING THE PATIENT'S CONSENT

Recording valid and informed consent can be achieved by making an annotation in the patient's clinical records and/or having the patient read and sign a consent form. Box 7.1 lists the broad categories of complications that have been associated with HVLA thrust techniques and can be used as a checklist in the patient's clinical records.

References

1 Woolf SH, Chan EC, Harris R, et al. Promoting informed choice: Transforming health care to dispense knowledge for decision making. Ann Intern Med 2005;143(4):293–300.

2 Rushton A, Rivett D, Carlesso L, et al. International framework for examination of the cervical region for potential of cervical arterial dysfunction prior to orthopaedic manual therapy intervention. Available at: <www.ifompt.com>; 2012.

3 Sim J. Informed consent: Ethical implications for physiotherapy. Physiotherapy 1986;72:584.

4 Sim J. Informed consent and manual therapy. Man Ther 1996;2:104–6.

5 Delany C. Informed consent: Broadening the focus. Aust J Physiother 2003;49:159–61.

6 Osteopathy Board of Australia. Informed Consent: Guidelines for Osteopaths. Melbourne, Australia: Osteopathy Board of Australia; 2013.

7 Albert T, Chadwick S. How readable are practice leaflets. BMJ 1992;305(6864):1266–8.

8 Gagliano M. A literature review on the efficacy of video in patient education. J Med Educ 1988;63(10):785–92.

9 Delany C. Cervical manipulation – How might informed consent be obtained before treatment? J Law Med 2002;10(2):174–86.

10 Daniels G, Vogel S. Consent in osteopathy: A cross sectional survey of patients' information and process preferences. Int J Osteopath Med 2012;15(3):92–102.

11 Braddock C, Fihn S, Levinson W, et al. How doctors and patients discuss routine clinical decisions. Informed decision making in the out-patient setting. J Gen Intern Med 1997;12(6):339–45.

HVLA thrust techniques

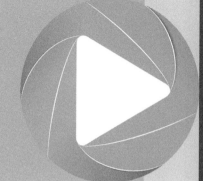

INTRODUCTION

Part B includes 41 manipulative techniques applied to the spine, thorax and pelvis. All techniques are described using a variable height manipulation couch.

This part of the book relates to specific high-velocity low-amplitude (HVLA) thrust techniques. HVLA thrust techniques are also known by a number of different names, e.g. adjustment, high-velocity thrust, mobilization with impulse, grade V mobilization. Despite the different nomenclature, the common feature in techniques of this type is that they are designed to achieve a joint cavitation (pop or cracking sound). The cause of the popping or cracking sound is open to some speculation.

Information gained from a thorough history, clinical examination and segmental analysis will direct the practitioner towards any possible somatic dysfunction and/or pathology. The use of HVLA thrust techniques is dependent on a diagnosis of somatic dysfunction.

Somatic dysfunction is identified by the S-T-A-R-T of diagnosis:
- S relates to symptom reproduction.
- T relates to tissue tenderness.
- A relates to asymmetry.
- R relates to range of motion.
- T relates to tissue texture changes.

The manual is designed in a format that presents a standardized approach to each region of the spine, thorax and pelvis. If the instructions are followed conscientiously, the novice manipulator will be well placed to achieve a positive outcome from the procedure. The nature of manipulative practice is such that there are many different ways to achieve joint cavitation. Many clinicians achieve extremely high levels of expertise and competence in the use of HVLA thrust techniques. This is the result of many years of individual clinical experience and practice.

This manual is designed to be a safe and effective starting point upon which practitioners can build basic, and then more refined, technical skills. The text lays out the primary and secondary joint leverages required to facilitate effective localization of forces to a specific segment before application of the thrust. If the instructions are followed, the resultant thrust is likely to achieve joint gliding and cavitation with the use of minimal force. The joint to be thrust should remain free to move and not be locked by the prethrust positioning so that the practitioner can direct a gliding thrust along the joint plane.

Appropriate prethrust tension is then developed by using a minimal leverage positioning approach. The prethrust positioning is not at end-range or at the motion restriction barrier. The goal in prethrust positioning is to use the least amount of leverage that will enable the practitioner to safely and effectively achieve a cavitation at the targeted segment in a position that is comfortable for the patient. No text can teach the subtle nuances of HVLA thrust techniques. For example, the sense of appropriate prethrust tension is difficult to describe and acquire. If a practitioner is uncertain about the optimum prethrust tension, a number of light trial thrusts may be used before the application of the final thrust. Experienced practitioners often use compression as an additional lever. Extensive practice under the supervision of skilled and experienced clinicians is strongly recommended.

Positioning can be achieved by either facet apposition or the utilization of ligamentous myofascial tension. Modifications of positioning for the stiffer or more flexible spine may be necessary and have been described in Chapter 4. The majority of techniques are described using facet apposition positioning. In broad terms, facet apposition locking uses combinations of sidebending and rotation. An understanding of the biomechanics associated with coupled movements of the spine in different postures allows the operator to decide on optimal leverages. Although rotation and sidebending are the principal leverages used, the more experienced manipulator may include elements of flexion, extension, translation, compression or traction to enhance localization of forces and patient comfort.

When a practitioner has acquired some skill and experience in applying HVLA thrust techniques, they may consider using momentum-induced thrusts with some patients. A momentum-induced thrust is where the impulse is associated with movement as opposed to where an impulse is applied from a stationary position. A momentum-induced thrust approach should be considered with very flexible patients or where a patient has difficulty relaxing. It takes a period of time and practice to acquire the psychomotor skill to apply momentum-induced thrusts safely and effectively and avoid large amplitude thrust procedures.

Patient relaxation is an essential prerequisite for effective HVLA thrust techniques. This may be facilitated by the use of respiration and other distraction methods.

After making a diagnosis of somatic dysfunction and before proceeding with a thrust, it is recommended that the following checklist be used for each of the techniques described in this section:

- Have I excluded all contraindications?
- Have I explained to the patient what I am going to do?
- Do I have informed consent?
- Is the patient well positioned and comfortable? (minimal leverage positioning)
- Am I in a comfortable and balanced position?
- Do I need to modify any prethrust physical or biomechanical factors? (refer Box C3, Part C)
- Have I achieved appropriate prethrust tissue tension? (not end-range)
- Am I relaxed and confident to proceed?
- Is the patient relaxed and willing for me to proceed?

8

Cervical and cervicothoracic spine

CERVICAL SPINE HOLDS AND GRIPS

The hold or wrist position selected for any particular technique is that which enables the operator to effectively localize forces to a specific segment of the spine and deliver a high-velocity low-amplitude (HVLA) thrust in a controlled manner. Patient comfort must be a major consideration in selecting the most appropriate hold.

Chin Hold

- Operator's left forearm must be over, or slightly in front of, the patient's left ear (Fig. 8.1).
- Operator's fingers lightly clasp the patient's chin (Fig. 8.2).
- Operator's chest should be in contact with the vertex of the patient's head.

- Operator's right hand applies applicator to contact point.

Cradle Hold

- Patient's left ear rests in the palm of operator's left hand.
- Operator's left hand is spread out for maximum contact.
- Operator's right hand applies applicator to contact point and gives support to the patient's occiput.
- The weight of the patient's head and neck is balanced between the operator's left and right hands (Figs. 8.3, 8.4).

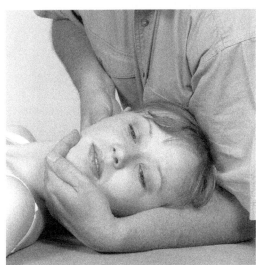

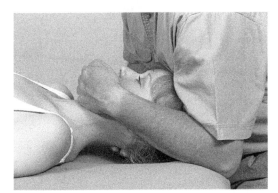

Figure 8.1

Figure 8.2

Wrist Position

Operators can select from either the pistol grip (Fig. 8.5) or wrist extension grip (Fig. 8.6).

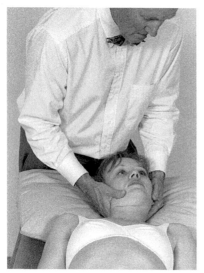

Figure 8.3

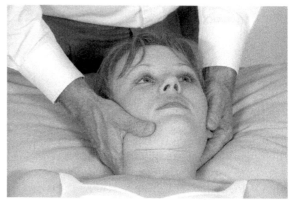

Figure 8.4

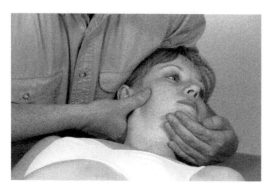

Figure 8.5 Pistol grip. Note the radius in line with first metacarpal.

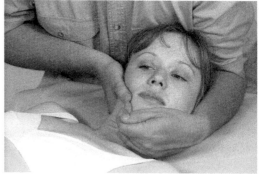

Figure 8.6 Wrist extension grip. Note the wrist extension.

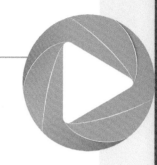

Atlanto-occipital joint C0–1
Ligamentous myofascial positioning:
Contact point on occiput

Chin hold
Patient supine
Anterior and superior thrust in a curved plane
Ligamentous myofascial positioning

Assume somatic dysfunction (S-T-A-R-T) is identified and you wish to use a thrust in the plane of the C0–C1 apophysial joint to produce cavitation on the right (Fig. 8.7).

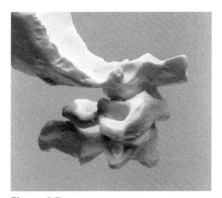

Figure 8.7

Key

✳ Stabilization

● Applicator

➡ Plane of thrust (operator)

⇨ Direction of body movement
(patient)

Note: The dimensions for the arrows
are not a pictorial representation of
the amplitude or force of the thrust.

1. Contact point

Right posterior occiput. Medial and
posterior to the mastoid process.

2. Applicator

Lateral border, proximal or middle phalanx
of the operator's right index finger.

3. Patient positioning

Supine with the neck in a neutral relaxed
position. If necessary, remove pillow or
adjust pillow height. The neck should not
be in any significant amount of flexion or
extension.

4. Operator stance

Head of couch, feet spread slightly. Adjust
couch height so that the operator can stand

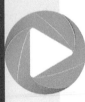

as erect as possible and avoid crouching over the patient, as this will limit the technique and restrict delivery of the thrust.

5. Palpation of contact point

Place fingers of both hands gently under the occiput. Lift the head slightly, and gently rotate it to the left, taking the weight of the head in your left hand. Remove your right hand from the occiput, and palpate the contact point on the occiput with the tip of your index or middle finger. Ensure that you are medial to, and not on, the mastoid process. Slowly but firmly slide your right index finger, in close approximation to the suboccipital musculature, downwards (towards the couch) along the occiput until it approximates the middle or proximal phalanx. Several sliding pressures may be necessary to establish close approximation to the contact point. It is important to obtain a contact point as far along the underside of the occiput as possible and into the suboccipital musculature. This thrust uses a curved plane of movement to produce a cavitation, and this positioning ensures that the applicator will not slip during the thrust.

6. Fixation of contact point

Keep your right index finger firmly pressed on the contact point while you flex the other fingers and thumb of the right hand so as to clasp the back of the occiput and head, thereby locking the applicator in position. You must now keep the applicator on the contact point until the technique is complete. Keeping the hands in position, return the head to the neutral position.

7. Chin hold

Keep your right hand in position and slide the left hand, slowly and carefully, forwards until the fingers lightly clasp the chin. Ensure that your left forearm is over or slightly anterior to the ear. Placing the forearm on or behind the ear puts the neck

into too much flexion. The head is now controlled by balancing forces between the right palm and the left forearm. Maintain the applicator in position.

8. Vertex contact

Move your body forwards slightly so that your chest is in contact with the vertex of the patient's head. The head is now securely cradled between the left forearm, the flexed left elbow, the right palm and your chest. Vertex contact is often useful in a heavy, stiff or difficult case but can, on occasions, be omitted.

9. Positioning for thrust

Step to the right and stand across the right corner of the couch, keeping the hands firmly in position and taking care not to lose pressure on the contact point. Gently introduce a little rotation of the head to the left. Straighten your right wrist so that the radius and first metacarpal are in line. While maintaining firm applicator pressure, allow the right index finger to roll slightly on the contact point as you move your right elbow towards the patient's right shoulder. This facilitates optimal alignment for the thrust, which is in a curved plane because of the shape of the apophysial joint. It is important that your applicator is well beneath the occiput so that you do not slip when applying the thrust along a curved facet plane. Keep your right elbow close to the couch in order to keep the contact point on the occiput (Fig. 8.8).

Add extension and slight sidebending to the right to provide a feeling of tension at the contact point. The extension and right sidebending are introduced by pivoting slightly via the legs and trunk so that your trunk and upper body rotate to the left. Do not attempt to introduce sidebending by moving the hands or arms, as this will lead to loss of contact and inaccurate technique. This technique does not use facet apposition locking. The prethrust tension is achieved by

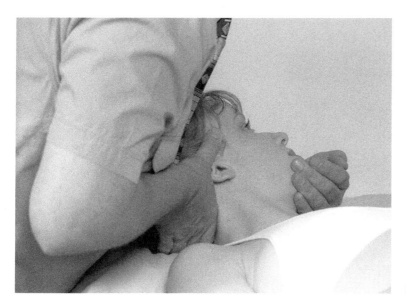

Figure 8.8

positioning the occipito-atlantal joint towards the end-range of available joint gliding using a minimal leverage approach while avoiding excessive rotation and sidebending leverages. Extensive practice is necessary to develop an appreciation of the required tension.

10. Adjustments to achieve appropriate prethrust tension

Ensure the patient remains relaxed. Maintaining all holds, make any necessary minor changes in flexion, extension, sidebending or rotation until you can sense a state of appropriate tension and leverage at the contact point. The patient should not be aware of any pain or discomfort. You should introduce these final adjustments by slight movements of the ankles, knees, hips and trunk, not by altering the position of your hands or arms.

11. Immediately prethrust

Relax and adjust your balance as necessary. Keep your head up; looking down impedes the thrust and can cause embarrassing proximity to the patient. An effective HVLA thrust technique is best achieved if the operator and patient are relaxed and not holding themselves rigid. This is a common impediment to achieving effective cavitation.

Ensure the patient's head and neck remain on the pillow, as this facilitates the arrest of the technique and limits excessive amplitude of thrust.

12. Delivering the thrust

This is a difficult technique to master, as the thrust must be applied along a curved plane. Apply an HVLA thrust to the occiput, using both hands, in an anterior and superior direction along a curved plane that follows the shape of the occipito-atlantal articulation (Fig. 8.9).

The thrust, although very rapid, must never be excessively forcible. The aim should be to use the absolute minimum of force necessary to achieve joint cavitation. A common fault arises from the use of excessive amplitude with insufficient velocity of thrust.

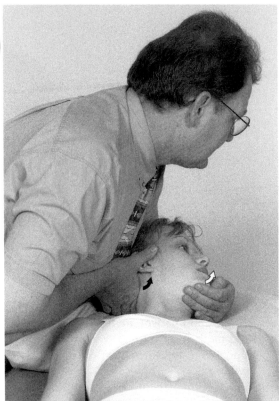

Figure 8.9

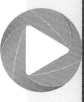

Summary

Atlanto-occipital joint C0–C1: Contact point on occiput

Chin hold

Patient supine

Ligamentous myofascial positioning

Contact point: Right posterior occiput

Applicator: Lateral border, proximal or middle phalanx

Patient positioning: Supine with the neck in a neutral relaxed position

Operator stance: Head of couch, feet spread slightly

Palpation of contact point: Ensure that you are medial to, and not on, the mastoid process

Fixation of contact point

Chin hold: Ensure your left forearm is over or slightly anterior to the ear

Vertex contact: Optional

Positioning for thrust: Step to the right, and stand across the right corner of the couch. Optimal alignment for the thrust is in a curved plane. Keep your right elbow close to the couch in order to keep the contact point on the occiput (Fig. 8.8)

Adjustments to achieve appropriate prethrust tension

Immediately prethrust: Relax and adjust your balance

Delivering the thrust: The thrust must be applied, using both hands, along a curved plane that follows the shape of the occipito-atlantal articulation (Fig. 8.9)

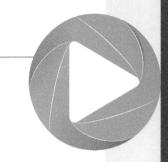

Atlanto-occipital joint C0–1:
Ligamentous myofascial positioning contact point on atlas

Chin hold
Patient supine
Anterior and superior thrust in a curved plane
Ligamentous myofascial positioning

Assume somatic dysfunction (S-T-A-R-T) is identified and you wish to use a thrust in the plane of the C0–C1 apophysial joint to produce cavitation on the right (Fig. 8.10).

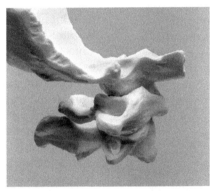

Figure 8.10

Key

✳ Stabilization

● Applicator

➡ Plane of thrust (operator)

⇨ Direction of body movement (patient)

Note: The dimensions for the arrows are not a pictorial representation of the amplitude or force of the thrust.

1. Contact point
Right posterior arch of atlas.

2. Applicator
Lateral border, proximal or middle phalanx of operator's right index finger.

3. Patient positioning
Supine with the neck in a neutral relaxed position. If necessary, remove pillow or adjust pillow height. The neck should not be in any significant amount of flexion or extension.

4. Operator stance

Head of couch, feet spread slightly. Adjust couch height so that the operator can stand as erect as possible and avoid crouching over the patient, as this will limit the technique and restrict delivery of the thrust.

5. Palpation of contact point

Place fingers of both hands gently under the occiput. Lift the head slightly and gently rotate it to the left, taking the weight of the head in your left hand. Remove your right hand from occiput and palpate the contact point on the right posterior arch of the atlas with the tip of your index or middle finger. Slowly but firmly slide your right index finger, in close approximation to the suboccipital musculature, downwards (towards the couch) along the posterior arch of the atlas until it approximates the middle or proximal phalanx. Several sliding pressures may be necessary to establish close approximation to the contact point.

6. Fixation of contact point

Keep your right index finger firmly pressed on the contact point while you flex the other fingers and thumb of the right hand so as to clasp the back of the occiput and head, thereby locking the applicator in position. You must now keep the applicator on the contact point until the technique is complete. Keeping the hands in position, return the head to the neutral position.

7. Chin hold

Keep your right hand in position and slide the left hand, slowly and carefully, forwards until the fingers lightly clasp the chin. Ensure that your left forearm is over or slightly anterior to the ear. Placing the forearm on or behind the ear puts the neck into too much flexion. The head is now controlled by balancing forces between the right palm and left forearm. Maintain the applicator in position.

8. Vertex contact

Move your body forwards slightly so that your chest is in contact with the vertex of the patient's head. The head is now securely cradled between the left forearm, the flexed left elbow, the right palm, and your chest. Vertex contact is essential in this technique.

9. Positioning for thrust

Step to the right and stand across the right corner of the couch, keeping the hands firmly in position and taking care not to lose pressure on the contact point. Gently introduce a little rotation of the head to the left. Straighten your right wrist so that the radius and first metacarpal are in line. While maintaining firm applicator pressure, allow the right index finger to roll slightly on the contact point as you move your right elbow towards the patient's right shoulder. This facilitates optimal alignment for the thrust, which is in a curved plane because of the shape of the apophysial joint. It is important that your applicator has a firm contact on the atlas so that you do not slip when applying the thrust along a curved facet plane. Keep your right elbow close to the couch in order to keep the contact point on the atlas (Fig. 8.11).

Add extension and slight sidebending to the right to provide a feeling of tension at the contact point. The extension and right sidebending are introduced by pivoting slightly via the legs and trunk so your trunk and upper body rotate to the left. Do not attempt to introduce sidebending by moving the hands or arms, as this will lead to loss of contact and inaccurate technique. This technique does not use facet apposition locking. The prethrust tension is achieved by positioning the occipito-atlantal joint towards the end-range of available joint gliding using a minimal leverage approach while avoiding excessive rotation and sidebending leverages. Extensive practice is necessary to develop an appreciation of the required tension.

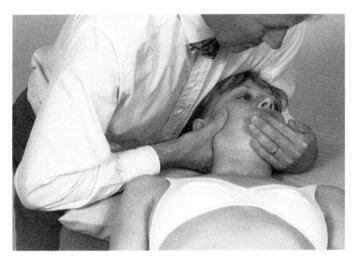

Figure 8.11

10. Adjustments to achieve appropriate prethrust tension

Ensure the patient remains relaxed. Maintaining all holds, make any necessary minor changes in flexion, extension, sidebending, or rotation until you can sense a state of appropriate tension and leverage at the contact point. The patient should not be aware of any pain or discomfort. You should introduce these final adjustments by slight movements of the ankles, knees, hips, and trunk, not by altering the position of your hands or arms.

11. Immediately prethrust

Relax and adjust your balance as necessary. Keep your head up; looking down impedes the thrust and can cause embarrassing proximity to the patient. An effective HVLA thrust technique is best achieved if the operator and patient are relaxed and not holding themselves rigid. This is a common impediment to achieving effective cavitation.

Ensure the patient's head and neck remain on the pillow, as this facilitates the arrest of the technique and limits excessive amplitude of thrust.

12. Delivering the thrust

This is a difficult technique to master, as the thrust must be applied along a curved plane. Apply an HVLA thrust to the posterior arch of the atlas in an anterior and superior direction along a curved plane, which follows the shape of the occipito-atlantal articulation. Do not apply simultaneous rapid increase of cervical rotation, extension, or sidebending with the left hand (Fig. 8.12).

The thrust, although very rapid, must never be excessively forcible. The aim should be to use the absolute minimum force necessary to achieve joint cavitation. A common fault arises from the use of excessive amplitude with insufficient velocity of thrust.

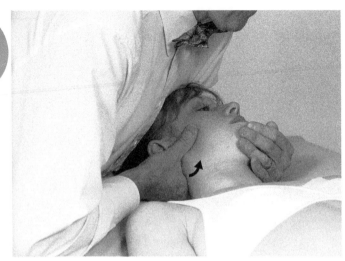

Figure 8.12

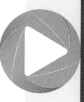

Summary

Atlanto-occipital joint C0–C1: Contact point on atlas

Chin hold

Patient supine

Ligamentous myofascial positioning

- **Contact point:** Right posterior arch of atlas

- **Applicator:** Lateral border, proximal or middle phalanx

- **Patient positioning:** Supine with the neck in a neutral relaxed position

- **Operator stance:** Head of couch, feet spread slightly

- **Palpation of contact point**

- **Fixation of contact point**

- **Chin hold:** Ensure your left forearm is over or slightly anterior to the ear

- **Vertex contact:** Essential in this technique

- **Positioning for thrust:** Step to the right and stand across the right corner of the couch. Optimal alignment for the thrust is in a curved plane. Keep your right elbow close to the couch in order to keep the contact point on the atlas (Fig. 8.11)

- **Adjustments to achieve appropriate prethrust tension**

- **Immediately prethrust:** Relax and adjust your balance

- **Delivering the thrust:** The thrust must be applied along a curved plane, which follows the shape of the occipito-atlantal articulation (Fig. 8.12)

Atlanto-axial joint C1–2:
Ligamentous myofascial positioning

Chin hold
Patient supine
Rotation thrust
Ligamentous myofascial positioning

Assume somatic dysfunction (S-T-A-R-T) is identified and you wish to use a thrust in the plane of the atlanto-axial (C1–2) apophysial joint to produce cavitation on the right (Figs. 8.13, 8.14).

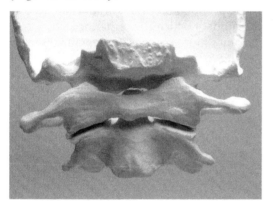

Figure 8.13

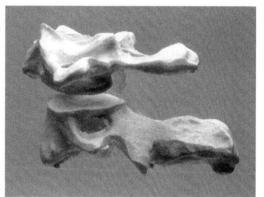

Figure 8.14

Key

✳ Stabilization

● Applicator

➡ Plane of thrust (operator)

⇨ Direction of body movement (patient)

Note: The dimensions for the arrows are not a pictorial representation of the amplitude or force of the thrust.

1. Contact point
Right posterior arch of atlas.

2. Applicator
Lateral border, proximal or middle phalanx of operator's right index finger.

3. Patient positioning
Supine with the neck in a neutral relaxed position. If necessary, remove pillow or adjust pillow height. The neck should not be in any significant amount of flexion or extension.

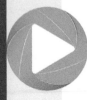

4. Operator stance

Head of couch, feet spread slightly. Adjust couch height so that the operator can stand as erect as possible and avoid crouching over the patient, as this will limit the technique and restrict delivery of the thrust.

5. Palpation of contact point

Place fingers of both hands gently under the occiput. Lift the head slightly and gently rotate it to the left, taking the weight of the head in your left hand. Remove your right hand from the occiput and palpate the region of the right posterior arch of the atlas with the tip of your index or middle finger. Slowly but firmly slide your right index finger downwards (towards the couch) along the posterior arch of the atlas until it approximates the middle or proximal phalanx. Several sliding pressures may be necessary to establish close approximation to the contact point.

6. Fixation of contact point

Keep your right index finger firmly pressed upon the contact point while you flex the other fingers and thumb of the right hand so as to clasp the back of the neck and occiput, thereby locking the applicator in position. You must now keep the applicator on the contact point until the technique is complete. Keeping the hands in position, return the head to the neutral position.

7. Chin hold

Keep your right hand in position and slide the left hand, slowly and carefully, forwards until the fingers lightly clasp the chin. Ensure that your left forearm is over, or slightly anterior to, the ear. Placing the forearm on or behind the ear puts the neck into too much flexion. The head is now controlled by balancing forces between the right palm and left forearm. Maintain the applicator in position.

8. Vertex contact

Move your body forwards slightly so that your chest is in contact with the vertex of the patient's head. The head is now securely cradled between the left forearm, the flexed left elbow, the right palm, and your chest. Vertex contact is often useful in a heavy, stiff, or difficult case but can, on occasions, be omitted.

9. Positioning for thrust

Step to the right and stand across the right corner of the couch, keeping the hands firmly in position and taking care not to lose pressure on the contact point. Gently introduce rotation of the head to the left, to the point at which the posterior arch becomes more obvious under your contact point. Straighten your right wrist so that the radius and first metacarpal are in line. While maintaining firm applicator pressure, allow the right index finger to roll slightly on the contact point as you move your right elbow towards the patient's right shoulder to reach that point when your line of thrust is directed towards the corner of the patient's mouth. The thrust plane is into rotation. Ensure that you maintain a firm contact point on the posterior arch of the atlas and that your applicator is in line with your forearm.

a. *Primary leverage of rotation.* Maintaining all holds and contact points, complete rotation of the head and neck to the left until slight tension is palpated in the tissues at your contact point (Fig. 8.15). This is not end-range, and the aim is to use a minimal leverage approach. Maintain firm pressure against the contact point. A common mistake is to use insufficient head and neck rotation.

b. *Secondary leverage.* This technique uses minimal secondary leverage. This technique does not use facet apposition locking. Extensive practice is necessary to develop an appreciation of the required tension.

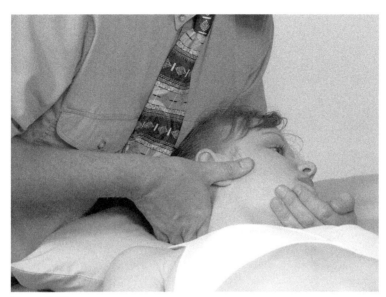

Figure 8.15

10. Adjustments to achieve appropriate prethrust tension

This is almost a pure rotation thrust but the appropriate tension can be achieved by adjusting flexion, extension, and sidebending. The patient should not be aware of any pain or discomfort. Introduce any sidebending, flexion, or extension by pivoting slightly via the legs and trunk. Do not attempt to introduce these leverages by moving the hands or arms, as this will lead to loss of contact and inaccurate technique.

11. Immediately prethrust

Relax and adjust your balance as necessary. Keep your head up; looking down impedes the thrust and can cause embarrassing proximity to the patient. An effective HVLA thrust technique is best achieved if the operator and patient are relaxed and not holding themselves rigid. This is a common impediment to achieving effective cavitation.

Ensure the patient's head and neck remain on the pillow, as this facilitates the arrest of the technique and limits excessive amplitude of thrust.

12. Delivering the thrust

Apply an HVLA thrust to the posterior arch of the atlas directed towards the corner of the patient's mouth. Simultaneously, apply a rapid low-amplitude increase of head rotation to the left by supinating the left forearm (Fig. 8.16). This rotation movement of the head is very small but of high velocity. This ensures that the occiput and atlas move as one unit during the thrust. The atlas rotates about the odontoid peg of the axis and cavitation occurs at the right C1–2 articulation. A very rapid contraction of the flexors and adductors of the right shoulder induces the thrust. The thrust, although very rapid, must never be excessively forcible. The aim should be to use the absolute minimum force necessary to achieve joint cavitation. A common fault arises from the use of excessive amplitude with insufficient velocity of thrust.

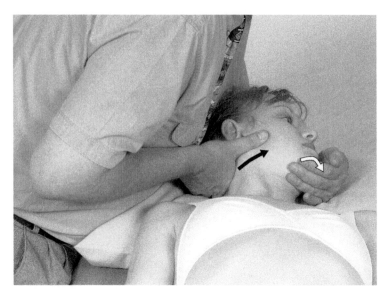

Figure 8.16

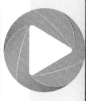

Summary

Atlanto-axial joint C1–2: Chin hold

Patient supine

Rotation thrust

Ligamentous myofascial positioning

- **Contact point:** Right posterior arch of atlas

- **Applicator:** Lateral border, proximal or middle phalanx

- **Patient positioning:** Supine with the neck in a neutral relaxed position

- **Operator stance:** Head of couch, feet spread slightly

- **Palpation of contact point**

- **Fixation of contact point**

- **Chin hold:** Ensure your left forearm is over or slightly anterior to the ear

- **Vertex contact:** Optional

- **Positioning for thrust:** Step to the right and stand across the right corner of the couch. Use primary leverage of rotation with minimal secondary leverage. Your direction of thrust is towards the patient's mouth and into rotation (Fig. 8.15)

- **Adjustments to achieve appropriate prethrust tension**

- **Immediately prethrust:** Relax and adjust your balance

- **Delivering the thrust:** The thrust is directed towards the corner of the patient's mouth. Simultaneously, apply a rapid low-amplitude increase of head rotation to the left. The occiput and atlas move as one unit during the thrust (Fig. 8.16)

Atlanto-axial joint C1–2:
Ligamentous myofascial positioning

Cradle hold
Patient supine
Rotation thrust
Ligamentous myofascial positioning

Assume somatic dysfunction (S-T-A-R-T) is identified and you wish to use a thrust in the plane of the atlanto-axial (C1–2) apophysial joint to produce cavitation on the right (Figs. 8.17, 8.18).

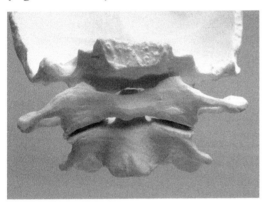

Figure 8.17

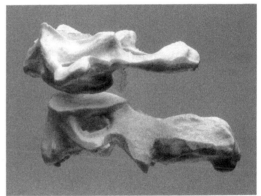

Figure 8.18

Key

✳ Stabilization

● Applicator

➡ Plane of thrust (operator)

⇨ Direction of body movement (patient)

Note: The dimensions for the arrows are not a pictorial representation of the amplitude or force of the thrust.

1. Contact point
Right posterior arch of atlas.

2. Applicator
Lateral border, proximal or middle phalanx of operator's right index finger.

3. Patient positioning
Supine with the neck in a neutral relaxed position. If necessary, remove pillow or adjust pillow height. The neck should not be in any significant amount of flexion or extension.

4. Operator stance

Head of couch, feet spread slightly. Adjust couch height so that the operator can stand as erect as possible and avoid crouching over the patient, as this will limit the technique and restrict delivery of the thrust.

5. Palpation of contact point

Place fingers of both hands gently under the occiput. Lift the head slightly, and gently rotate it to the left, taking the weight of the head in your left hand. Remove your right hand from the occiput and palpate the region of the right posterior arch of the atlas with the tip of your index or middle finger. Slowly but firmly slide your right index finger downwards (towards the couch) along the posterior arch of the atlas until it approximates the middle or proximal phalanx. Several sliding pressures may be necessary to establish close approximation to the contact point.

6. Fixation of contact point

Keep your right index finger firmly pressed upon the contact point while you flex the other fingers and thumb of the right hand so as to clasp the back of the neck and occiput, thereby locking the applicator in position. You must now keep the applicator on the contact point until the technique is complete. Keeping the hands in position, return the head to the neutral position.

7. Cradle hold

Keep your left hand under the head and spread the fingers out for maximum contact. Keep the patient's ear resting in the palm of your left hand. Flex the left wrist, allowing you to cradle the patient's head in your palm, flexed wrist and anterior aspect of forearm. Keep your right index finger firmly on the contact point and press the right palm against the occiput. The weight of the patient's head and neck is now balanced between your left and right hands with the cervical

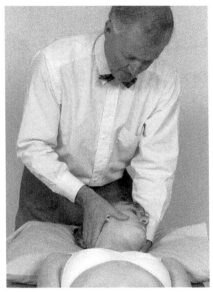

Figure 8.19

positioning controlled by the converging pressures of your two hands and arms.

8. Vertex contact

None in this technique.

9. Positioning for thrust

The elbows are held close to or only slightly away from your sides. This is an essential feature of the cradle hold method. Stand easily upright at the head of the couch and do not step to the right as in the chin hold method.

a. *Primary leverage of rotation.* Maintaining all holds and contact points, complete the rotation of the head and neck to the left until tension is palpated at the contact point. Supination of the left wrist and forearm and simultaneous pronation of the right wrist and forearm achieve the rotation movement (Fig. 8.19). This is not end-range, and the aim is to use a minimal leverage approach. Do not lose firm pressure on the contact point. Do not force rotation, but a common mistake is to use insufficient primary leverage of head and neck rotation.

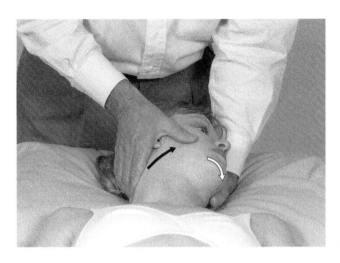

Figure 8.20

b. *Secondary leverage.* This technique uses minimal secondary leverage. This technique does not use facet apposition locking. Extensive practice is necessary to develop an appreciation of the required tension.

10. Adjustments to achieve appropriate prethrust tension

This is almost a pure rotation thrust, but the appropriate tension can be achieved by adjusting flexion, extension and sidebending. The patient should not be aware of any pain or discomfort. The operator makes final minor adjustments by introducing any sidebending, flexion or extension with slight movements of the wrists, arms and shoulders.

11. Immediately prethrust

Relax and adjust your balance, as necessary. Keep your head up; looking down impedes the thrust and can cause embarrassing proximity to the patient. An effective HVLA thrust technique is best achieved if the operator and patient are relaxed and not holding themselves rigid. This is a common impediment to achieving effective cavitation.

Ensure the patient's head and neck remain on the pillow, as this facilitates the arrest of the technique and limits excessive amplitude of thrust.

12. Delivering the thrust

Apply an HVLA thrust to the posterior arch of the atlas directed towards the corner of the patient's mouth. This thrust is generated by rapid pronation of your right forearm. Simultaneously, apply a rapid low-amplitude increase of head rotation to the left by supinating the left forearm (Fig. 8.20). This rotation movement of the head is very small but of high velocity. This ensures that the occiput and atlas move as one unit during the thrust. The atlas rotates about the odontoid peg of the axis and cavitation occurs at the right C1–2 articulation. This is an HVLA 'flick' type thrust. Coordination between the left and right hands and forearms is critical.

The thrust, although very rapid, must never be excessively forcible. The aim should be to use the absolute minimum force necessary to achieve joint cavitation. A common fault arises from the use of excessive amplitude with insufficient velocity of thrust.

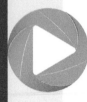

Summary

Atlanto-axial joint C1–2: Cradle hold

Patient supine

Rotation thrust

Ligamentous myofascial positioning

- **Contact point:** Right posterior arch of atlas

- **Applicator:** Lateral border, proximal or middle phalanx

- **Patient positioning:** Supine with the neck in a neutral, relaxed position

- **Operator stance:** Head of couch, feet spread slightly

- **Palpation of contact point**

- **Fixation of contact point**

- **Cradle hold:** The weight of the patient's head and neck is balanced between your left and right hands with cervical positioning controlled by the converging pressures

- **Vertex contact:** None

- **Positioning for thrust:** Stand upright at the head of the couch. The elbows are held close to or only slightly away from your sides. Use primary leverage of rotation with minimal secondary leverage. Your direction of thrust is towards the patient's mouth and into rotation (Fig. 8.19)

- **Adjustments to achieve appropriate prethrust tension**

- **Immediately prethrust:** Relax and adjust your balance

- **Delivering the thrust:** The thrust is directed towards the corner of the patient's mouth. Simultaneously, apply a rapid low-amplitude increase of head rotation to the left. The occiput and atlas move as one unit during the thrust (Fig. 8.20)

Cervical spine C2–7:
Up-slope gliding

Chin hold

Patient supine

Assume somatic dysfunction (S-T-A-R-T) is identified and you wish to use an upwards and forwards gliding thrust, parallel to the apophysial joint plane, to produce cavitation at C4–5 on the right (Figs. 8.21, 8.22).

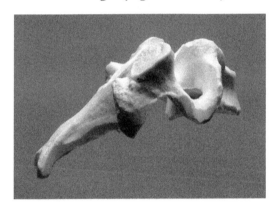

Figure 8.21

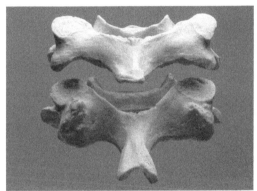

Figure 8.22

Key

✳ Stabilization

● Applicator

➡ Plane of thrust (operator)

⇨ Direction of body movement (patient)

Note: The dimensions for the arrows are not a pictorial representation of the amplitude or force of the thrust.

1. Contact point

Posterolateral aspect of right C4 articular pillar.

2. Applicator

Lateral border, proximal or middle phalanx of operator's right index finger.

3. Patient positioning

Supine with the neck in a neutral relaxed position. If necessary, remove pillow or adjust pillow height. The neck should not be in any significant amount of flexion or extension.

4. Operator stance

Head of couch, feet spread slightly. Adjust couch height so that you can stand as erect

121

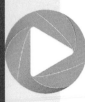

as possible and avoid crouching over the patient, as this will limit the technique and restrict delivery of the thrust.

5. Palpation of contact point

Place fingers of both hands gently under the occiput. Rotate the head to the left, taking its weight in your left hand. Remove your right hand from the occiput and palpate the right articular pillar of C4 with the tip of your index or middle finger. Slowly but firmly slide your right index finger downwards (towards the couch) along the articular pillar until it approximates the middle or proximal phalanx. Several sliding pressures may be necessary to establish close approximation to the contact point.

6. Fixation of contact point

Keep your right index finger firmly pressed upon the contact point while you flex the other fingers and thumb of the right hand so as to clasp the back of the neck and thereby lock the applicator in position. You must now keep the applicator on the contact point until the technique is complete. Keeping the hands in position, return the head to the neutral position.

7. Chin hold

Keeping your right hand in position, slide the left hand slowly and carefully forwards until the fingers lightly clasp the chin. Ensure that your left forearm is over or slightly anterior to the ear. Placing the forearm on or behind the ear puts the neck into too much flexion. The head is now controlled by balancing forces between the right palm and left forearm. Maintain the applicator in position.

8. Vertex contact

Move your body forwards slightly so that your chest is in contact with the vertex of the patient's head. The head is now securely cradled between your left forearm, the flexed left elbow, the right palm and your chest. Vertex contact is often useful in a heavy, stiff or difficult case but can, on occasions, be omitted.

9. Positioning for thrust

Step to the right and stand across the right corner of the couch, keeping the hands firmly in position and taking care not to lose pressure on the contact point. Straighten the right wrist so that the radius and first metacarpal are in line. Maintaining applicator pressure, allow the right index finger to roll slightly on the contact point to align your right wrist and forearm with the thrust plane, which is upwards and towards the midline in the direction of the patient's left eye. Keep the right elbow close to the couch in order to maintain the contact point on the posterolateral aspect of the articular pillar.

a. *Primary leverage of rotation.* Maintaining all holds and contact points, complete the rotation of the head and neck to the left until tension is palpated at the contact point (Fig. 8.23). Do not lose firm pressure at the contact point. A common mistake is to use insufficient primary leverage of head and neck rotation.

b. *Secondary leverage.* Add a very small degree of sidebending to the right, down to and including the C3–4 segment but leaving C4–5 free to move. The operator pivoting slightly, via the legs and trunk, introduces the right sidebending so that the trunk and upper body rotate to the left, enabling the hands and arms to remain in position (Fig. 8.24). Do not attempt to introduce sidebending by moving the hands or arms, as this will lead to loss of contact and inaccurate technique.

10. Adjustments to achieve appropriate prethrust tension

Ensure your patient remains relaxed. Maintaining all holds, make any necessary

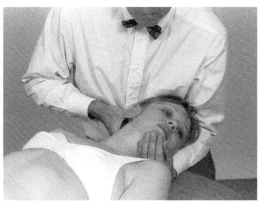

Figure 8.23

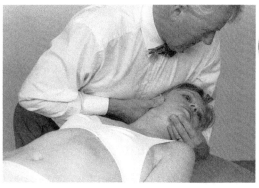

Figure 8.24

changes in flexion, extension, sidebending or rotation until you can sense a state of appropriate tension and leverage. The patient should not be aware of any pain or discomfort. You make these final adjustments by slight movements of your ankles, knees, hips and trunk, not by altering the position of the hands or arms.

11. Immediately prethrust

Relax and adjust your balance as necessary. Keep your head up; looking down impedes the thrust and can cause embarrassing proximity to the patient. An effective HVLA thrust technique is best achieved if both the operator and patient are relaxed and not holding themselves rigid. This is a common impediment to achieving effective cavitation.

Ensure the patient's head and neck remain on the pillow, as this facilitates the arrest of the technique and limits excessive amplitude of thrust.

12. Delivering the thrust

Apply an HVLA thrust to the right articular pillar of C4. The thrust is upwards and towards the midline in the direction of the patient's left eye, parallel to the apophysial joint plane. Simultaneously, apply a slight, rapid increase of rotation of the head and

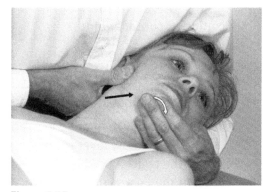

Figure 8.25

neck to the left, but do not increase the sidebending leverage (Fig. 8.25). The increase of rotation to the left is accomplished by slight supination of the left wrist and forearm. The thrust is induced by a very rapid contraction of the flexors and adductors of the right shoulder and, if necessary, trunk and lower limb movement.

The thrust, although very rapid, must never be excessively forcible. The aim should be to use the absolute minimum force necessary to achieve joint cavitation. A common fault arises from the use of excessive amplitude with insufficient velocity of thrust.

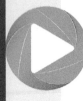

Summary

Cervical spine C2–7: Up-slope gliding

Chin hold

Patient supine

- **Contact point:** Posterolateral aspect of right C4 articular pillar

- **Applicator:** Lateral border, proximal or middle phalanx

- **Patient positioning:** Supine with the neck in a neutral relaxed position

- **Operator stance:** Head of couch, feet spread slightly

- **Palpation of contact point**

- **Fixation of contact point**

- **Chin hold:** Ensure your left forearm is over or slightly anterior to the ear

- **Vertex contact:** Optional

- **Positioning for thrust:** Step to the right and stand across the right corner of the couch. Introduce primary leverage of rotation left (Fig. 8.23) and a small degree of secondary leverage of sidebending right. Keep the right elbow close to the couch in order to maintain the contact point on the posterolateral aspect of the C4 articular pillar (Fig. 8.24)

- **Adjustments to achieve appropriate prethrust tension**

- **Immediately prethrust:** Relax and adjust your balance

- **Delivering the thrust:** The thrust is directed towards the patient's left eye. Simultaneously, apply a slight, rapid increase of rotation of the head and neck to the left with no increase of sidebending to the right (Fig. 8.25)

8.6

Cervical spine C2–7:
Up-slope gliding

Chin hold

Patient supine – variation

Assume somatic dysfunction (S-T-A-R-T) is identified and you wish to use an upward and forward gliding thrust, parallel to the apophysial joint plane, to produce cavitation at C4–5 on the right (Figs. 8.26, 8.27).

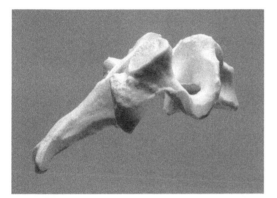

Figure 8.26

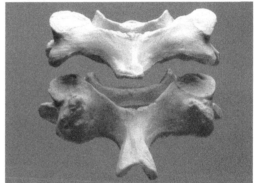

Figure 8.27

Key

✳ Stabilization

● Applicator

➡ Plane of thrust (operator)

⇨ Direction of body movement (patient)

Note: The dimensions for the arrows are not a pictorial representation of the amplitude or force of the thrust.

1. Contact point
Posterolateral aspect of right C4 articular pillar.

2. Applicator
Lateral border, proximal or middle phalanx of operator's right index finger.

3. Patient positioning
Supine with the neck in a neutral relaxed position. If necessary, remove pillow or adjust pillow height. The neck should not be in any significant amount of flexion or extension.

4. Operator stance

Head of couch, feet spread slightly. Adjust couch height so that you can stand as erect as possible and avoid crouching over the patient, as this will limit the technique and restrict delivery of the thrust.

5. Palpation of contact point

Place fingers of both hands gently under the occiput. Rotate the head to the left, taking its weight in your left hand. Remove your right hand from the occiput and palpate the right articular pillar of C4 with the tip of your index or middle finger. Slowly but firmly slide your right index finger downwards (towards the couch) along the articular pillar until it approximates the middle or proximal phalanx. Several sliding pressures may be necessary to establish close approximation to the contact point.

6. Fixation of contact point

Keep your right index finger firmly pressed upon the contact point while you flex the other fingers and thumb of the right hand so as to clasp the back of the neck and thereby lock the applicator in position. You must now keep the applicator on the contact point until the technique is complete. Keeping the hands in position, return the head to the neutral position.

7. Chin hold

Step to the right while allowing your applicator to roll on the contact point. Keeping your right hand in position, slide the left hand slowly and carefully forwards until the fingers lightly clasp the chin (Fig. 8.28). Ensure that your left forearm is over or slightly anterior to the ear. Placing the forearm on or behind the ear puts the neck into too much flexion. The head is now controlled by balancing forces between the right palm and left forearm. Maintain the applicator in position.

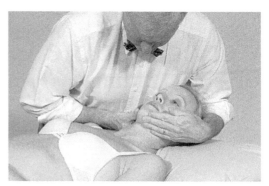

Figure 8.28

8. Vertex contact

Move your body forwards slightly so that your chest is in contact with the vertex of the patient's head. The head is now securely cradled between your left forearm, the flexed left elbow, the right palm and your chest. Vertex contact is often useful in a heavy, stiff or difficult case but can, on occasions, be omitted.

9. Positioning for thrust

Keeping the hands firmly in position and taking care not to lose pressure on the contact point, straighten the right wrist so that the radius and first metacarpal are in line. Maintaining applicator pressure, allow the right index finger to roll slightly on the contact point to align your right wrist and forearm with the thrust plane, which is upwards and towards the midline in the direction of the patient's left eye. Keep the right elbow close to the couch in order to maintain the contact point on the posterolateral aspect of the articular pillar.

a. *Primary leverage of rotation.* Maintaining all holds and contact points, complete the rotation of the head and neck to the left until tension is palpated at the contact point (Fig. 8.29). Do not lose firm pressure at the contact point. A common mistake is to use insufficient

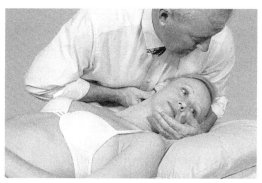

Figure 8.29

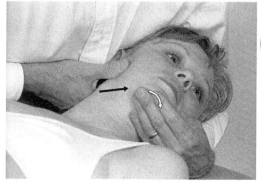

Figure 8.31

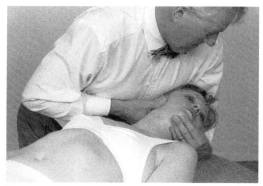

Figure 8.30

10. Adjustments to achieve appropriate prethrust tension

Ensure your patient remains relaxed. Maintaining all holds, make any necessary changes in flexion, extension, sidebending or rotation until you can sense a state of appropriate tension and leverage. The patient should not be aware of any pain or discomfort. You make these final adjustments by slight movements of your ankles, knees, hips and trunk, not by altering the position of the hands or arms.

11. Immediately prethrust

Relax and adjust your balance as necessary. Keep your head up; looking down impedes the thrust and can cause embarrassing proximity to the patient. An effective HVLA thrust technique is best achieved if both the operator and patient are relaxed and not holding themselves rigid. This is a common impediment to achieving effective cavitation.

Ensure the patient's head and neck remain on the pillow, as this facilitates the arrest of the technique and limits excessive amplitude of thrust.

primary leverage of head and neck rotation.

b. *Secondary leverage.* Add a very small degree of sidebending to the right, down to and including the C3–4 segment but leaving C4–5 free to move. The operator pivoting slightly, via the legs and trunk, introduces the right sidebending so that the trunk and upper body rotate to the left, enabling the hands and arms to remain in position (Fig. 8.30). Do not attempt to introduce sidebending by moving the hands or arms as this will lead to loss of contact and inaccurate technique.

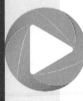

12. **Delivering the thrust**

Apply an HVLA thrust to the right articular pillar of C4. The thrust is upwards and towards the midline in the direction of the patient's left eye, parallel to the apophysial joint plane. Simultaneously, apply a slight, rapid increase of rotation of the head and neck to the left but do not increase the sidebending leverage (Fig. 8.31). The increase of rotation to the left is accomplished by slight supination of the left wrist and forearm. The thrust is induced by a very rapid contraction of the flexors and adductors of the right shoulder and, if necessary, trunk and lower limb movement.

The thrust, although very rapid, must never be excessively forcible. The aim should be to use the absolute minimum force necessary to achieve joint cavitation. A common fault arises from the use of excessive amplitude with insufficient velocity of thrust.

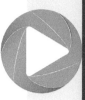

Summary

Cervical spine C2–7: Up-slope gliding

Chin hold

Patient supine

- **Contact point:** Posterolateral aspect of right C4 articular pillar

- **Applicator:** Lateral border, proximal or middle phalanx

- **Patient positioning:** Supine with the neck in a neutral relaxed position

- **Operator stance:** Head of couch, feet spread slightly

- **Palpation of contact point**

- **Fixation of contact point**

- **Chin hold:** Step to the right before taking up chin hold (Fig. 8.28). Take up chin hold and ensure your left forearm is over or slightly anterior to the ear

- **Vertex contact:** Optional

- **Positioning for thrust:** Introduce primary leverage of rotation left (Fig. 8.29) and a small degree of secondary leverage of sidebending right. Keep the right elbow close to the couch in order to maintain the contact point on the posterolateral aspect of the C4 articular pillar (Fig. 8.30)

- **Adjustments to achieve appropriate prethrust tension**

- **Immediately prethrust:** Relax and adjust your balance

- **Delivering the thrust:** The thrust is directed towards the patient's left eye. Simultaneously, apply a slight, rapid increase of rotation of the head and neck to the left with no increase of sidebending to the right (Fig. 8.31)

Cervical spine C2–7:
Up-slope gliding

Cradle hold

Patient supine

Assume somatic dysfunction (S-T-A-R-T) is identified and you wish to use an upward and forward gliding thrust, parallel to the apophysial joint plane, to produce cavitation at C4–5 on the right (Figs. 8.32, 8.33).

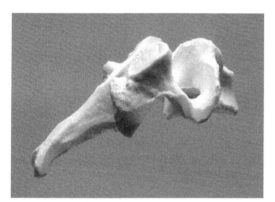

Figure 8.32

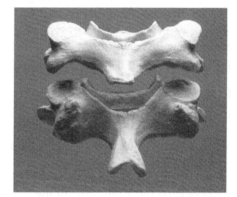

Figure 8.33

Key

✳ Stabilization

● Applicator

➡ Plane of thrust (operator)

⇨ Direction of body movement (patient)

Note: The dimensions for the arrows are not a pictorial representation of the amplitude or force of the thrust.

1. Contact point

Posterolateral aspect of the right articular pillar of C4.

2. Applicator

Lateral border, proximal or middle phalanx of operator's right index finger.

3. Patient positioning

Supine with the neck in a neutral relaxed position. If necessary, remove or adjust pillow height. The technique should not normally be executed in any significant degree of flexion or extension.

4. Operator stance

Head of couch, feet spread slightly. Adjust couch height so that you can stand as erect

131

as possible and avoid crouching over the patient, as this will limit the technique and restrict delivery of the thrust.

5. Palpation of contact point

Place fingers of both hands gently under the occiput. Lift the head to throw the articular pillars into prominence. Rotate the head slightly to the left, taking its weight in your left hand. Remove your right hand from the occiput and palpate the right articular pillar of C4 with the tip of your right index finger. Slowly but firmly slide your right forefinger downwards (towards the couch) along the articular pillar until it approximates the middle or proximal phalanx. Several sliding pressures may be necessary to establish close approximation to the contact point.

6. Fixation of contact point

Keep your right index finger firmly pressed upon the contact point while you flex the other fingers and thumb of the right hand so as to clasp the back of the neck and thereby lock the applicator in position. You must now keep the applicator on the contact point until the technique is complete. Keeping the hands in position, return the head to the neutral position.

7. Cradle hold

Keep your left hand under the head and spread the fingers out for maximum contact. Keep the patient's ear resting in the palm of your left hand. Flex the left wrist, which allows you to cradle the patient's head in your palm, flexed wrist and anterior aspect of forearm. Keep your right index finger firmly on the contact point and press the right palm against the occiput. The weight of the patient's head and neck is now balanced between your left and right hands with the cervical positioning controlled by the converging pressures of your two hands and arms. When treating the lower cervical segments, the middle or distal phalanx may be used as the applicator.

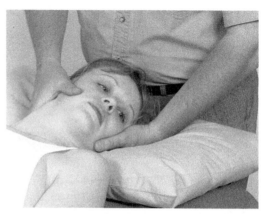

Figure 8.34

8. Vertex contact

None in this technique.

9. Positioning for thrust

The elbows are held close to or only slightly away from your sides. This is an essential feature of the cradle hold method. Stand easily upright at the head of the couch and do not step to the right as in the chin hold method.

a. *Primary leverage of rotation.* Maintaining all holds and contact points, complete the rotation of the head and neck to the left until tension is palpated at the contact point. Supination of the left wrist and forearm and simultaneous pronation of the right wrist and forearm achieve the rotation movement (Fig. 8.34). Do not lose firm pressure on the contact point. Do not force rotation; take it up fully but carefully. A common mistake is to use insufficient primary leverage of head and neck rotation.

b. *Secondary leverage.* Add a very small degree of sidebending to the right, down to and including the C3–4 segment but leaving C4–5 free to move. This is achieved by moving the right arm a little forward and the left arm a little back or by rotating the trunk and upper body to the left (Fig. 8.35). *Note:* Strong sidebending will lock the neck.

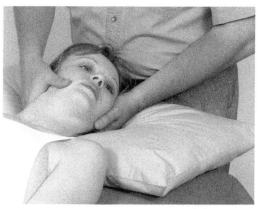

Figure 8.35

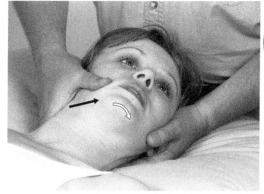

Figure 8.36

10. Adjustments to achieve appropriate prethrust tension

Ensure your patient remains relaxed. Maintaining all holds, make any necessary changes in flexion, extension, sidebending or rotation until you can sense a state of appropriate tension and leverage. The patient should not be aware of any pain or discomfort. You make these final adjustments by slight movements of your ankles, knees, hips and trunk, not by altering the position of the hands or arms.

11. Immediately prethrust

Relax and adjust your balance as necessary. Keep your head up; looking down impedes the thrust and can cause embarrassing proximity to the patient. An effective HVLA thrust technique is best achieved if both the operator and patient are relaxed and not holding themselves rigid. This is a common impediment to achieving effective cavitation.

Ensure the patient's head and neck remain on the pillow, as this facilitates the arrest of the technique and limits excessive amplitude of thrust.

12. Delivering the thrust

Apply an HVLA thrust to the right articular pillar of C4. The thrust is upwards and towards the midline in the direction of the patient's left eye, parallel to the apophysial joint plane (Fig. 8.36). This thrust is generated by rapid pronation of your right forearm. Simultaneously, apply a slight rapid increase of rotation of the head and neck to the left, but do not increase sidebending leverages. The increase of rotation to the left is accomplished by slight supination of the left wrist and forearm and is coordinated to match the thrust upon the contact point. This is an HVLA 'flick' type thrust. Coordination between the left and right hands and forearms is critical.

The thrust, although very rapid, must never be excessively forcible. The aim should be to use the absolute minimum force necessary to achieve joint cavitation. A common fault arises from the use of excessive amplitude with insufficient velocity of thrust.

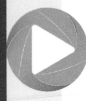

Summary

Cervical spine C2–7: Up-slope gliding

Cradle hold

Patient supine

- **Contact point:** Posterolateral aspect of the right C4 articular pillar

- **Applicator:** Lateral border, proximal or middle phalanx

- **Patient positioning:** Supine with the neck in a neutral relaxed position

- **Operator stance:** Head of couch, feet spread slightly

- **Palpation of contact point**

- **Fixation of contact point**

- **Cradle hold:** The weight of the patient's head and neck is balanced between your left and right hands with cervical positioning controlled by the converging pressures

- **Vertex contact:** None

- **Positioning for thrust:** Stand upright at the head of the couch. The elbows are held close to or only slightly away from your sides. Introduce primary leverage of rotation to the left (Fig. 8.34) and a small degree of secondary leverage of sidebending right (Fig. 8.35). Maintain the contact point on the posterolateral aspect of the C4 articular pillar

- **Adjustments to achieve appropriate prethrust tension**

- **Immediately prethrust:** Relax and adjust your balance

- **Delivering the thrust:** The thrust is directed towards the patient's left eye. Simultaneously, apply a slight, rapid increase of rotation of the head and neck to the left with no increase of sidebending to the right (Fig. 8.36)

Cervical spine C2–7:
Up-slope gliding

Cradle hold

Patient supine

Reversed primary and secondary leverage

In certain circumstances, the operator might wish to perform an up-slope gliding thrust but minimize the extent of head and neck rotation. Assume somatic dysfunction (S-T-A-R-T) is identified and you wish to use an upward and forward gliding thrust, parallel to the apophysial joint plane, to produce cavitation at C4–5 on the right (Figs. 8.37, 8.38).

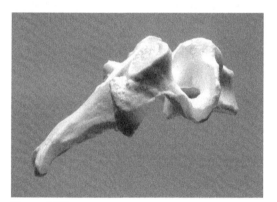

Figure 8.37

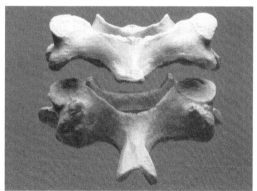

Figure 8.38

Key

✳ Stabilization

● Applicator

➡ Plane of thrust (operator)

⇨ Direction of body movement (patient)

Note: The dimensions for the arrows are not a pictorial representation of the amplitude or force of the thrust.

1. Contact point
Posterolateral aspect of the right articular pillar of C4.

2. Applicator
Lateral border, proximal or middle phalanx of operator's right index finger.

3. Patient positioning
Supine with the neck in a neutral relaxed position. If necessary, remove or adjust pillow height. The technique should not normally be executed in any significant degree of flexion or extension.

4. Operator stance

Head of couch, feet spread slightly. Adjust couch height so that you can stand as erect as possible and avoid crouching over the patient, as this will limit the technique and restrict delivery of the thrust.

5. Palpation of contact point

Place fingers of both hands gently under the occiput. Lift the head to throw the articular pillars into prominence. Rotate the head slightly to the left, taking its weight in your left hand. Remove your right hand from the occiput, and palpate the right articular pillar of C4 with the tip of your right index finger. Slowly but firmly slide your right forefinger downwards (towards the couch) along the articular pillar until it approximates the middle or proximal phalanx. Several sliding pressures may be necessary to establish close approximation to the contact point.

6. Fixation of contact point

Keep your right index finger firmly pressed upon the contact point while you flex the other fingers and thumb of the right hand so as to clasp the back of the neck and thereby lock the applicator in position. You must now keep the applicator on the contact point until the technique is complete. Keeping the hands in position, return the head to the neutral position.

7. Cradle hold

Keep your left hand under the head and spread the fingers out for maximum contact. Keep the patient's ear resting in the palm of your left hand. Flex the left wrist, which allows you to cradle the patient's head in your palm, flexed wrist and anterior aspect of forearm. Keep your right index finger firmly on the contact point and press the right palm against the occiput. The weight of the patient's head and neck is now balanced between your left and right hands, with the cervical positioning controlled by

the converging pressures of your two hands and arms. When treating the lower cervical segments, the middle or distal phalanx may be used as the applicator.

8. Vertex contact

None in this technique.

9. Positioning for thrust

The intent with this technique is to perform an up-slope gliding thrust but to limit the amount of head and neck rotation. This modification requires a greater emphasis upon the use of sidebending to achieve joint locking. It is critical that the direction of thrust be parallel to the apophysial joint plane in an up-slope direction. There should be no exaggeration of the sidebending leverage.

The elbows are held close to or only slightly away from your sides. This is an essential feature of the cradle hold method. Stand easily upright at the head of the couch, and do not step to the right as in the chin hold method.

a. *Primary leverage of sidebending.* Maintaining all holds and contact points, gently introduce sidebending of the head and neck to the right until tension is palpated at the contact point (Fig. 8.39). To introduce the right sidebending, the operator pivots slightly via the legs and trunk so that the trunk and upper body rotate to the left, enabling the hands and arms to remain in position. Do not lose firm contact with your contact point on the articular pillar of C4. A common mistake is to use insufficient primary leverage of head and neck sidebending.

b. *Secondary leverage.* Add a little rotation to the left, down to and including the C3–4 segment but leaving C4–5 free to move (Fig. 8.40). This requires extensive practice before one develops a refined 'tension sense'. Movement of your hands and forearms introduces the rotation.

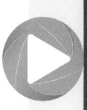

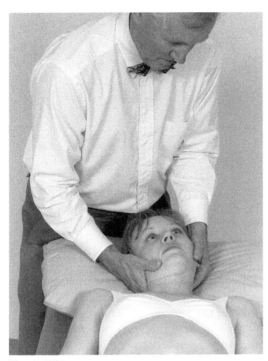

Figure 8.39

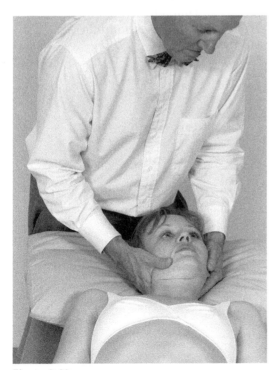

Figure 8.40

10. Adjustments to achieve appropriate prethrust tension

Ensure your patient remains relaxed. Maintaining all holds, make any necessary changes in flexion, extension, sidebending or rotation until you can sense a state of appropriate tension and leverage. The patient should not be aware of any pain or discomfort. You make these final adjustments by slight movements of your ankles, knees, hips and trunk, not by altering the position of the hands or arms.

11. Immediately prethrust

Relax and adjust your balance as necessary. Keep your head up; looking down impedes the thrust and can cause embarrassing proximity to the patient. An effective HVLA thrust technique is best achieved if both the operator and patient are relaxed and not holding themselves rigid. This is a common impediment to achieving effective cavitation.

Ensure the patient's head and neck remain on the pillow, as this facilitates the arrest of the technique and limits excessive amplitude of thrust.

12. Delivering the thrust

Apply an HVLA thrust to the right articular pillar of C4. The thrust is upwards and towards the midline in the direction of the patient's left eye, parallel to the apophysial joint plane (Fig. 8.41). This thrust is generated by rapid pronation of your right forearm. Simultaneously, apply a slight rapid increase of rotation of the head and neck to the left. A key element in this technique is to avoid exaggeration of the primary leverage of sidebending when the thrust is applied. The increase of rotation to the left is accomplished by slight supination of left wrist and forearm and coordinated to match the thrust upon the contact point. This is an HVLA 'flick' type thrust. Coordination between the left and right hands and forearms is critical.

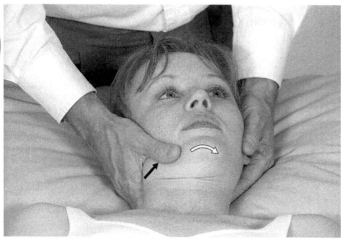

Figure 8.41

It must be appreciated that the use of sidebending as a primary leverage is predicated upon the operator's desire to limit the amount of head and neck rotation. Generally, when sidebending is used as a primary leverage, the aim will be to thrust in a down-slope direction. Exaggeration of the sidebending leverage in this technique must be avoided. Sidebending enhances locking but does not assist with an up-slope gliding thrust. The thrust in this technique is accompanied by slight exaggeration of the secondary leverage of rotation and is directed towards the patient's opposite eye.

The thrust, although very rapid, must never be excessively forcible. The aim should be to use the absolute minimum force necessary to achieve joint cavitation. A common fault arises from the use of excessive amplitude with insufficient velocity of thrust.

Summary

Cervical spine C2–7: Up-slope gliding

Cradle hold

Patient supine

Reversed primary and secondary leverage

- **Contact point:** Posterolateral aspect of the right C4 articular pillar

- **Applicator:** Lateral border, proximal or middle phalanx

- **Patient positioning:** Supine with the neck in a neutral, relaxed position

- **Operator stance:** Head of couch, feet spread slightly

- **Palpation of contact point**

- **Fixation of contact point**

- **Cradle hold:** The weight of the patient's head and neck is now balanced between your left and right hands with cervical positioning controlled by the converging pressures

- **Vertex contact:** None

- **Positioning for thrust:** Stand upright at the head of the couch. The elbows are held close to or only slightly away from your sides. Introduce primary leverage of sidebending to the right (Fig. 8.39) and a small degree of secondary leverage of rotation left (Fig. 8.40). Maintain the contact point on the posterolateral aspect of the C4 articular pillar

- **Adjustments to achieve appropriate prethrust tension**

- **Immediately prethrust:** Relax and adjust your balance

- **Delivering the thrust:** The thrust is directed towards the patient's left eye. Simultaneously, apply a slight rapid increase of rotation of the head and neck to the left with no increase of sidebending to the right (Fig. 8.41). A key element in this technique is to avoid exaggeration of the primary leverage of sidebending when the thrust is applied. The use of sidebending as a primary leverage is predicated upon the operator's desire to limit the amount of head and neck rotation

8.9

Cervical spine C2–7:
Up-slope gliding

Patient sitting
Operator standing in front

Assume somatic dysfunction (S-T-A-R-T) is identified and you wish to use an upward and forward thrust, parallel to the apophysial joint plane, to produce joint cavitation at C4–5 on the left (Figs. 8.42, 8.43).

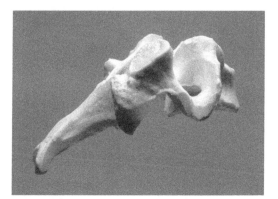

Figure 8.42

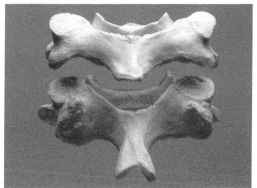

Figure 8.43

Key

✳ Stabilization

● Applicator

➡ Plane of thrust (operator)

⇨ Direction of body movement (patient)

Note: The dimensions for the arrows are not a pictorial representation of the amplitude or force of the thrust.

1. Contact point
Posterolateral aspect of the left articular pillar of C4.

2. Applicator
Palmar aspect, proximal or middle phalanx of operator's right index or middle finger.

3. Patient positioning
Sitting with the neck in a neutral relaxed position. The neck should not be in any significant amount of flexion or extension.

4. Operator stance
Stand in front and to the right of the patient, feet spread slightly. Adjust couch height so that you can stand as erect as possible and avoid crouching over the

141

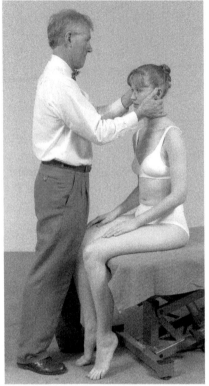

Figure 8.44

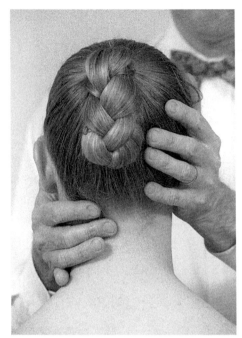

Figure 8.45

patient, as this will limit the technique and restrict delivery of the thrust (Fig. 8.44).

5. Palpation of contact point

Place the fingers and palm of your left hand against the patient's right occiput and neck, gently covering the patient's right ear. Use the index or middle finger of your right hand to palpate the patient's left articular pillar of C4. Slowly but firmly slide your applicator along the articular pillar of C4 until it approximates the proximal or middle phalanx (Fig. 8.45). Several sliding pressures may be necessary to establish close approximation to the contact point.

6. Fixation of contact point

Keep your right index or middle finger firmly pressed upon the contact point while you spread the other fingers and thumb of

the right hand to securely support the head, mandible and neck, thereby locking the applicator in position. You must now keep the applicator on the contact point until the technique is complete. The weight of the head and neck is now balanced between your left and right hands, with the cervical spine positioning controlled by the converging pressures of your two hands.

7. Positioning for thrust

The elbows are held close to or only slightly away from your sides.

a. *Primary leverage.* Ensure that the patient's head is securely supported between your two hands. Maintaining all holds and contact points, rotate the head and neck to the right until tension is palpated at the contact point (Fig. 8.46). Do not lose contact between your applicator and the articular pillar of C4. Do not force rotation; take it up fully but carefully. A common mistake is to use insufficient

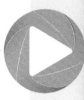

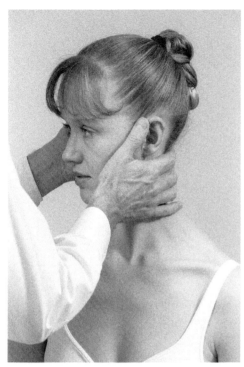

Figure 8.46

primary leverage of head and neck rotation.

b. *Secondary leverage.* Add a very small degree of sidebending to the left, down to and including the C3–4 segment but leaving C4–5 free to move. *Note:* strong sidebending will lock the neck. Slight movements of the operator's forearms, shoulders and trunk introduce the sidebending.

8. Adjustments to achieve appropriate prethrust tension

Ensure your patient remains relaxed. It is important to keep your elbows close to your sides. Maintaining all holds, make any necessary changes in flexion, extension, sidebending or rotation until you can sense a state of appropriate tension and leverage. The patient should not be aware of any pain or discomfort. You make these final adjustments by slight movements of your legs and trunk, not by altering the position of the hands or arms.

9. Immediately prethrust

Relax and adjust your balance as necessary. Keep your head up; looking down impedes the thrust and can cause embarrassing proximity to the patient. An effective HVLA thrust technique is best achieved if both the operator and patient are relaxed and not holding themselves rigid. This is a common impediment to achieving effective cavitation.

10. Delivering the thrust

Apply an HVLA thrust to the left articular pillar of C4. The thrust is upwards and towards the midline in the direction of the patient's right eye, parallel to the apophysial joint plane (Fig. 8.47). Simultaneously, apply a slight, rapid increase of rotation to the right, but do not increase sidebending leverages. This is an HVLA 'flick' type thrust. Coordination between the left and right hands and arms is critical.

The thrust, although very rapid, must never be excessively forcible. The aim should be to use the absolute minimum force necessary to achieve joint cavitation. A common fault arises from the use of excessive amplitude with insufficient velocity of thrust.

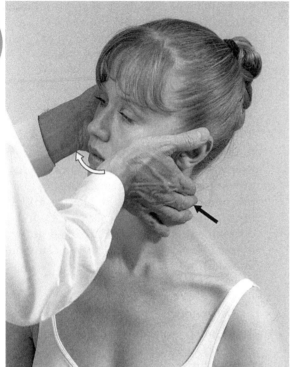

Figure 8.47

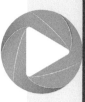

Summary

Cervical spine C2–7: Up-slope gliding

Patient sitting

Operator standing in front

- **Contact point:** Posterolateral aspect of the left C4 articular pillar

- **Applicator:** Palmar aspect, proximal or middle phalanx

- **Patient positioning:** Sitting with the neck in a neutral, relaxed position

- **Operator stance:** In front and to the right of the patient, feet spread slightly (Fig. 8.44)

- **Palpation of contact point**

- **Fixation of contact point:** Keep your right index or middle finger firmly pressed upon the contact point while you spread the other fingers and thumb of the right hand to securely support the head, mandible and neck (Fig. 8.45)

- **Positioning for thrust:** Stand upright with the elbows held close to or only slightly away from your sides. Introduce primary leverage of rotation to the right (Fig. 8.46) and a small degree of secondary leverage of sidebending left. Maintain the contact point on the posterolateral aspect of the C4 articular pillar

- **Adjustments to achieve appropriate prethrust tension**

- **Immediately prethrust:** Relax and adjust your balance

- **Delivering the thrust:** The thrust is directed towards the patient's right eye. Simultaneously, apply a slight, rapid increase of rotation of the head and neck to the right with no increase of sidebending to the left (Fig. 8.47). Coordination between both hands and arms is critical

Cervical spine C2–7:
Up-slope gliding

Patient sitting

Operator standing to the side

Assume somatic dysfunction (S-T-A-R-T) is identified and you wish to use an upward and forward gliding thrust, parallel to the apophysial joint plane, to produce cavitation at C4–5 on the left (Figs. 8.48, 8.49).

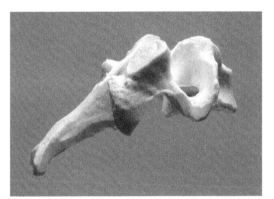

Figure 8.48

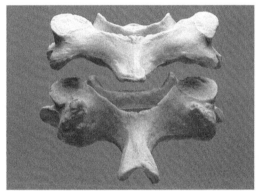

Figure 8.49

Key

✳ Stabilization

● Applicator

➡ Plane of thrust (operator)

⇨ Direction of body movement (patient)

Note: The dimensions for the arrows are not a pictorial representation of the amplitude or force of the thrust.

1. Contact point

Posterolateral aspect of the left articular pillar of C4.

2. Applicator

Palmar aspect, proximal or middle phalanx of operator's right index or middle finger.

3. Patient positioning

Sitting with the neck in a neutral relaxed position. The neck should not be in any significant amount of flexion or extension.

4. Operator stance

Stand to the right of the patient, feet spread slightly. Adjust couch height so that you can stand as erect as possible and avoid crouching over the patient, as this will limit

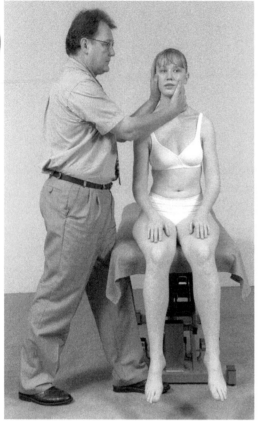

Figure 8.50

the technique and restrict delivery of the thrust (Fig. 8.50).

5. Palpation of contact point

Place the fingers and palm of your left hand over the right side of the patient's head and neck, gently covering the right ear. Reach in front of the patient with your right hand and palpate the left articular pillar of C4 with the tip of your right index or middle finger. Slowly but firmly slide your applicator along the articular pillar of C4 until it approximates the proximal or middle phalanx. Several sliding pressures may be necessary to establish close approximation to the contact point.

6. Fixation of contact point

Keep your right index or middle finger firmly pressed upon the contact point while you spread the other fingers and thumb of the right hand to securely support the head, mandible and neck, thereby locking the applicator in position. You must now keep the applicator on the contact point until the technique is complete. The weight of the head and neck is now balanced between your left and right hands, with the cervical spine positioning controlled by the converging pressures of your two hands.

7. Positioning for thrust

The elbows are held close to or only slightly away from your sides.

a. *Primary leverage.* Ensure that the patient's head is securely supported between your two hands. Maintaining all holds and contact points, rotate the head and neck to the right until tension is palpated at the contact point (Fig. 8.51). Do not lose contact between your applicator and the articular pillar of C4. Do not force rotation; take it up fully but carefully. A common mistake is to use insufficient primary leverage of head and neck rotation.

b. *Secondary leverage.* Add a very small degree of sidebending to the left, down to and including the C3–4 segment but leaving C4–5 free to move. *Note:* strong sidebending will lock the neck. Slight movements of the operator's forearms, shoulders and trunk introduce the sidebending.

8. Adjustments to achieve appropriate prethrust tension

Ensure your patient remains relaxed. It is important to keep your elbows close to your sides. Maintaining all holds, make any necessary changes in flexion, extension, sidebending or rotation until you can sense a state of appropriate tension and leverage. The patient should not be aware of any pain

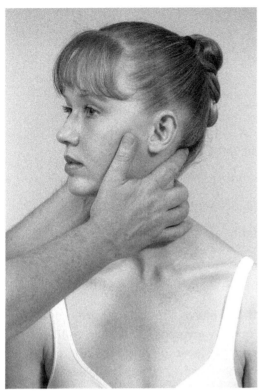

Figure 8.51

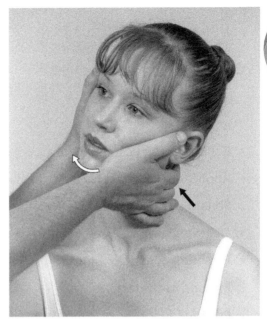

Figure 8.52

or discomfort. You make these final adjustments by slight movements of your legs and trunk, not by altering the position of the hands or arms.

9. Immediately prethrust

Relax and adjust your balance as necessary. Keep your head up; looking down impedes the thrust and can cause embarrassing proximity to the patient. An effective HVLA thrust technique is best achieved if both the operator and patient are relaxed and not holding themselves rigid. This is a common impediment to achieving effective cavitation.

10. Delivering the thrust

Apply an HVLA thrust to the left articular pillar of C4. The thrust is upwards and towards the midline in the direction of the patient's right eye, parallel to the apophysial joint plane (Fig. 8.52). Simultaneously, apply a slight, rapid increase of rotation to the right, but do not increase sidebending leverages. This is an HVLA 'flick' type thrust. Coordination between the left and right hands and arms is critical.

The thrust, although very rapid, must never be excessively forcible. The aim should be to use the absolute minimum force necessary to achieve joint cavitation. A common fault arises from the use of excessive amplitude with insufficient velocity of thrust.

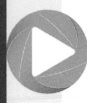

Summary

Cervical spine C2–7: Up-slope gliding

Patient sitting

Operator standing to the side

- **Contact point:** Posterolateral aspect of the left C4 articular pillar

- **Applicator:** Palmar aspect, proximal or middle phalanx

- **Patient positioning:** Sitting with the neck in a neutral relaxed position

- **Operator stance:** To the right of the patient, feet spread slightly (Fig. 8.50)

- **Palpation of contact point**

- **Fixation of contact point**

- **Positioning for thrust:** Stand upright with the elbows held close to or only slightly away from your sides. Introduce primary leverage of rotation to the right (Fig. 8.51) and a small degree of secondary leverage of sidebending left. Maintain the contact point on the posterolateral aspect of the left C4 articular pillar

- **Adjustments to achieve appropriate prethrust tension**

- **Immediately prethrust:** Relax and adjust your balance

- **Delivering the thrust:** The thrust is directed towards the patient's right eye. Simultaneously, apply a slight, rapid increase of rotation of the head and neck to the right with no increase of sidebending left (Fig. 8.52). Coordination between both hands and arms is critical

8.11

Cervical spine C2–7:
Down-slope gliding

Chin hold

Patient supine

Assume somatic dysfunction (S-T-A-R-T) is identified and you wish to use a downward and backward gliding thrust, parallel to the apophysial joint plane, to produce cavitation at C4–5 on the right (Figs. 8.53, 8.54).

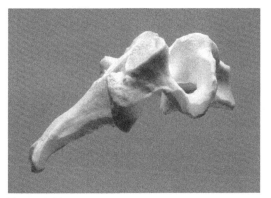

Figure 8.53

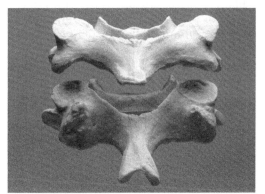

Figure 8.54

Key

✳ Stabilization

● Applicator

➡ Plane of thrust (operator)

⇨ Direction of body movement (patient)

Note: The dimensions for the arrows are not a pictorial representation of the amplitude or force of the thrust.

1. Contact point
Lateral aspect of the right articular pillar of C4.

2. Applicator
Lateral border, proximal or middle phalanx of operator's right index finger.

3. Patient positioning
Supine with the neck in a neutral relaxed position. If necessary, remove pillow or adjust pillow height. The neck should not be in any significant amount of flexion or extension.

4. Operator stance

Head of couch, feet spread slightly. Adjust couch height so that you can stand as erect as possible and avoid crouching over the patient, as this will limit the technique and restrict delivery of the thrust.

5. Palpation of contact point

Place fingers of both hands gently under the occiput. Rotate the head to the left, taking its weight in your left hand. Remove your right hand from the occiput and palpate the right articular pillar of C4 with the tip of your index or middle finger. Slowly but firmly slide your right index finger downwards (towards the couch) along the articular pillar until it approximates the middle or proximal phalanx. Several sliding pressures may be necessary to establish close approximation to the contact point.

6. Fixation of contact point

Keep your right index finger firmly pressed upon the contact point while you flex the other fingers and thumb of the right hand so as to clasp the back of the neck and thereby lock the applicator in position. You must now keep the applicator on the contact point until the technique is complete. Keeping the hands in position, return the head to the neutral position.

7. Chin hold

Keeping your right hand in position, slide the left hand slowly and carefully forwards until the fingers lightly clasp the chin. Ensure that your left forearm is over or slightly anterior to the ear. Placing the forearm on or behind the ear puts the neck into too much flexion. The head is now controlled by balancing forces between the right palm and left forearm. Maintain the applicator in position.

8. Vertex contact

Move your body forwards slightly so that your chest is in contact with the vertex of the patient's head. The head is now securely cradled between your left forearm, the flexed left elbow, the right palm and your chest. Vertex contact is often useful in a heavy, stiff or difficult case but can, on occasions, be omitted.

9. Positioning for thrust

Step slightly to the right, keeping the hands firmly in position and taking care not to lose pressure on the contact point. This introduces an element of cervical sidebending to the right. Straighten your right wrist so that the radius and first metacarpal are in line. Align your body and right arm for the thrust plane, which is caudad in the direction of the patient's left shoulder and downwards towards the couch.

a. *Primary leverage of sidebending.* Maintaining all holds and contact points, sidebend the patient's head and neck to the right until tension is palpated at the contact point (Fig. 8.55). The operator pivoting slightly, via the legs and trunk, introduces the right sidebending so that the trunk and upper body rotate to the left, enabling the hands and arms to remain in position. Do not attempt to introduce sidebending by moving the hands or arms alone, as this will lead to loss of contact and inaccurate technique. Do not lose firm contact with your contact point on the articular pillar of C4. A common mistake is to use insufficient primary leverage of head and neck sidebending.

b. *Secondary leverage.* Add a little rotation to the left, down to and including the C3–4 segment but leaving C4–5 free to move (Fig. 8.56). This requires extensive practice before one develops a refined 'tension sense'. Movement of your hands and forearms introduces the rotation.

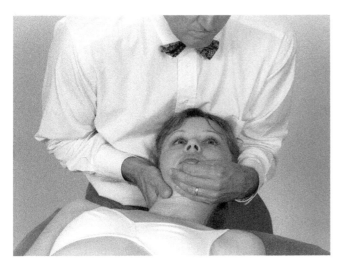

Figure 8.55

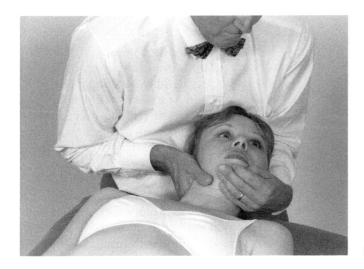

Figure 8.56

10. Adjustments to achieve appropriate prethrust tension

Ensure your patient remains relaxed. Maintaining all holds, make any necessary changes in flexion, extension, sidebending or rotation until you can sense a state of appropriate tension and leverage. The patient should not be aware of any pain or discomfort. You make these final adjustments by slight movements of your ankles, knees, hips and trunk, not by altering the position of the hands or arms.

11. Immediately prethrust

Relax and adjust your balance as necessary. Keep your head up; looking down impedes the thrust and can cause embarrassing proximity to the patient. An effective HVLA thrust technique is best achieved if both the operator and patient are relaxed and not

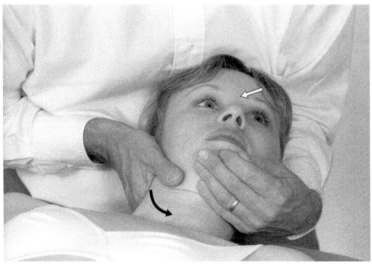

Figure 8.57

holding themselves rigid. This is a common impediment to achieving effective cavitation.

12. Delivering the thrust

Apply an HVLA thrust to the right articular pillar of C4. The direction of thrust is caudad in the direction of the patient's left shoulder and downwards towards the couch, parallel to the apophysial joint plane. Simultaneously, apply a slight, rapid increase of sidebending of the head and neck to the right, but do not increase the rotation leverage (Fig. 8.57). The increase of sidebending is induced by a slight rotation of the operator's trunk and upper body to the left. A very rapid contraction of the flexors and adductors of the right shoulder joint induce the thrust; if necessary, trunk and lower limb movement may be incorporated.

The thrust, although very rapid, must never be excessively forcible. The aim should be to use the absolute minimum force necessary to achieve joint cavitation. A common fault arises from the use of excessive amplitude with insufficient velocity of thrust.

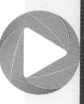

Summary

Cervical spine C2–7: Down-slope gliding

Chin hold

Patient supine

- **Contact point:** Lateral aspect of the right C4 articular pillar

- **Applicator:** Lateral border, proximal or middle phalanx

- **Patient positioning:** Supine with the neck in a neutral relaxed position

- **Operator stance:** Head of couch, feet spread slightly

- **Palpation of contact point**

- **Fixation of contact point**

- **Chin hold:** Ensure your left forearm is over or slightly anterior to the ear

- **Vertex contact:** Optional but often useful

- **Positioning for thrust:** Step slightly to the right. Introduce primary leverage of sidebending right (Fig. 8.55) and a small degree of secondary leverage of rotation left (Fig. 8.56). Align your body and right arm for the thrust plane, which is caudad in the direction of the patient's left shoulder and downwards towards the couch

- **Adjustments to achieve appropriate prethrust tension**

- **Immediately prethrust:** Relax and adjust your balance

- **Delivering the thrust:** The thrust is directed towards the patient's left shoulder and downwards towards the couch. Simultaneously, apply a slight, rapid increase of sidebending of the head and neck to the right with no increase of rotation to the left (Fig. 8.57)

8.12

Cervical spine C2–7:
Down-slope gliding

Cradle hold

Patient supine

Assume somatic dysfunction (S-T-A-R-T) is identified and you wish to use a downward and backward gliding thrust, parallel to the apophysial joint plane, to produce cavitation at C4–5 on the right (Figs. 8.58, 8.59).

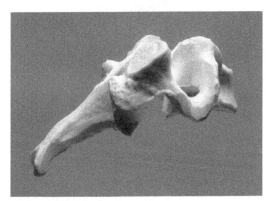

Figure 8.58

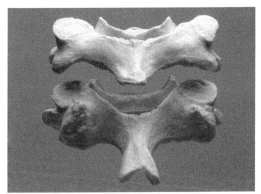

Figure 8.59

Key

✳ Stabilization

● Applicator

➡ Plane of thrust (operator)

⇨ Direction of body movement (patient)

Note: The dimensions for the arrows are not a pictorial representation of the amplitude or force of the thrust.

1. Contact point
The lateral aspect of the right articular pillar of C4.

2. Applicator
Lateral border, proximal or middle phalanx of operator's right index finger.

3. Patient positioning
Supine with the neck in a neutral relaxed position. If necessary, remove pillow or adjust pillow height. The neck should not be in any significant amount of flexion or extension.

4. Operator stance

Head of couch, feet spread slightly. Adjust couch height so that you can stand as erect as possible and avoid crouching over the patient, as this will limit the technique and restrict delivery of the thrust.

5. Palpation of contact point

Place fingers of both hands gently under the occiput. Rotate the head to the left, taking its weight in your left hand. Remove your right hand from the occiput and palpate the right articular pillar of C4 with the tip of your index or middle finger. Slowly but firmly slide your right index finger downwards (towards the couch) along the articular pillar until it approximates the middle or proximal phalanx. Several sliding pressures may be necessary to establish close approximation to the contact point.

6. Fixation of contact point

Keep the right index finger firmly pressed on the contact point while you flex the other fingers and thumb of the right hand so as to clasp the back of the neck and thereby lock the applicator in position. You must now keep the applicator on the contact point until the technique is complete. Keeping the hands in position, return the head to the neutral position.

7. Cradle hold

Keep the left hand under the head and spread the fingers out for maximum contact; keep the patient's ear resting in the palm of your left hand. Flex the left wrist, allowing you to cradle the patient's head in your palm, flexed wrist and anterior aspect of forearm. Keep your right index finger firmly on the contact point and press the right palm against the occiput. The weight of the patient's head and neck is now balanced between your left and right hands, with the cervical positioning controlled by the converging pressures of your two hands and

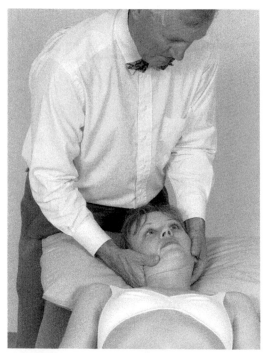

Figure 8.60

arms. When treating the lower cervical segments, the middle or distal phalanx may be used as the applicator.

8. Vertex contact

None in this technique.

9. Positioning for thrust

The elbows are held close to or only slightly away from your sides. This is an essential feature of the cradle hold method. Stand easily upright at the head of the couch, and do not step to the right as in the chin hold method.

a. *Primary leverage of sidebending.*
Maintaining all holds and contact points, gently introduce sidebending of the head and neck to the right until tension is palpated at the contact point (Fig. 8.60). To introduce the right sidebending, the operator pivots slightly via the legs and trunk so that the trunk and upper body rotate to the left, enabling the hands

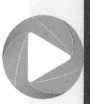

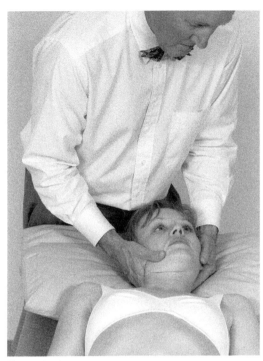

Figure 8.61

and arms to remain in position. Do not lose firm contact with your contact point on the articular pillar of C4. A common mistake is to use insufficient primary leverage of head and neck sidebending.

b. *Secondary leverage.* Add a little rotation to the left, down to and including the C3–4 segment but leaving C4–5 free to move (Fig. 8.61). This requires extensive practice before one develops a refined 'tension sense'. Movement of your hands and forearms introduces the rotation.

10. Adjustments to achieve appropriate prethrust tension

Ensure your patient remains relaxed. Maintaining all holds, make any necessary changes in flexion, extension, sidebending or rotation until you can sense a state of appropriate tension and leverage. The patient should not be aware of any pain or discomfort. You make these final adjustments by slight movements of your ankles, knees, hips and trunk, not by altering the position of the hands or arms.

11. Immediately prethrust

Relax and adjust your balance as necessary. Keep your head up; looking down impedes the thrust and can cause embarrassing proximity to the patient. An effective HVLA thrust technique is best achieved if both the operator and patient are relaxed and not holding themselves rigid. This is a common impediment to achieving effective cavitation.

Ensure the patient's head and neck remain on the pillow, as this facilitates the arrest of the technique and limits excessive amplitude of thrust.

Note that the final thrust is directed in a downward and backward direction parallel to the facet joint plane. The thrust is directed towards the patient's left shoulder, as illustrated. The primary leverage is sidebending to the right and the secondary (lesser leverage) is rotation to the left.

12. Delivering the thrust

Apply an HVLA thrust to the right articular pillar of C4. The direction of thrust is caudad in the direction of the patient's left shoulder and downwards towards the couch, parallel to the apophysial joint plane (Fig. 8.62). The operator rotating the trunk and upper body to the left, enabling the hands and arms to remain in position on the cervical spine, generates the thrust. Simultaneously, apply a very slight, rapid increase of sidebending of the head and neck to the right but do not increase the rotation leverage.

The thrust, although very rapid, must never be excessively forcible. The aim should be to use the absolute minimum force necessary to achieve joint cavitation. A common fault arises from the use of excessive amplitude with insufficient velocity of thrust.

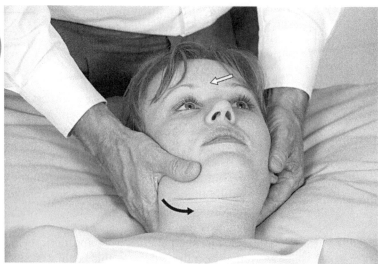

Figure 8.62

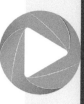

Summary

Cervical spine C2–7: Down-slope gliding

Cradle hold

Patient supine

- **Contact point:** Lateral aspect of the right C4 articular pillar

- **Applicator:** Lateral border, proximal or middle phalanx

- **Patient positioning:** Supine with the neck in a neutral, relaxed position

- **Operator stance:** Head of couch, feet spread slightly

- **Palpation of contact point**

- **Fixation of contact point**

- **Cradle hold:** The weight of the patient's head and neck is balanced between your left and right hands with cervical positioning controlled by the converging pressures

- **Vertex contact:** None

- **Positioning for thrust:** Stand upright at the head of the couch. The elbows are held close to or only slightly away from your sides. Introduce primary leverage of sidebending to the right (Fig. 8.60) and a small degree of secondary leverage of rotation left (Fig. 8.61). Maintain the contact point on the lateral aspect of the right C4 articular pillar

- **Adjustments to achieve appropriate prethrust tension**

- **Immediately prethrust:** Relax and adjust your balance

- **Delivering the thrust:** The thrust is directed towards the patient's left shoulder and downwards towards the couch. Simultaneously, apply a slight, rapid increase of sidebending of the head and neck to the right with no increase of rotation to the left (Fig. 8.62)

8.13

Cervical spine C2–7:
Down-slope gliding

Patient sitting

Operator standing to the side

Assume somatic dysfunction (S-T-A-R-T) is identified and you wish to use a downward and backward gliding thrust, parallel to the apophysial joint plane, to produce cavitation at C4–5 on the right (Figs. 8.63, 8.64).

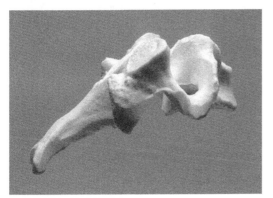

Figure 8.63

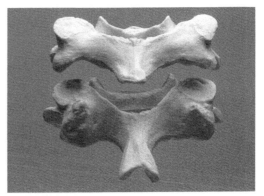

Figure 8.64

Key

❋ Stabilization

● Applicator

➡ Plane of thrust (operator)

⇨ Direction of body movement (patient)

Note: The dimensions for the arrows are not a pictorial representation of the amplitude or force of the thrust.

1. Contact point

Lateral aspect of the right articular pillar of C4.

2. Applicator

Palmar aspect, proximal or middle phalanx of operator's left index or middle finger.

3. Patient positioning

Sitting with the neck in a neutral relaxed position. The neck should not be in any significant amount of flexion or extension.

4. Operator stance

Stand to the left of the patient, feet spread slightly. Adjust couch height so that you can stand as erect as possible and avoid crouching over the patient, as this will limit

163

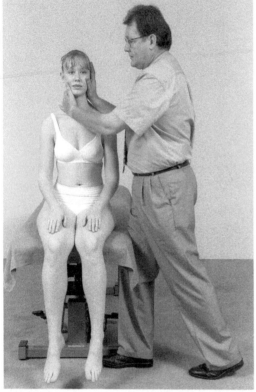

Figure 8.65

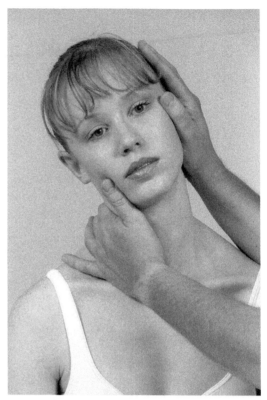

Figure 8.66

the technique and restrict delivery of the thrust (Fig. 8.65).

5. Palpation of contact point

Place the fingers and palm of your right hand over the left side of the patient's head and neck, gently covering the left ear. Reach in front of the patient with your left hand and palpate the right articular pillar of C4 with the tip of your left index or middle finger. Slowly but firmly slide your applicator along the articular pillar of C4 until it approximates the proximal or middle phalanx. Several sliding pressures may be necessary to establish close approximation to the contact point.

6. Fixation of contact point

Keep your left index or middle finger firmly pressed upon the contact point while you

spread the other fingers and thumb of the left hand to securely support the head, mandible and neck, thereby locking the applicator in position. You must now keep the applicator on the contact point until the technique is complete. The weight of the head and neck is now balanced between your right and left hands, with the cervical spine positioning controlled by the converging pressures of your two hands.

7. Positioning for thrust

The elbows are held close to or only slightly away from your sides.

a. *Primary leverage.* Ensure that the patient's head is securely supported between your two hands. Maintaining all holds and contact points, sidebend the head and neck to the right until tension is palpated at the contact point (Fig. 8.66). Do not lose contact between your applicator and the articular pillar of C4. Do not force sidebending; take it up fully but carefully. A common mistake is to use insufficient primary leverage of head and neck sidebending.

b. *Secondary leverage.* Add a very small degree of rotation to the left, down to and including the C3–4 segment but leaving C4–5 free to move. Slight movements of the operator's hands and arms introduce the rotation.

8. Adjustments to achieve appropriate prethrust tension

Ensure your patient remains relaxed. It is important to keep your elbows close to your sides. Maintaining all holds, make any necessary changes in flexion, extension, sidebending or rotation until you can sense a state of appropriate tension and leverage. The patient should not be aware of any pain or discomfort.

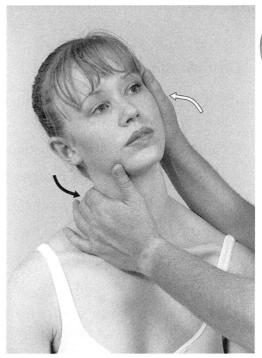

Figure 8.67

9. Immediately prethrust

Relax and adjust your balance as necessary. Keep your head up; looking down impedes the thrust and can cause embarrassing proximity to the patient. An effective HVLA thrust technique is best achieved if both the operator and patient are relaxed and not holding themselves rigid. This is a common impediment to achieving effective cavitation.

10. Delivering the thrust

Apply an HVLA thrust to the right articular pillar of C4. The thrust is caudad and towards the patient's left shoulder, parallel to the apophysial joint plane (Fig. 8.67). Simultaneously, apply a slight, rapid increase of sidebending to the right but do not increase rotation leverage. This is an HVLA 'flick' type thrust. Coordination between the left and right hands and arms is critical.

The thrust, although very rapid, must never be excessively forcible. The aim should be to use the absolute minimum force necessary to achieve joint cavitation. A common fault arises from the use of excessive amplitude with insufficient velocity of thrust.

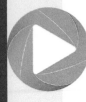

Summary

Cervical spine C2–7: Down-slope gliding

Patient sitting

Operator standing to the side

- **Contact point:** Lateral aspect of the right C4 articular pillar

- **Applicator:** Palmar aspect, proximal or middle phalanx

- **Patient positioning:** Sitting with the neck in a neutral, relaxed position

- **Operator stance:** To the left of the patient, feet spread slightly (Fig. 8.65)

- **Palpation of contact point**

- **Fixation of contact point**

- **Positioning for thrust:** Stand upright with the elbows held close to or only slightly away from your sides. Introduce primary leverage of sidebending to the right (Fig. 8.66) and a small degree of secondary leverage of rotation left. Maintain the contact point on the lateral aspect of the right C4 articular pillar

- **Adjustments to achieve appropriate prethrust tension**

- **Immediately prethrust:** Relax and adjust your balance

- **Delivering the thrust:** The thrust is caudad and towards the patient's left shoulder. Simultaneously, apply a slight, rapid increase of sidebending of the head and neck to the right with no increase of rotation to the left (Fig. 8.67). Coordination between both hands and arms is critical

8.14

Cervicothoracic spine C7–T3:
Rotation gliding

Patient prone
Operator at side of couch

Assume somatic dysfunction (S-T-A-R-T) is identified and you wish to use a rotation gliding thrust, parallel to the apophysial joint plane, to produce cavitation at the T2–3 apophysial joint (Figs. 8.68, 8.69).

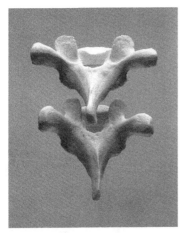

Figure 8.68

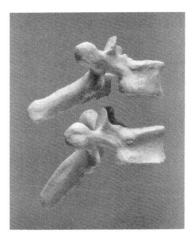

Figure 8.69

Key

 Stabilization

● Applicator

➡ Plane of thrust (operator)

⇨ Direction of body movement (patient)

Note: The dimensions for the arrows are not a pictorial representation of the amplitude or force of the thrust.

1. Contact point
Right side of spinous process of T3.

2. Applicator
Thumb of right hand.

3. Patient positioning
Patient lying prone with the head and neck turned to the left and arms hanging over the edge of the couch or against the patient's sides (Fig. 8.70). Introduce a small amount of sidebending to the right by gently moving the patient's head to the right while in the rotated position. Do not introduce too much sidebending.

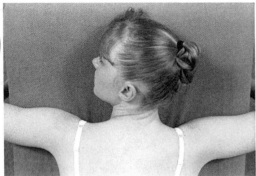

Figure 8.70

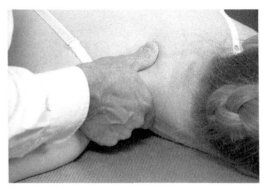

Figure 8.71

4. Operator stance

Stand on the right side of the patient facing towards the head of the couch.

5. Palpation of contact point

Locate the spinous process of T3. Place the thumb of your right hand gently but firmly against the right side of this spinous process. Spread the fingers of your right hand to rest over the patient's right trapezius muscle, with your fingertips resting on the patient's right clavicle (Fig. 8.71). Ensure that you have good contact and will not slip off the spinous process of T3 when you apply a force against it. Maintain this contact point.

6. Positioning for thrust

Keeping your position at the side of the couch, gently place your left hand against the left side of the patient's head. This hand will control the rotation and sidebending leverages. Increase rotation of the patient's head and neck to the left by applying gentle pressure to the patient's head until a sense of tension is palpated at the contact point. Move your right forearm so that it lines up with your thumb against the spinous process of T3 and forms an angle of approximately 90° at the elbow (Fig. 8.72).

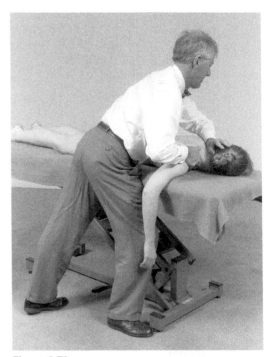

Figure 8.72

7. Adjustments to achieve appropriate prethrust tension

Ensure the patient remains relaxed. Maintaining all holds, make any necessary changes in extension, sidebending or rotation until you can sense a state of appropriate tension and leverage. The patient should not be aware of any pain or discomfort. Make these final adjustments by altering the

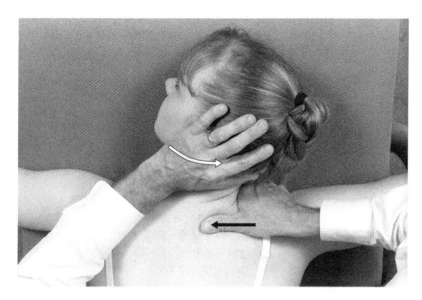

Figure 8.73

pressure and direction of forces between the left hand against the patient's head and your right thumb at the contact point.

8. Immediately prethrust

Relax and adjust your balance as necessary. Keep your head up and ensure that your contacts are firm and your body position is well controlled. An effective HVLA thrust technique is best achieved if the operator and patient are relaxed and not holding themselves rigid. This is a common impediment to achieving effective cavitation.

9. Delivering the thrust

Apply an HVLA thrust to the spinous process of T3 in the direction of the patient's left shoulder joint. Simultaneously,

apply a slight, rapid increase of head and neck rotation to the left with your left hand (Fig. 8.73). The thrust induces local rotation of the T3 vertebra, focusing forces at the T2–3 segment. You must not overemphasize the thrust with your left hand against the patient's head. Your left hand stabilizes the leverages and maintains the position of the head against the thrust imposed upon the contact point. The thrust is induced by a very rapid contraction of the shoulder adductors.

The thrust, although very rapid, must never be excessively forcible. The aim should be to use the absolute minimum force necessary to achieve joint cavitation. A common fault arises from the use of excessive amplitude with insufficient velocity of thrust.

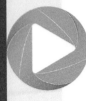

Summary

Cervicothoracic spine C7–T3: Rotation gliding

Patient prone

Operator at side of couch

- **Contact point:** Right side of T3 spinous process

- **Applicator:** Thumb of right hand

- **Patient positioning:** Prone with the head rotated to the left and arms hanging over the edge of the couch or against the patient's sides (Fig. 8.70). Introduce a small amount of sidebending to the right. Do not introduce too much sidebending

- **Operator stance:** Right side of the patient facing towards the head of the couch

- **Palpation of contact point:** Place the thumb of your right hand against the right side of the spinous process of T3. Spread the fingers of your right hand to rest over the patient's trapezius muscle and clavicle (Fig. 8.71)

- **Positioning for thrust:** Place your left hand against the left side of the patient's head. Increase rotation of the head and neck to the left until a sense of tension is palpated at the contact point. Move your right forearm so that it lines up with your thumb against the spinous process of T3 and forms an angle of approximately 90° at the elbow (Fig. 8.72)

- **Adjustments to achieve appropriate prethrust tension**

- **Immediately prethrust:** Relax and adjust your balance

- **Delivering the thrust:** Thrust is directed towards the patient's left shoulder joint. Simultaneously, apply a slight rapid increase of head and neck rotation to the left with your left hand (Fig. 8.73). You must not overemphasize the thrust with your left hand against the patient's head

8.15

Cervicothoracic spine C7–T3:
Rotation gliding

Patient prone
Operator at head of couch

Assume somatic dysfunction (S-T-A-R-T) is identified and you wish to use a rotation gliding thrust, parallel to the apophysial joint plane, to produce cavitation at the T2–3 apophysial joint (Figs. 8.74, 8.75).

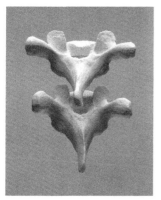

Figure 8.74

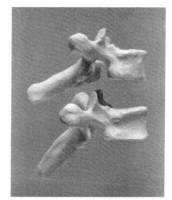

Figure 8.75

Key

※ Stabilization

● Applicator

➡ Plane of thrust (operator)

⇨ Direction of body movement (patient)

Note: The dimensions for the arrows are not a pictorial representation of the amplitude or force of the thrust.

1. Contact point
Transverse process of T3 on the left.

2. Applicator
Hypothenar eminence of left hand.

3. Patient positioning
Patient prone with the point of the chin resting on the couch and the arms hanging over the edge of the couch or against the patient's sides. Introduce a small amount of sidebending to the right by gently lifting and moving the patient's chin to the right (Fig. 8.76). Do not introduce too much sidebending.

4. Operator stance

Head of the couch, feet spread slightly. Stand as erect as possible and avoid crouching over the patient, as this will limit the technique and restrict delivery of the thrust.

5. Palpation of contact point

Locate the transverse process of T3 on the left. Place the hypothenar eminence of your left hand gently but firmly against the transverse process of T3 on the left. Ensure that you have good contact and will not slip across the skin or superficial musculature when you apply a caudad and downward force towards the couch against the transverse process of T3. Maintain this contact point.

6. Positioning for thrust

Keeping your position at the head of the couch, gently place your right hand against the left side of the patient's head and neck with your fingers pointing towards the patient's right shoulder. While maintaining the right sidebending introduced earlier, begin to rotate the cervical and upper thoracic spine to the left by applying gentle pushing pressure to the left side of the patient's head and neck with your right hand (Fig. 8.77). Maintaining all holds and pressures, complete the rotation of the patient's head and neck until a sense of tension is palpated at your left hypothenar eminence. Keep firm pressure against the contact point.

7. Adjustments to achieve appropriate prethrust tension

Ensure the patient remains relaxed. Maintaining all holds, make any necessary changes in extension, sidebending or rotation until you can sense a state of appropriate tension and leverage. The patient should not be aware of any pain or discomfort. You make these final adjustments by altering the pressure and

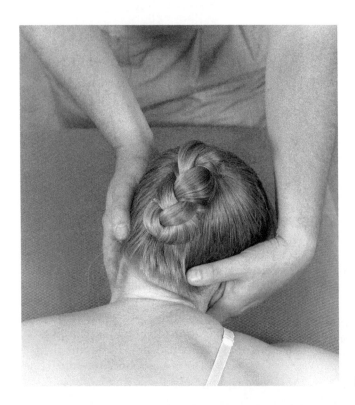

Figure 8.76

direction of forces between the right hand against the patient's head and neck and your left hypothenar eminence against the contact point.

8. Immediately prethrust

Relax and adjust your balance as necessary. Keep your head up and ensure that your

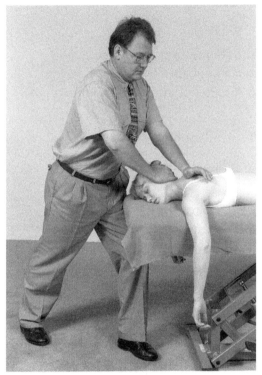

Figure 8.77

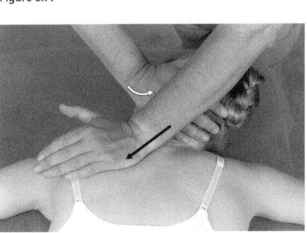

contacts are firm and that your body position is well controlled. An effective HVLA thrust technique is best achieved if the operator and patient are relaxed and not holding themselves rigid. This is a common impediment to achieving effective cavitation.

9. Delivering the thrust

Apply an HVLA thrust to the left transverse process of T3 down towards the couch and in the direction of the patient's left axilla. Simultaneously, apply a slight, rapid increase of head and neck rotation to the left with your right hand (Fig. 8.78). The thrust induces local rotation of the T3 vertebra, focusing forces at the T2–3 segment. You must not overemphasize the thrust with your right hand against the patient's head and neck. Your right hand stabilizes the leverages and maintains the position of the head and cervical spine against the thrust imposed upon the contact point. The thrust is induced by a very rapid contraction of the triceps, shoulder adductors and internal rotators.

The thrust, although very rapid, must never be excessively forcible. The aim should be to use the absolute minimum force necessary to achieve joint cavitation. A common fault arises from the use of excessive amplitude with insufficient velocity of thrust.

Figure 8.78

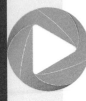

Summary

Cervicothoracic spine C7–T3: Rotation gliding

Patient prone

Operator at head of couch

- **Contact point:** Left T3 transverse process

- **Applicator:** Hypothenar eminence of the left hand

- **Patient positioning:** Patient prone with the chin resting on the couch and the arms hanging over the edge of the couch or against the patient's sides. Introduce sidebending to the right (Fig. 8.76). Do not introduce too much sidebending

- **Operator stance:** Head of the couch, feet spread slightly

- **Palpation of contact point:** Place your hypothenar eminence against the transverse process of T3 on the left

- **Positioning for thrust:** Place your right hand against the left side of the patient's head and neck. Rotate the cervical and upper thoracic spine to the left by applying pushing pressure to the left side of the patient's head and neck with your right hand until a sense of tension is palpated at the contact point (Fig. 8.77)

- **Adjustments to achieve appropriate prethrust tension**

- **Immediately prethrust:** Relax and adjust your balance

- **Delivering the thrust:** The thrust is in the direction of the patient's left axilla and down towards the couch. Simultaneously, apply a slight rapid increase of head and neck rotation to the left with your right hand (Fig. 8.78). You must not overemphasize the thrust with your right hand against the patient's head

Cervicothoracic spine C7–T3:
Rotation gliding

Patient prone
Operator at head of couch – variation

Assume somatic dysfunction (S-T-A-R-T) is identified and you wish to use a rotation gliding thrust, parallel to the apophysial joint plane, to produce cavitation at the T2–3 apophysial joint (Figs. 8.79, 8.80).

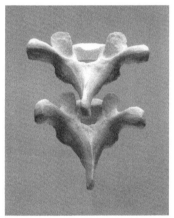

Figure 8.79

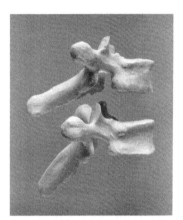

Figure 8.80

Key

✱ Stabilization

● Applicator

➡ Plane of thrust (operator)

⇨ Direction of body movement (patient)

Note: The dimensions for the arrows are not a pictorial representation of the amplitude or force of the thrust.

1. Contact point
Transverse process of T3 on the left.

2. Applicator
Hypothenar eminence of left hand.

3. Patient positioning
Patient prone with the point of the chin resting on the couch and the arms hanging over the edge of the couch or against the patient's sides. Introduce slight head and neck flexion. Now introduce a small amount of sidebending to the right by gently lifting and moving the patient's head to the right (Fig. 8.81).

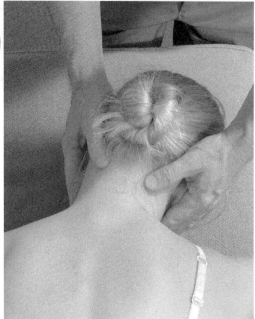

Figure 8.81

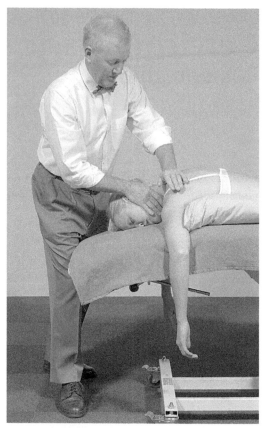

Figure 8.82

4. Operator stance

To the right of the head of the couch, feet spread slightly. Stand as erect as possible and avoid crouching over the patient, as this will limit the technique and restrict delivery of the thrust.

5. Palpation of contact point

Locate the transverse process of T3 on the left. Place the hypothenar eminence of your left hand gently but firmly against the transverse process of T3 on the left. Ensure that you have good contact and will not slip across the skin or superficial musculature when you apply a caudad and downward force towards the couch against the transverse process of T3. Maintain this contact point.

6. Positioning for thrust

Keeping your position at the head of the couch, gently place your right hand against

the left side of the patient's head and neck with your fingers pointing towards the couch. While maintaining the right sidebending introduced earlier, begin to rotate the cervical and upper thoracic spine to the left by applying gentle pulling pressure to the left side of the patient's head and neck with your right hand (Fig. 8.82). Maintaining all holds and pressures, complete the rotation of the patient's head and neck until a sense of tension is palpated at your left hypothenar eminence. Keep firm pressure against the contact point.

7. Adjustments to achieve appropriate prethrust tension

Ensure the patient remains relaxed. Maintaining all holds, make any necessary

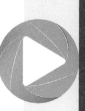

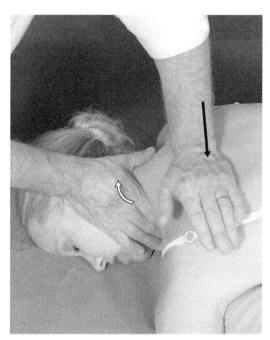

Figure 8.83

8. Immediately prethrust

Relax and adjust your balance as necessary. Keep your head up and ensure that your contacts are firm and that your body position is well controlled. An effective HVLA thrust technique is best achieved if the operator and patient are relaxed and not holding themselves rigid. This is a common impediment to achieving effective cavitation.

9. Delivering the thrust

Apply an HVLA thrust to the left transverse process of T3 down towards the couch and in the direction of the patient's left axilla. Simultaneously, apply a slight, rapid increase of head and neck rotation to the left with your right hand (Fig. 8.83). The thrust induces local rotation of the T3 vertebra, focusing forces at the T2–3 segment. You must not overemphasize the thrust with your right hand against the patient's head and neck. Your right hand stabilizes the leverages and maintains the position of the head and cervical spine against the thrust imposed upon the contact point. The thrust is induced by a very rapid contraction of the triceps, shoulder adductors and internal rotators.

changes in flexion, extension, sidebending or rotation until you can sense a state of appropriate tension and leverage. The patient should not be aware of any pain or discomfort. You make these final adjustments by altering the pressure and direction of forces between the right hand against the patient's head and neck and your left hypothenar eminence against the contact point.

The thrust, although very rapid, must never be excessively forcible. The aim should be to use the absolute minimum force necessary to achieve joint cavitation. A common fault arises from the use of excessive amplitude with insufficient velocity of thrust.

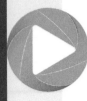

Summary

Cervicothoracic spine C7–T3: Rotation gliding

Patient prone
Operator at head of couch

- **Contact point:** Left T3 transverse process

- **Applicator:** Hypothenar eminence of the left hand

- **Patient positioning:** Patient prone with the chin resting on the couch and the arms hanging over the edge of the couch or against the patient's sides. Introduce slight head and neck flexion. Introduce sidebending to the right (Fig. 8.81). Do not introduce too much sidebending

- **Operator stance:** To the right of the head of the couch, feet spread slightly

- **Palpation of contact point:** Place your hypothenar eminence against the transverse process of T3 on the left

- **Positioning for thrust:** Place your right hand against the left side of the patient's head and neck with your fingers pointing towards the couch. Rotate the cervical and upper thoracic spine to the left by applying pulling pressure to the left side of the patient's head and neck with your right hand until a sense of tension is palpated at the contact point (Fig. 8.82)

- **Adjustments to achieve appropriate prethrust tension**

- **Immediately prethrust:** Relax and adjust your balance

- **Delivering the thrust:** The thrust is in the direction of the patient's left axilla and down towards the couch. Simultaneously, apply a slight rapid increase of head and neck rotation to the left with your right hand (Fig. 8.83). You must not overemphasize the thrust with your right hand against the patient's head

Cervicothoracic spine C7–T3:
Sidebending gliding

Patient sitting

Assume somatic dysfunction (S-T-A-R-T) is identified and you wish to use a sidebending gliding thrust, parallel to the apophysial joint plane, to produce cavitation at the T2–3 apophysial joint (Figs. 8.84, 8.85).

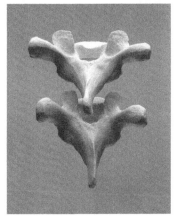

Figure 8.84

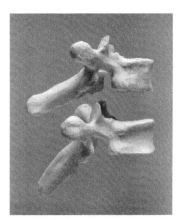

Figure 8.85

Key

❋ Stabilization

● Applicator

➡ Plane of thrust (operator)

⇨ Direction of body movement (patient)

Note: The dimensions for the arrows are not a pictorial representation of the amplitude or force of the thrust.

1. Contact point
Left side of the spinous process of T2.

2. Applicator
Thumb of left hand.

3. Patient positioning
Patient sitting with back towards the operator.

4. Operator stance
Stand behind the patient.

5. Palpation of contact point
Locate the spinous process of T2. Place the thumb of your left hand gently but firmly against the left side of this spinous process. Spread the fingers of your left hand to rest

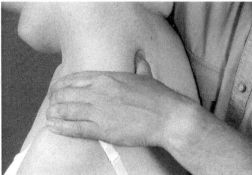

Figure 8.86

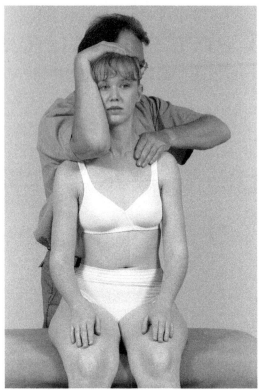

Figure 8.87

over the patient's left trapezius muscle, with your fingertips resting on the patient's left clavicle (Fig. 8.86). Ensure that you have good contact and will not slip off the spinous process of T2 when you apply a force against it. Maintain this contact point.

6. Positioning for thrust

Keeping your position behind the patient place your right hand and forearm alongside the right side of the patient's head and neck and gently rest the palm of your hand over the top of the patient's head (Fig. 8.87). Ensure that your forearm remains anterior to, and just over, the patient's ear. This hand will introduce and control the rotation and sidebending leverages.

Use your left hand to slightly rotate the patient's trunk to the left while using your right hand to introduce head and neck rotation to the right until a sense of tension is palpated at the contact point (Fig. 8.88). Now gently introduce cervical sidebending to the left by allowing the patient's body weight to fall slightly to the right. Keeping the patient's head centred over the sacrum, guide the neck into left sidebending with your right arm against the right side of the patient's head. A vertex compression force can be added to assist in localizing forces to the T2–3 segment. Ensure that your applicator thumb forms a straight line with your left forearm.

7. Adjustments to achieve appropriate prethrust tension

Ensure the patient remains relaxed. Maintaining all holds, make any necessary changes in flexion, extension, sidebending or rotation until you can sense a state of appropriate tension and leverage. The patient should not be aware of any pain or discomfort. Make these final adjustments by balancing the pressure and direction of forces between the left hand against the contact point and the right hand and forearm against the patient's head and neck.

8. Immediately prethrust

Relax and adjust your balance as necessary. Keep your head up and ensure that your contacts are firm and that the patient's body weight and position are well controlled. An effective HVLA thrust technique is best

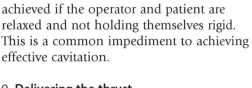

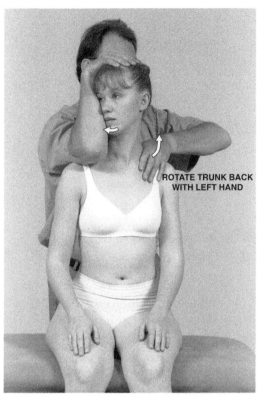

Figure 8.88

achieved if the operator and patient are relaxed and not holding themselves rigid. This is a common impediment to achieving effective cavitation.

9. Delivering the thrust

Apply an HVLA thrust to the left side of the spinous process of T2 in the direction of the patient's right axilla. At the same time, slightly increase head and neck sidebending to the left with your right arm (Fig. 8.89). The thrust on the spinous process of T2 and the slight increase in neck sidebending to the left focus forces at the T2–3 segment and causes cavitation at that level. The thrust is induced by a very rapid contraction of the shoulder adductors.

The thrust, although very rapid, must never be excessively forcible. The aim should be to use the absolute minimum force necessary to achieve joint cavitation. A common fault arises from the use of excessive amplitude with insufficient velocity of thrust.

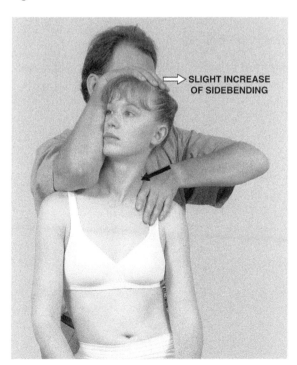

Figure 8.89

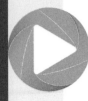

Summary

Cervicothoracic spine C7–T3: Sidebending gliding

Patient sitting

- **Contact point:** Left side of the T2 spinous process

- **Applicator:** Thumb of left hand

- **Patient positioning:** Patient sitting with back towards the operator

- **Operator stance:** Behind the patient

- **Palpation of contact point:** Place your left thumb against the left side of the T2 spinous process. Spread the fingers of your left hand to rest over the patient's trapezius muscle and clavicle (Fig. 8.86)

- **Positioning for thrust:** Place your right hand and forearm alongside the right side of the patient's head and neck (Fig. 8.87). Use your left hand to slightly rotate the patient's trunk to the left whilst using your right hand to introduce head and neck rotation to the right (Fig. 8.88). Introduce left sidebending to the cervical spine, localizing forces to the T2–3 segment. Ensure that your applicator thumb forms a straight line with your left forearm

- **Adjustments to achieve appropriate prethrust tension**

- **Immediately prethrust:** Relax and adjust your balance

- **Delivering the thrust:** The thrust is directed towards the patient's right axilla. Simultaneously, apply a slight, rapid increase of head and neck sidebending to the left (Fig. 8.89)

Cervicothoracic spine C7–T3:
Sidebending gliding

Patient sitting

Ligamentous myofascial positioning

Assume somatic dysfunction (S-T-A-R-T) is identified and you wish to use a sidebending gliding thrust, parallel to the apophysial joint plane, to produce cavitation at the T2–3 apophysial joint (Figs. 8.90, 8.91).

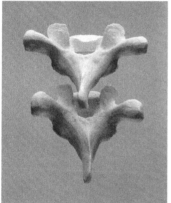

Figure 8.90

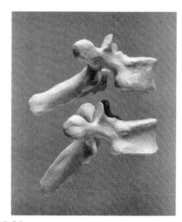

Figure 8.91

Key

✳ Stabilization

● Applicator

➡ Plane of thrust (operator)

⇨ Direction of body movement (patient)

Note: The dimensions for the arrows are not a pictorial representation of the amplitude or force of the thrust.

1. **Contact point**
Left side of the spinous process of T2.

2. **Applicator**
Thumb of left hand.

3. **Patient positioning**
Patient sitting with back towards the operator.

4. **Operator stance**
Stand behind the patient.

5. **Palpation of contact point**
Locate the spinous process of T2. Place the thumb of your left hand gently but firmly against the left side of this spinous process.

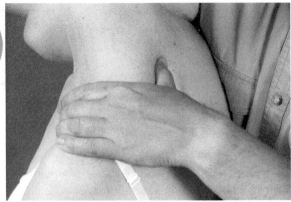

Figure 8.92

6. Positioning for thrust

Keeping your position behind the patient, place your right hand and forearm alongside the right side of the patient's head and neck and gently rest the palm of your hand over the top of the patient's head (Fig. 8.93). Ensure that your forearm remains anterior to, and just over, the patient's ear. This hand will introduce and control the rotation and sidebending leverages.

Use your right hand to introduce a small amount of head and neck extension (Fig. 8.94). Now introduce cervical sidebending to the left by allowing the patient's body weight to fall slightly to the right. Keeping the patient's head centred over the sacrum, guide the neck into left sidebending with your right arm against the right side of the patient's head. A vertex compression force can be added to assist in localizing forces to the T2–3 segment. Ensure that your applicator thumb forms a straight line with your left forearm.

7. Adjustments to achieve appropriate prethrust tension

Ensure the patient remains relaxed. Maintaining all holds, make any necessary changes in flexion, extension, sidebending or rotation until you can sense a state of appropriate tension and leverage. The patient should not be aware of any pain or discomfort. Make these final adjustments by

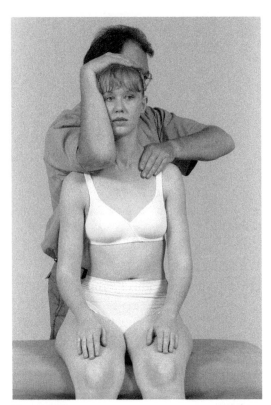

Figure 8.93

Spread the fingers of your left hand to rest over the patient's left trapezius muscle, with your fingertips resting on the patient's left clavicle (Fig. 8.92). Ensure that you have good contact and will not slip off the spinous process of T2 when you apply a force against it. Maintain this contact point.

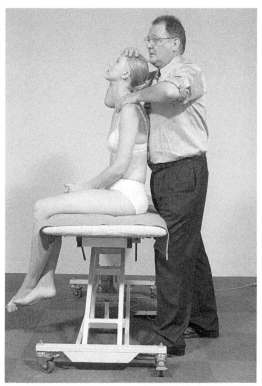

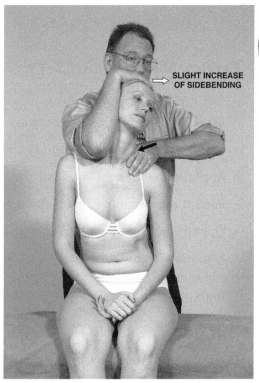

SLIGHT INCREASE
OF SIDEBENDING

Figure 8.94

Figure 8.95

balancing the pressure and direction of forces between the left hand against the contact point and the right hand and forearm against the patient's head and neck.

8. Immediately prethrust

Relax and adjust your balance as necessary. Keep your head up and ensure that your contacts are firm and that the patient's body weight and position are well controlled. An effective HVLA thrust technique is best achieved if the operator and patient are relaxed and not holding themselves rigid. This is a common impediment to achieving effective cavitation.

9. Delivering the thrust

This technique uses ligamentous myofascial positioning and not facet apposition locking. This approach generally requires a greater emphasis on the exaggeration of primary

leverage than is the case with facet apposition locking techniques.

Apply an HVLA thrust to the left side of the spinous process of T2 in the direction of the patient's right axilla. At the same time, increase head and neck sidebending to the left with your right arm (Fig. 8.95). The thrust on the spinous process of T2 and the increase in neck sidebending to the left focus forces at the T2–3 segment and causes cavitation at that level. The thrust is induced by a very rapid contraction of the shoulder adductors.

The thrust, although very rapid, must never be excessively forcible. The aim should be to use the absolute minimum force necessary to achieve joint cavitation. A common fault arises from the use of excessive amplitude with insufficient velocity of thrust.

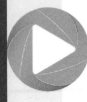

Summary

Cervicothoracic spine C7–T3: Sidebending gliding

Patient sitting

Ligamentous myofascial positioning

- **Contact point:** Left side of the T2 spinous process

- **Applicator:** Thumb of left hand

- **Patient positioning:** Patient sitting with back towards the operator

- **Operator stance:** Behind the patient

- **Palpation of contact point:** Place your left thumb against the left side of the T2 spinous process. Spread the fingers of your left hand to rest over the patient's trapezius muscle and clavicle (Fig. 8.92)

- **Positioning for thrust:** Place your right hand and forearm alongside the right side of the patient's head and neck (Fig. 8.93). Use your right hand to introduce a small amount of head and neck extension (Fig. 8.94). Introduce left sidebending to the cervical spine localizing forces to the T2–3 segment. Ensure that your applicator thumb forms a straight line with your left forearm

- **Adjustments to achieve appropriate prethrust tension**

- **Immediately prethrust:** Relax and adjust your balance

- **Delivering the thrust:** The thrust is directed towards the patient's right axilla. Simultaneously, apply a rapid increase of head and neck sidebending to the left (Fig. 8.95)

Cervicothoracic spine C7–T3:
Sidebending gliding

Patient sidelying

Assume somatic dysfunction (S-T-A-R-T) is identified and you wish to use a sidebending gliding thrust, parallel to the apophysial joint plane, to produce cavitation at the T2–3 apophysial joint (Figs. 8.96, 8.97).

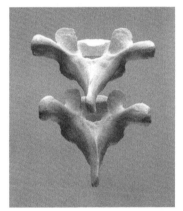

Figure 8.96

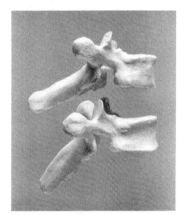

Figure 8.97

Key

✳ Stabilization

● Applicator

➡ Plane of thrust (operator)

⇨ Direction of body movement (patient)

Note: The dimensions for the arrows are not a pictorial representation of the amplitude or force of the thrust.

1. **Contact point**
Right side of the spinous process of T2.

2. **Applicator**
Thumb of left hand.

3. **Patient positioning**
Patient lying on the left side. Flex the patient's knees and hips for stability.

4. **Operator stance**
Stand facing the patient and gently place your right arm under the head, lightly spreading your fingers around the patient's occiput. The head should now be cradled in your right arm with your upper arm against the patient's forehead and your forearm and hand supporting the head and neck.

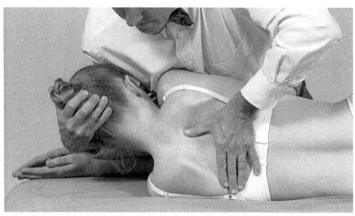

Figure 8.98

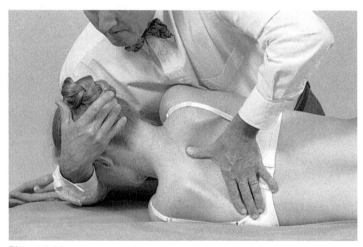

Figure 8.99

5. Palpation of contact point

Locate the spinous process of T2. Place the thumb of your left hand gently but firmly against the right side of this spinous process. Spread the fingers of your left hand to enable firm contact of your thumb. This will ensure that you have good contact and will not slip off the spinous process when you apply a force against it. Maintain this contact point, but do not press too hard, as it can be uncomfortable.

6. Positioning for thrust

Using your right arm, sidebend the patient's head and neck to the right until a sense of tension is palpable at the contact point. This sidebending is achieved by gently lifting the patient's head, within the cradle of your right arm (Fig. 8.98).

Gently introduce cervical rotation to the left until a sense of tension is palpated at the contact point (Fig. 8.99). If necessary, you may add a compression force to the

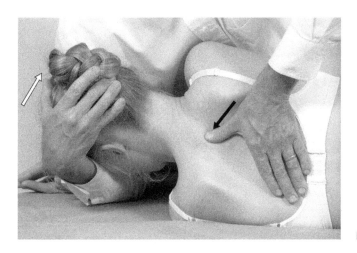

Figure 8.100

patient's shoulder girdle, from your chest, to stabilize the upper torso before applying the thrust.

7. Adjustments to achieve appropriate prethrust tension

Ensure the patient remains relaxed. Maintaining all holds, make any necessary changes in flexion, extension, sidebending or rotation until you can sense a state of appropriate tension and leverage at the contact point. The patient should not be aware of any pain or discomfort. Make these final adjustments by balancing the pressure and direction of forces between the left hand against the contact point and the right hand and forearm against the patient's head and neck.

8. Immediately prethrust

Relax and adjust your balance as necessary. Keep your head up and ensure that your contacts are firm and that your body position is well controlled. An effective HVLA thrust technique is best achieved if the operator and patient are relaxed and not holding themselves rigid. This is a common impediment to achieving effective cavitation.

9. Delivering the thrust

Apply an HVLA thrust to the spinous process of T2 down towards the couch in the direction of the patient's left shoulder. The thrust is accompanied by a simultaneous downwards application of force with your chest to the patient's right shoulder girdle. At the same time, introduce a slight increase in head and neck sidebending to the right with your right arm (Fig. 8.100). The thrust on the spinous process of T2 and slight increase in neck sidebending to the right focus forces at the T2–3 segment and causes cavitation at that level. Do not apply excessive sidebending at the time of the thrust, as this can cause strain and discomfort.

The thrust, although very rapid, must never be excessively forcible. The aim should be to use the absolute minimum force necessary to achieve joint cavitation. A common fault arises from the use of excessive amplitude with insufficient velocity of thrust.

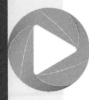

Summary

Cervicothoracic spine C7–T3: Sidebending gliding

Patient sidelying

- **Contact point:** Right side of T2 spinous process

- **Applicator:** Thumb of left hand

- **Patient positioning:** Patient lying on the left side. Flex the patient's knees and hips for stability

- **Operator stance:** Facing the patient. Place your right arm under the patient's head, supporting the patient's occiput

- **Palpation of contact point:** Place the thumb of your left hand against the right side of the spinous process of T2

- **Positioning for thrust:** Using your right arm, sidebend the patient's head and neck to the right (Fig. 8.98). Introduce cervical rotation to the left until a sense of tension is palpated at the contact point (Fig. 8.99)

- **Adjustments to achieve appropriate prethrust tension**

- **Immediately prethrust:** Relax and adjust your balance

- **Delivering the thrust:** The thrust is in the direction of the patient's left shoulder and down towards the couch. The thrust is accompanied by a downwards application of force with your chest to the patient's right shoulder girdle. Simultaneously, apply a slight rapid increase of head and neck sidebending to the right with your right arm (Fig. 8.100). Do not apply excessive sidebending

8.20

Cervicothoracic spine C7–T3:
Sidebending gliding

Patient sidelying

Ligamentous myofascial positioning

Assume somatic dysfunction (S-T-A-R-T) is identified and you wish to use a sidebending gliding thrust, parallel to the apophysial joint plane, to produce cavitation at the T2–3 apophysial joint (Figs. 8.101, 8.102).

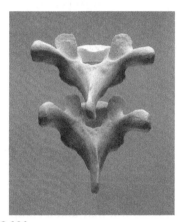

Figure 8.101

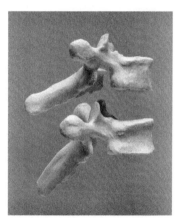

Figure 8.102

Key

❊ Stabilization

● Applicator

➡ Plane of thrust (operator)

⇨ Direction of body movement (patient)

Note: The dimensions for the arrows are not a pictorial representation of the amplitude or force of the thrust.

1. **Contact point**
Right side of the spinous process of T2.

2. **Applicator**
Thumb of left hand.

3. **Patient positioning**
Patient lying on the left side. Flex the patient's knees and hips for stability.

4. Operator stance

Stand facing the patient and gently place your right arm under the head, lightly spreading your fingers around the patient's occiput. The head should now be cradled in your right arm with your upper arm against the patient's forehead and your forearm and hand supporting the head and neck.

5. Palpation of contact point

Locate the spinous process of T2. Place the thumb of your left hand gently but firmly against the right side of this spinous process. Spread the fingers of your left hand to enable firm contact of your thumb and position your left forearm over the posterior aspect of the patient's thorax and lumbar spine. This will ensure that you have good contact and will not slip off the spinous process when you apply a force against it. Maintain this contact point, but do not press too hard, as it can be uncomfortable.

6. Positioning for thrust

Using your right arm, extend the patient's head and neck (Fig. 8.103). Now introduce sidebending to the right until a sense of tension is palpable at the contact point. This sidebending is achieved by gently lifting the patient's head, within the cradle of your right arm (Fig. 8.104).

If necessary, you may add a compression force to the patient's shoulder girdle, from your chest, to stabilize the upper torso before applying the thrust.

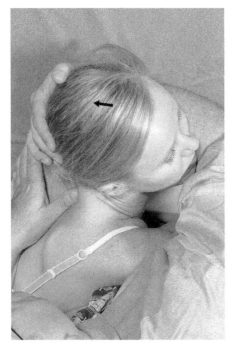

Figure 8.103

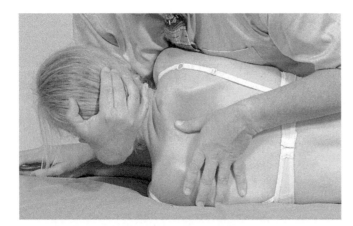

Figure 8.104

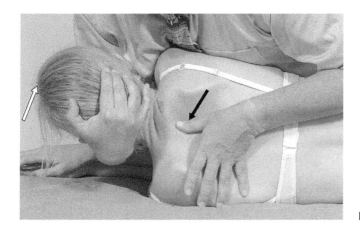

Figure 8.105

7. Adjustments to achieve appropriate prethrust tension

Ensure the patient remains relaxed. Maintaining all holds, make any necessary changes in flexion, extension, sidebending or rotation until you can sense a state of appropriate tension and leverage at the contact point. The patient should not be aware of any pain or discomfort. Make these final adjustments by balancing the pressure and direction of forces between the left hand against the contact point and the right hand and forearm against the patient's head and neck.

8. Immediately prethrust

Relax and adjust your balance as necessary. Keep your head up and ensure that your contacts are firm and that your body position is well controlled. An effective HVLA thrust technique is best achieved if the operator and patient are relaxed and not holding themselves rigid. This is a common impediment to achieving effective cavitation.

9. Delivering the thrust

This technique uses ligamentous myofascial positioning and not facet apposition locking. This approach generally requires a greater emphasis on the exaggeration of primary leverage than is the case with facet apposition locking techniques.

Apply an HVLA thrust to the spinous process of T2 down towards the couch in the direction of the patient's left shoulder. The thrust is accompanied by a simultaneous downwards application of force with your chest to the patient's right shoulder girdle. At the same time, introduce an increase in head and neck sidebending to the right with your right arm (Fig. 8.105). The thrust on the spinous process of T2 and increase in neck sidebending to the right focus forces at the T2–3 segment and causes cavitation at that level. Do not apply excessive sidebending at the time of the thrust as this can cause strain and discomfort.

The thrust, although very rapid, must never be excessively forcible. The aim should be to use the absolute minimum force necessary to achieve joint cavitation. A common fault arises from the use of excessive amplitude with insufficient velocity of thrust.

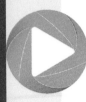

Summary

Cervicothoracic spine C7–T3: Sidebending gliding

Patient sidelying

Ligamentous myofascial positioning

- **Contact point:** Right side of T2 spinous process

- **Applicator:** Thumb of left hand

- **Patient positioning:** Patient lying on the left side. Flex the patient's knees and hips for stability

- **Operator stance:** Facing the patient. Place your right arm under the patient's head, supporting the patient's occiput

- **Palpation of contact point:** Place the thumb of your left hand against the right side of the spinous process of T2

- **Positioning for thrust:** Using your right arm, extend the patient's head and neck (Fig. 8.103). Introduce sidebending to the right until a sense of tension is palpable at the contact point (Fig. 8.104)

- **Adjustments to achieve appropriate prethrust tension**

- **Immediately prethrust:** Relax and adjust your balance

- **Delivering the thrust:** The thrust is in the direction of the patient's left shoulder and down towards the couch. The thrust is accompanied by a downwards application of force with your chest to the patient's right shoulder girdle. Simultaneously, apply a rapid increase of head and neck, sidebending to the right with your right arm (Fig. 8.105). Do not apply excessive sidebending

8.21

Cervicothoracic spine C7–T3:
Extension gliding

Patient sitting

Ligamentous myofascial positioning

Assume somatic dysfunction (S-T-A-R-T) is identified and you wish to use an extension gliding thrust, parallel to the apophysial joint plane, to produce joint cavitation at T2–3 (Figs. 8.106, 8.107).

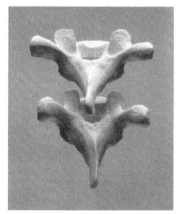

Figure 8.106

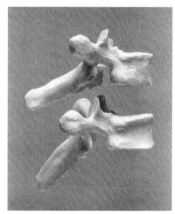

Figure 8.107

Key

 Stabilization

● Applicator

➡ Plane of thrust (operator)

⇨ Direction of body movement (patient)

Note: The dimensions for the arrows are not a pictorial representation of the amplitude or force of the thrust.

1. Contact points
a. Spinous process of T3.
b. Patient's forearms.

2. Applicators
a. Operator's sternum, with a cushion or small rolled towel, applied to the T3 spinous process (Fig. 8.108).
b. Operator's hands applied to the patient's forearms.

3. Patient positioning
Sitting with arms comfortably by side.

4. Operator stance
Stand directly behind the patient with your feet apart and one leg behind the other. Bend your knees slightly to lower your body.

195

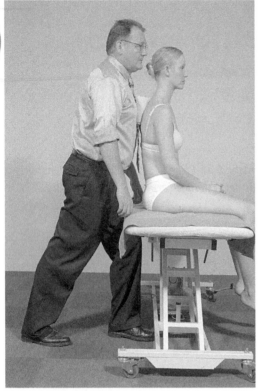

Figure 8.108

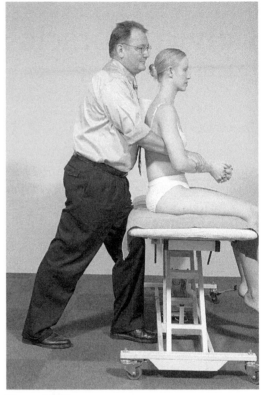

Figure 8.109

5. Positioning for thrust

Place the thrusting part of your sternum, with a cushion or small rolled towel, firmly against the spinous process of T3. Place your hands between the patient's chest and upper arms to take hold of the patients' forearms (Fig. 8.109). Maintaining your grip on the forearms, ask the patient to put their hands behind their neck with fingers intertwined (Fig. 8.110). This results in your forearms contacting the patient's axillae. Lean forwards with the thrusting part of your chest against the spinous process of T3 and introduce a backwards and compressive force to the patient's arms and axillae. These combined movements introduce local extension to the thoracic spine. By balancing these different leverages, the tension can be localized to the T2–3 segment. Maintaining all holds and pressures, bring the patient backwards until your body weight is evenly distributed between both feet.

6. Adjustments to achieve appropriate prethrust tension

Ensure your patient remains relaxed. Maintaining all holds, make any necessary changes in flexion, extension, sidebending or rotation until you can sense a state of appropriate tension and leverage at the T2–3 segment. The patient should not be aware of any pain or discomfort. Make these final adjustments by slight movements of the ankles, knees, hips and trunk. A common mistake is to lose the chest and axillae compression during the final adjustments.

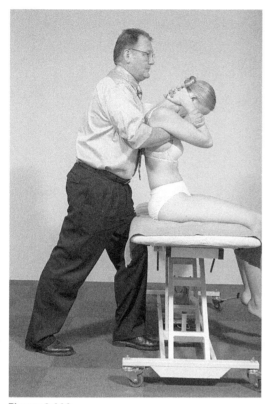

Figure 8.110

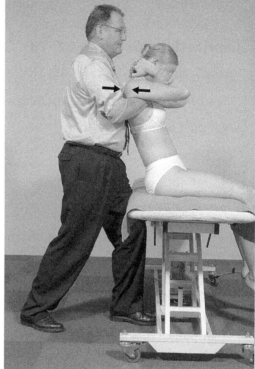

Figure 8.111

7. Immediately prethrust

Relax and adjust your balance as necessary. Keep your head up and ensure that your contacts are firm and the patient's body weight is well controlled. An effective HVLA thrust technique is best achieved if the operator and patient are relaxed and not holding themselves rigid. This is a common impediment to achieving effective cavitation.

8. Delivering the thrust

This technique uses ligamentous myofascial positioning and not facet apposition locking. This approach generally requires a greater emphasis on the exaggeration of primary leverage than is the case with facet apposition locking techniques.

The shoulder girdles and thorax of the patient are now a solid mass against which a thrust may be applied. Apply an HVLA thrust towards you via your hands and forearms. Simultaneously, apply an HVLA thrust directly forwards against the spinous process of T3 via your sternum (Fig. 8.111).

The thrust, although very rapid, must never be excessively forcible. The aim should be to use the absolute minimum force necessary to achieve joint cavitation. Common faults arise from the use of excessive amplitude, insufficient velocity of thrust and lifting the patient off the couch. When delivering the thrust, particular care must be taken to not allow the patient's arms to move away from the chest wall.

This technique has some modifications:
- Respiration can be used to make the technique more effective.
- A certain degree of momentum is often necessary for success in the technique.

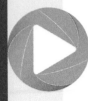

Summary

Cervicothoracic spine C7–T3: Extension gliding

Patient sitting

Ligamentous myofascial positioning

- **Contact points:**

  - **Spinous process of T3**

  - **Patient's forearms**

- **Applicators:**

  - **Operator's sternum applied to the T3 spinous process (Fig. 8.108)**

  - **Operator's hands applied to the patient's forearms**

- **Patient positioning:** Sitting with arms comfortably by side

- **Operator stance:** Directly behind the patient with your feet apart, knees bent slightly and one leg behind the other

- **Positioning for thrust:** Place your hands between the patient's chest and upper arm to take hold of the patients' forearms (Fig. 8.109). Maintaining your grip on the forearms, ask the patient to put their hands behind their neck with fingers intertwined (Fig. 8.110). Lean forwards with the thrusting part of your chest against the spinous process of T3 and introduce a backwards and compressive force to the patient's arms and axillae. Maintaining all holds and pressures, bring the patient backwards until your body weight is evenly distributed between both feet

- **Adjustments to achieve appropriate prethrust tension**

- **Immediately prethrust:** Relax and adjust your balance

- **Delivering the thrust:** The direction of thrust with your arms is towards you. Simultaneously, apply a thrust directly forwards against the spinous process of T3 with your sternum (Fig. 8.111)

- **Modifications to technique:**

  - **Respiration can be used to make the technique more effective**

  - **A certain degree of momentum is often necessary for success in the technique**

9

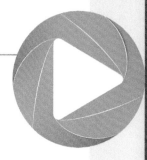

Thoracic spine and rib cage

PATIENT UPPER BODY POSITIONING FOR SITTING AND SUPINE TECHNIQUES

There are a variety of upper body holds available (Figs. 9.1–9.5). The hold selected for any particular technique is that which enables the operator to effectively localize forces to a specific segment of the spine or rib cage and deliver a high-velocity low-amplitude (HVLA) force in a controlled manner. Patient comfort must be a major consideration in selecting the most appropriate hold.

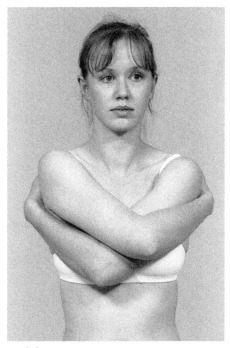

Figure 9.1

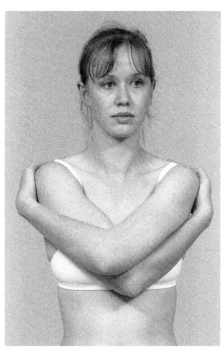

Figure 9.2

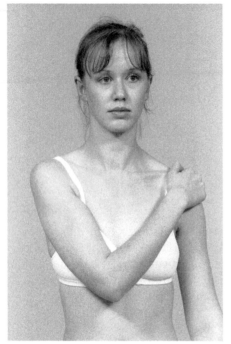

Figure 9.3

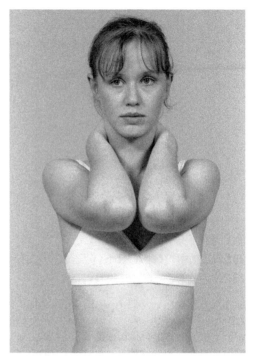

Figure 9.4

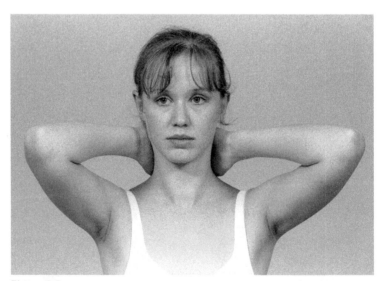

Figure 9.5

OPERATOR LOWER HAND POSITION FOR SUPINE TECHNIQUES

There are a variety of hand positions that can be adopted. The hand position selected for any particular technique is that which enables the operator to effectively localize forces to a specific segment of the spine or rib cage and deliver an HVLA force in a controlled manner. Patient comfort must be a major consideration in selecting the most appropriate hand position.

- Neutral hand position (Fig. 9.6)
- Clenched hand position (Fig. 9.7)
- Half closed fist (Fig. 9.8)
- Half closed fist with towel (Fig. 9.9)
- Closed fist (Fig. 9.10)
- Closed fist with towel (Fig. 9.11).

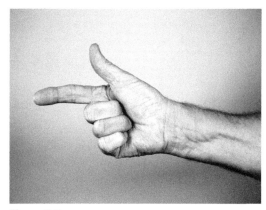

Figure 9.8

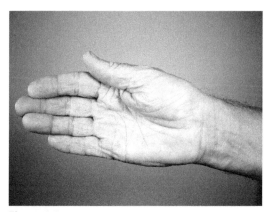

Figure 9.6

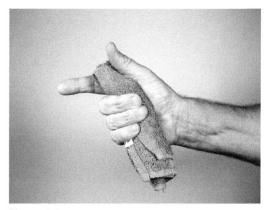

Figure 9.9

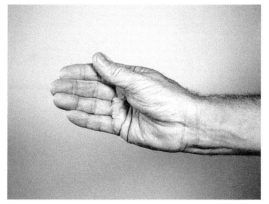

Figure 9.7

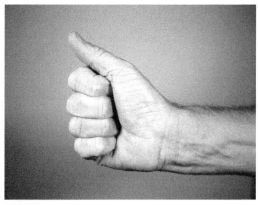

Figure 9.10

HVLA thrust techniques

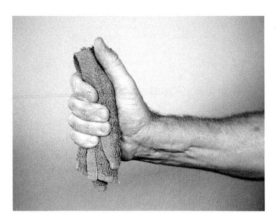

Figure 9.11

Thoracic spine T4–9:
Extension gliding

Patient sitting

Ligamentous myofascial positioning

Assume somatic dysfunction (S-T-A-R-T) is identified and you wish to use an extension gliding thrust, parallel to the apophysial joint plane, to produce joint cavitation at T5–6 (Figs. 9.12, 9.13).

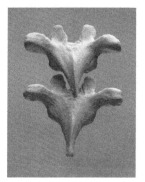

Figure 9.12

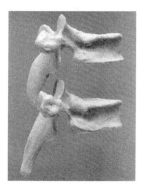

Figure 9.13

Key

✳ Stabilization

● Applicator

➡ Plane of thrust (operator)

⇨ Direction of body movement (patient)

Note: The dimensions for the arrows are not a pictorial representation of the amplitude or force of the thrust.

1. Contact points
a. Spinous process of T6.
b. Patient's elbows.

2. Applicators
a. Operator's sternum, with a cushion or small rolled towel, applied to the T6 spinous process (Fig. 9.14).
b. Operator's flexed fingers, hands and wrists applied to the patient's elbows.

3. Patient positioning
Sitting with arms crossed over the chest and hands passed around the shoulders. The arms should be firmly clasped around the body as far as the patient can comfortably reach.

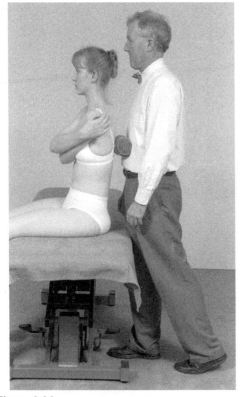

Figure 9.14

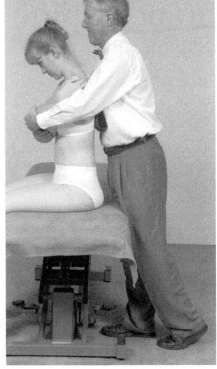

Figure 9.15

4. Operator stance

Stand directly behind the patient with your feet apart and one leg behind the other. Bend your knees slightly to lower your body.

5. Positioning for thrust

Place the thrusting part of your sternum, with a cushion or small rolled towel, firmly against the spinous process of T6. Place your hands over the patient's elbows. Lean forwards with the thrusting part of your chest against the spinous process of T6 (Fig. 9.15). Introduce a backwards (compressive) and upwards force to the patient's folded arms. These combined movements introduce local extension to the thoracic spine. By balancing these different leverages, the tension can be localized to the

T5–6 segment. Maintaining all holds and pressures, bring the patient backwards until your body weight is evenly distributed between both feet.

6. Adjustments to achieve appropriate prethrust tension

Ensure your patient remains relaxed. Maintaining all holds, make any necessary changes in flexion, extension, sidebending or rotation until you can sense a state of appropriate tension and leverage at the T5–6 segment. The patient should not be aware of any pain or discomfort. Make these final adjustments by slight movements of the ankles, knees, hips and trunk. A common mistake is to lose the chest compression during the final adjustments.

7. Immediately prethrust

Relax and adjust your balance as necessary. Keep your head up and ensure that your contacts are firm and the patient's body weight is well controlled. An effective HVLA thrust technique is best achieved if the operator and patient are relaxed and not holding themselves rigid. This is a common impediment to achieving effective cavitation.

8. Delivering the thrust

This technique uses ligamentous myofascial positioning and not facet apposition locking. This approach generally requires a greater emphasis on the exaggeration of primary leverage than is the case with facet apposition locking techniques.

The shoulder girdles and thorax of the patient are now a solid mass against which a thrust may be applied. Apply an HVLA thrust towards you and slightly upwards in a cephalad direction via your hands. Simultaneously, apply an HVLA thrust directly forwards against the spinous process of T6 via your sternum (Fig. 9.16).

The thrust, although very rapid, must never be excessively forcible. The aim should be to use the absolute minimum force necessary to achieve joint cavitation. A common fault arises from the use of excessive amplitude with insufficient velocity of thrust.

This technique has many modifications:
* Different shoulder girdle holds can be used.
* Respiration can be used to make the technique more effective.
* A certain degree of momentum is often necessary for success in the technique.

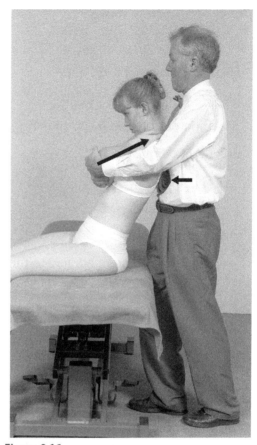

Figure 9.16

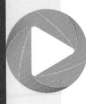

Summary

Thoracic spine T4–9: Extension gliding

Patient sitting

Ligamentous myofascial positioning

- **Contact points:**

  - Spinous process of T6

  - Patient's elbows

- **Applicators:**

  - Operator's sternum applied to the T6 spinous process (Fig. 9.14)

  - Operator's flexed fingers, hands and wrists applied to the patient's elbows

- **Patient positioning:** Sitting with arms crossed over chest

- **Operator stance:** Directly behind the patient with your feet apart, knees bent slightly and one leg behind the other

- **Positioning for thrust:** Lean forwards with the thrusting part of your chest against the spinous process of T6 (Fig. 9.15). Introduce a backwards (compressive) and upwards force to the patient's folded arms. Maintaining all holds and pressures, bring the patient backwards until your body weight is evenly distributed between both feet

- **Adjustments to achieve appropriate prethrust tension**

- **Immediately prethrust:** Relax and adjust your balance

- **Delivering the thrust:** The direction of thrust with your arms is towards you and slightly upwards. Simultaneously, apply a thrust directly forwards against the spinous process of T6 with your sternum (Fig. 9.16)

- **Modifications to technique:**

  - Different shoulder girdle holds can be used

  - Respiration can be used to make the technique more effective

  - A certain degree of momentum is often necessary for success in the technique

9.2

Thoracic spine T4–9:
Flexion gliding

Patient supine
Ligamentous myofascial positioning

Assume somatic dysfunction (S-T-A-R-T) is identified and you wish to use a flexion gliding thrust, parallel to the apophysial joint plane, to produce joint cavitation at T5–6 (Figs. 9.17, 9.18).

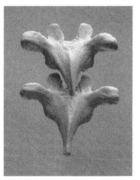

Figure 9.17

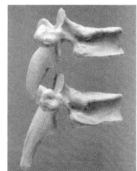

Figure 9.18

Key

＊ Stabilization

● Applicator

➡ Plane of thrust (operator)

⇨ Direction of body movement (patient)

Note: The dimensions for the arrows are not a pictorial representation of the amplitude or force of the thrust.

1. Contact points
a. Transverse processes of T6.
b. Patient's elbows.

2. Applicators
a. Palm of the operator's right hand, held in a clenched position.
b. Operator's lower sternum or upper abdomen.

3. Patient positioning
Supine with the arms crossed over the chest and hands passed around the shoulders. The arms should be firmly clasped round the body as far as the patient can comfortably reach (Fig. 9.19).

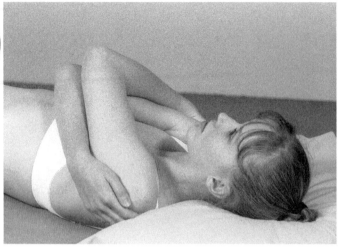

Figure 9.19

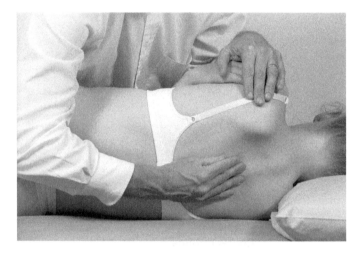

Figure 9.20

4. Operator stance

Stand on the right side of the patient, facing the head of the couch.

5. Positioning for thrust

Reach over the patient with your left hand to take hold of the left shoulder and gently pull it towards you. With your right hand, locate the transverse processes of T6. Now place the clenched palm of your right hand against the transverse processes of T6 (Fig. 9.20).

Keeping the right hand pressed against the transverse processes of T6, roll the

patient back to the supine position. As the patient approaches the supine position, transfer your left hand and forearm to support the patient's head, neck and upper thoracic spine (Fig. 9.21).

Allow the patient to roll fully into the supine position. Flex the patient's head, neck and upper thoracic spine until tension is localized to the T5–6 segment. Lean over the patient and rest your lower sternum or upper abdomen on the patient's elbows. Initially, a slow but firm pressure is applied with your lower sternum or upper abdomen downwards towards the couch. Maintaining

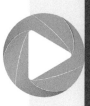

this downwards leverage, introduce a force in line with the patient's upper arms. By balancing these different leverages, tension can be localized to the T5–6 segment.

6. Adjustments to achieve appropriate prethrust tension

Ensure your patient remains relaxed. Maintaining all holds, make any necessary changes in flexion, extension, sidebending or rotation until you can sense a state of appropriate tension and leverage at the T5–6 segment. The patient should not be aware of any pain or discomfort. Make these final adjustments by slight movements of ankles, knees, hips and trunk. A common mistake is to lose the chest compression during the final adjustments.

7. Immediately prethrust

Relax and adjust your balance as necessary. Ensure that your contacts are firm and the patient's head, neck and upper thoracic spine are well controlled. An effective HVLA thrust technique is best achieved if the operator and patient are relaxed and not holding themselves rigid. This is a common impediment to achieving effective cavitation.

8. Delivering the thrust

This technique uses ligamentous myofascial positioning and not facet apposition locking.

This approach generally requires a greater emphasis on the exaggeration of primary leverage than is the case with facet apposition locking techniques.

The shoulder girdles and thorax of the patient are now a solid mass against which a thrust may be applied. Apply an HVLA thrust downwards towards the couch and in a cephalad direction via your lower sternum or upper abdomen. Simultaneously, apply an HVLA thrust with your right hand against the transverse processes in an upwards and caudad direction (Fig. 9.22).

A common fault is to emphasize the thrust via the patient's shoulder girdles at the expense of the thrust against the transverse processes. The hand contacting the transverse processes of T6 must actively participate in the generation of thrust forces.

The thrust, although very rapid, must never be excessively forcible. The aim should be to use the absolute minimum force necessary to achieve joint cavitation. A common fault arises from the use of excessive amplitude with insufficient velocity of thrust.

This technique has many modifications:
- Different shoulder girdle holds can be used.
- Different applicators can be used.
- Respiration can be used to make the technique more effective.

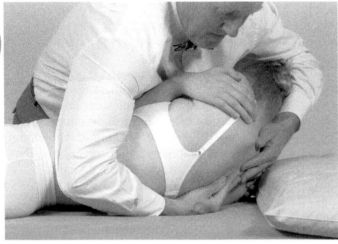

Figure 9.21

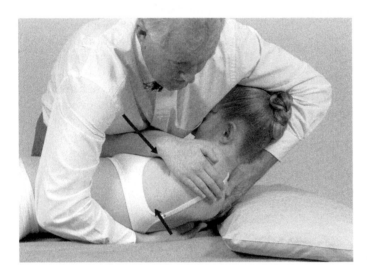

Figure 9.22

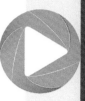

Summary

Thoracic spine T4–9: Flexion gliding

Patient supine

Ligamentous myofascial positioning

- **Contact points:**
  - Transverse processes of T6
  - Patient's elbows

- **Applicators:**
  - Palm of the operator's right hand, held in a clenched position
  - Operator's lower sternum or upper abdomen

- **Patient positioning:** Supine with arms crossed over chest (Fig. 9.19)

- **Operator stance:** To the right side of the patient, facing the couch

- **Positioning for thrust:** Take hold of the patient's left shoulder, and pull it towards you. Place the clenched palm of your right hand against the transverse processes of T6 (Fig. 9.20). Roll the patient back to the supine position. As the patient approaches the supine position, transfer your left hand and forearm to support the patient's head, neck and upper thoracic spine (Fig. 9.21). Allowing the patient to roll fully into the supine position, flex the head, neck and upper thoracic spine until tension is localized to the T5–6 segment. Apply a firm pressure with your lower sternum or upper abdomen downwards towards the couch. Maintaining this downwards leverage, introduce a force towards the patient's head in line with the patient's upper arms

- **Adjustments to achieve appropriate prethrust tension**

- **Immediately prethrust:** Relax and adjust your balance

- **Delivering the thrust:** The direction of thrust is downwards towards the couch and in a cephalad direction via your lower sternum or upper abdomen. Simultaneously, apply a thrust with your right hand against the transverse processes in an upwards and caudad direction (Fig. 9.22). The hand contacting the transverse processes of T6 must actively participate in the generation of thrust forces

- **Modifications to technique:**
  - Different shoulder girdle holds can be used
  - Different applicators can be used
  - Respiration can be used to make the technique more effective

Thoracic spine T4–9:
Rotation gliding

Patient supine

Ligamentous myofascial positioning

Assume somatic dysfunction (S-T-A-R-T) is identified and you wish to use a rotation gliding thrust, parallel to the apophysial joint plane, to produce joint cavitation at T5–6 (Figs. 9.23, 9.24).

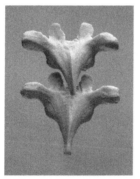

Figure 9.23

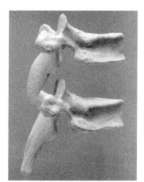

Figure 9.24

Key

❋ Stabilization

● Applicator

➡ Plane of thrust (operator)

⇨ Direction of body movement (patient)

Note: The dimensions for the arrows are not a pictorial representation of the amplitude or force of the thrust.

1. **Contact points**

a. Left transverse process of T6.

b. Patient's elbows and left forearm.

2. **Applicators**

a. Palm of the operator's right hand, held in a clenched position.

b. Operator's lower sternum or upper abdomen.

3. **Patient positioning**

Supine with the arms crossed over the chest and the hands passed around the shoulders. The left arm is placed over the right arm (Fig. 9.25). The arms should be firmly clasped around the body as far as the patient can comfortably reach.

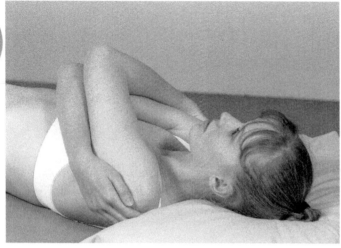

Figure 9.25

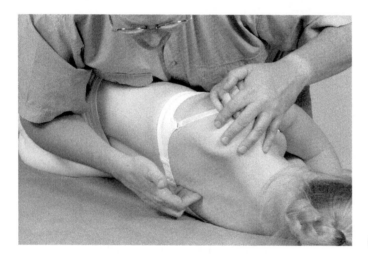

Figure 9.26

4. Operator stance

Stand on the right side of the patient, facing the couch.

5. Positioning for thrust

Reach over the patient with your left hand to take hold of the left shoulder and gently pull the patient's shoulder towards you (Fig. 9.26). With your right hand, locate the transverse processes of T6. Now place the thenar eminence of your right hand against the left transverse process of T6 (Fig. 9.27).

Keeping contact with the left transverse process of T6, roll the patient back towards the supine position. Rest your lower sternum or upper abdomen on the patient's elbows and left forearm (Fig. 9.28).

Initially, a slow but firm pressure is applied with your lower sternum or upper abdomen downwards towards the couch. Maintaining this downwards leverage, introduce left rotation of the patient's upper thorax by directing forces towards the patient's left shoulder along the line of the patient's left upper arm. By balancing these different leverages, tension can be localized to the T5–6 segment.

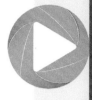

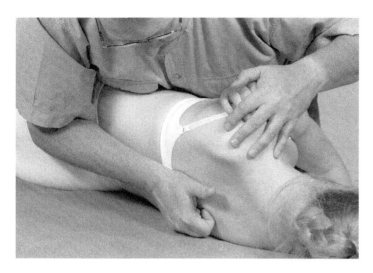

Figure 9.27

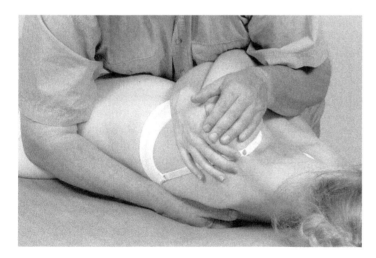

Figure 9.28

6. Adjustments to achieve appropriate prethrust tension

Ensure your patient remains relaxed. Maintaining all holds, make any necessary changes in flexion, extension, sidebending or rotation until you can sense a state of appropriate tension and leverage at the T5–6 segment. The patient should not be aware of any pain or discomfort. Make these final adjustments by slight movements of the ankles, knees, hips and trunk. A common mistake is to lose the chest compression during the final adjustments.

7. Immediately prethrust

Relax and adjust your balance as necessary. Keep your head up and ensure that your contacts are firm and the patient's body weight is well controlled. An effective HVLA thrust technique is best achieved if the operator and patient are relaxed and not holding themselves rigid. This is a common impediment to achieving effective cavitation.

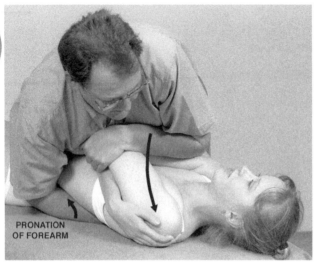

PRONATION
OF FOREARM

Figure 9.29

8. **Delivering the thrust**

This technique uses ligamentous myofascial positioning and not facet apposition locking. This approach generally requires a greater emphasis on the exaggeration of primary leverage than is the case with facet apposition locking techniques.

The shoulder girdles and thorax of the patient are now a solid mass against which a thrust may be applied. Apply an HVLA thrust downwards towards the couch and in the line of the patient's left upper arm via your lower sternum or upper abdomen. Simultaneously, apply an HVLA thrust with your right thenar eminence upwards against the left transverse process of T6 (Fig. 9.29). The force is produced by rapid pronation of your right forearm.

A common fault is to emphasize the thrust via the patient's shoulder girdles at the expense of the thrust against the left transverse process. The hand contacting the transverse process of T6 must actively participate in the generation of thrust forces.

The thrust, although very rapid, must never be excessively forcible. The aim should be to use the absolute minimum force necessary to achieve joint cavitation. A common fault arises from the use of excessive amplitude with insufficient velocity of thrust.

This technique has many modifications:
- Different shoulder girdle holds can be used.
- Different applicators can be used.
- Respiration can be used to make the technique more effective.

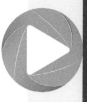

Summary

Thoracic spine T4–9: Rotation gliding

Patient supine

Ligamentous myofascial positioning

- **Contact points:**
  - Left transverse process of T6
  - Patient's elbows and left forearm

- **Applicators:**
  - Palm of the operator's right hand, held in a clenched position
  - Operator's lower sternum or upper abdomen

- **Patient positioning:** Supine with arms crossed over the chest (Fig. 9.25)

- **Operator stance:** To the right side of the patient, facing the couch

- **Positioning for thrust:** Take hold of the patient's left shoulder and pull it towards you (Fig. 9.26). Place the thenar eminence of your right hand against the left transverse process of T6 (Fig. 9.27). Roll the patient back towards the supine position. Rest your lower sternum or upper abdomen on the patient's elbows and left forearm (Fig. 9.28). Apply a slow firm pressure with your lower sternum or upper abdomen downwards towards the couch. Maintaining this downwards leverage, introduce left rotation of the patient's upper thorax by directing forces towards the patient's left shoulder along the line of the patient's left upper arm

- **Adjustments to achieve appropriate prethrust tension**

- **Immediately prethrust:** Relax and adjust your balance

- **Delivering the thrust:** The direction of thrust is downwards towards the couch and in the line of the patient's left upper arm via your lower sternum or upper abdomen. Simultaneously, apply a thrust with your right thenar eminence upwards against the left transverse process of T6 (Fig. 9.29). The force is produced by rapid pronation of your right forearm. The hand contacting the transverse process of T6 must actively participate in the generation of thrust forces

- **Modifications to technique:**
  - Different shoulder girdle holds can be used
  - Different applicators can be used
  - Respiration can be used to make the technique more effective

217

Thoracic spine T4–9:
Rotation gliding

Patient prone

Short-lever technique

Assume somatic dysfunction (S-T-A-R-T) is identified and you wish to use a rotation gliding thrust, parallel to the apophysial joint plane, to produce joint cavitation at T5–6 (Figs. 9.30, 9.31).

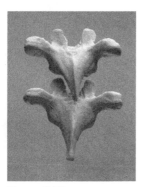

Figure 9.30

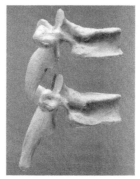

Figure 9.31

Key

✳ Stabilization

● Applicator

➡ Plane of thrust (operator)

⇨ Direction of body movement (patient)

Note: The dimensions for the arrows are not a pictorial representation of the amplitude or force of the thrust.

1. Contact points

Transverse processes of T5 (right applicator) and T6 (left applicator).

2. Applicators

Hypothenar eminence of left and right hands.

3. Patient positioning

Patient lying prone with the head and neck in a comfortable position and arms hanging over the edge of the couch.

4. Operator stance

Stand at the left side of the patient, feet spread slightly and facing the patient. Stand as erect as possible and avoid crouching, as

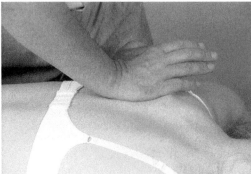

Figure 9.32

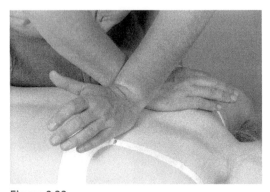

Figure 9.33

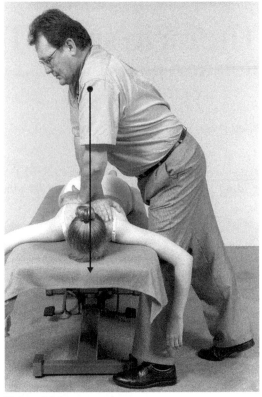

Figure 9.34

this will limit the technique and restrict delivery of the thrust.

5. Palpation of contact points

There are many different ways to perform this technique. This is one approach. Locate the transverse processes of T5 and T6. Place the hypothenar eminence of your right hand against the left transverse process of T5 and establish a firm contact (Fig. 9.32). Place the hypothenar eminence of your left hand against the right transverse process of T6 (Fig. 9.33). Ensure that you have good contact and will not slip across the skin or superficial musculature when you apply downwards and caudad or cephalad forces against the transverse processes. Maintain these contact points.

6. Positioning for thrust

This is a short-lever technique and the velocity of the thrust is critical. Move your centre of gravity over the patient by leaning your body weight forwards onto your arms and hypothenar eminences (Fig. 9.34). Shifting your centre of gravity forwards will direct a downwards pressure on the transverse processes. You must apply an additional force directed caudad with the left hand and cephalad with the right hand. The final direction of thrust is influenced by the degree of thoracic kyphosis and any pre-existing scoliosis. This technique does not use facet apposition locking. The prethrust tension is achieved by positioning the T5–6 segment towards the end-range of available joint gliding. Extensive practice is necessary to develop an appreciation of the required tension.

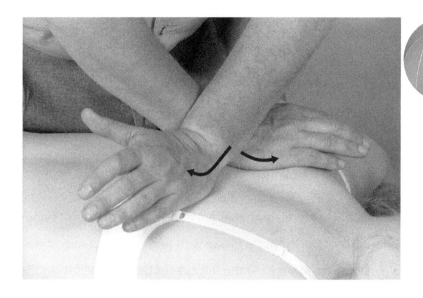

Figure 9.35

7. Adjustments to achieve appropriate prethrust tension

Ensure your patient remains relaxed. Maintaining all holds and pressure upon the transverse processes, make any necessary changes by introducing very slight components of extension, sidebending and rotation until you sense a state of appropriate tension and leverage at the T5–6 segment. The patient should not be aware of any pain or discomfort.

8. Immediately prethrust

Relax and adjust your balance as necessary. Keep your head up and ensure that your contacts are firm. An effective HVLA thrust technique is best achieved if the operator and patient are relaxed and not holding themselves rigid. This is a common impediment to achieving effective cavitation.

9. Delivering the thrust

Apply an HVLA thrust directed in a downwards and cephalad direction against the transverse process of T5 while simultaneously applying a thrust downwards and in a caudad direction against the transverse process of T6 (Fig. 9.35).

The thrust, although very rapid, must never be excessively forcible. The aim should be to use the absolute minimum force necessary to achieve joint cavitation. A common fault arises from the use of excessive amplitude with insufficient velocity of thrust.

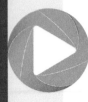

Summary

Thoracic spine T4–9: Rotation gliding

Patient prone

Short-lever technique

- **Contact points:** Transverse processes of T5 (right applicator) and T6 (left applicator)

- **Applicators:** Hypothenar eminence of left and right hands

- **Patient positioning:** Prone with arms hanging over the edge of the couch

- **Operator stance:** To the left side of the patient, facing the couch

- **Palpation of contact points:** Place the hypothenar eminence of your right hand against the left transverse process of T5 and establish a firm contact (Fig. 9.32). Place the hypothenar eminence of your left hand against the right transverse process of T6 (Fig. 9.33)

- **Positioning for thrust:** This is a short-lever technique and the velocity of the thrust is critical. Move your centre of gravity over the patient by leaning your body weight forwards onto your arms and hypothenar eminences (Fig. 9.34). Apply an additional force directed caudad with the left hand and cephalad with the right hand

- **Adjustments to achieve appropriate prethrust tension**

- **Immediately prethrust:** Relax and adjust your balance

- **Delivering the thrust:** The direction of thrust is in a downwards and cephalad direction against the transverse process of T5 while simultaneously applying a thrust downwards and in a caudad direction against the transverse process of T6 (Fig. 9.35)

Ribs R1–3: Patient prone

Gliding thrust

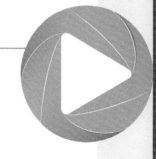

Assume somatic dysfunction (S-T-A-R-T) is identified and you wish to produce cavitation at the costotransverse joint of the second rib on the right (Figs. 9.36, 9.37).

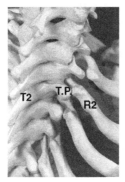

Figure 9.36

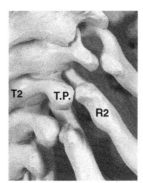

Figure 9.37

Key

✳ Stabilization

● Applicator

➡ Plane of thrust (operator)

⇨ Direction of body movement (patient)

Note: The dimensions for the arrows are not a pictorial representation of the amplitude or force of the thrust.

1. Contact point

Angle of the second rib on the right.

2. Applicator

Hypothenar eminence of the right hand.

3. Patient positioning

Patient prone with the point of the chin resting on the couch and the arms hanging over the edge of the couch. Introduce a small amount of sidebending to the left by gently lifting and moving the chin to the patient's left (Fig. 9.38). Do not introduce too much sidebending.

4. Operator stance

Head of the couch, feet spread slightly. Stand as erect as possible and avoid

223

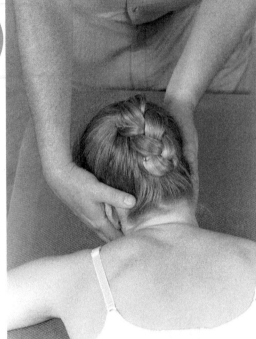

Figure 9.38

crouching over he patient, as this will limit the technique and restrict delivery of the thrust.

5. Palpation of contact point

Locate the angle of the second rib on the right. Place the hypothenar eminence of your right hand gently, but firmly, against the rib angle. Ensure that you have good contact and will not slip across the skin or superficial musculature when you apply a caudad and downwards force towards the couch against the angle of the second rib. Maintain this contact point.

6. Positioning for thrust

Keeping your position at the head of the couch, gently place your left hand against the right side of the patient's head and neck. While maintaining the left sidebending, introduce rotation to the right, in the cervical and upper thoracic spine, by applying gentle pressure to the right side of the patient's head and neck with your left

hand (Fig. 9.39). Maintaining all holds and pressures, complete the rotation of the patient's head and neck until a sense of tension is palpated at your right hypothenar eminence. Keep firm pressure against the contact point.

7. Adjustments to achieve appropriate prethrust tension

Ensure the patient remains relaxed. Maintaining all holds, make any necessary changes in extension, sidebending or rotation until you can sense a state of appropriate tension and leverage. The patient should not be aware of any pain or discomfort. You make these final adjustments by altering the pressure and direction of forces between the left hand against the patient's head and neck and your right hypothenar eminence against the contact point.

8. Immediately prethrust

Relax and adjust your balance as necessary. Keep your head up and ensure that your contacts are firm and your body position is well controlled. An effective HVLA thrust technique is best achieved if the operator and patient are relaxed and not holding themselves rigid. This is a common impediment to achieving effective cavitation.

9. Delivering the thrust

Apply an HVLA thrust to the angle of the second rib on the right directed downwards towards the couch and also in a caudad direction towards the patient's right iliac crest. Simultaneously, apply a slight, rapid increase of head and neck rotation to the right with your left hand (Fig. 9.40). You must not overemphasize the thrust with the left hand against the patient's head and neck. Your left hand stabilizes the leverages and maintains the position of the head and cervical spine against the thrust imposed upon the contact point. The thrust is

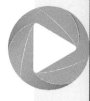

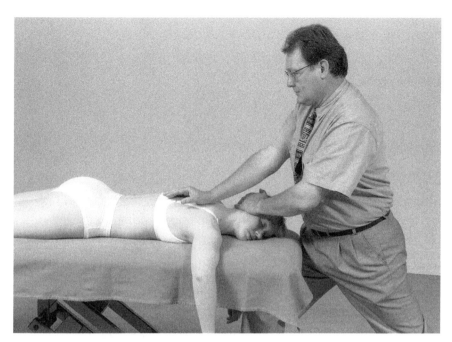

Figure 9.39

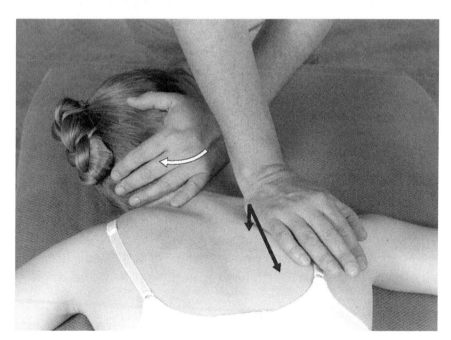

Figure 9.40

induced by a very rapid contraction of the triceps, shoulder adductors and internal rotators.

The thrust, although very rapid, must never be excessively forcible. The aim should be to use the absolute minimum force necessary to achieve joint cavitation. A common fault arises from the use of excessive amplitude with insufficient velocity of thrust.

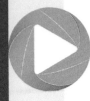

Summary

Ribs R1–3: Patient prone

Gliding thrust

- **Contact point:** Angle of the right second rib

- **Applicator:** Hypothenar eminence

- **Patient positioning:** Patient prone with the chin resting on the couch and arms hanging over the edge of the couch. Introduce sidebending to the left (Fig. 9.38). Do not introduce too much sidebending

- **Operator stance:** Head of the couch, feet spread slightly

- **Palpation of contact point:** Place your hypothenar eminence against the angle of the second rib on the right. Ensure that you have good contact and will not slip across the skin or superficial musculature when you apply a caudad and downwards force towards the couch against the angle of the second rib

- **Positioning for thrust:** Place your left hand against the right side of the patient's head and neck. Rotate the cervical and upper thoracic spine to the right, by applying pressure to the right side of the patient's head and neck with your left hand until a sense of tension is palpated at the contact point (Fig. 9.39)

- **Adjustments to achieve appropriate prethrust tension**

- **Immediately prethrust:** Relax and adjust your balance

- **Delivering the thrust:** The thrust to the angle of the second rib on the right is directed downwards towards the couch and also in a caudad direction towards the patient's right iliac crest. Simultaneously, apply a slight, rapid increase of head and neck rotation to the right with your left hand (Fig. 9.40). You must not overemphasize the thrust with the left hand against the patient's head and neck

9.6

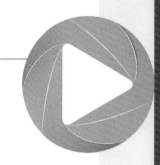

Ribs R4–10: Patient supine

Gliding thrust
Ligamentous myofascial positioning

Assume somatic dysfunction (S-T-A-R-T) is identified and you wish to produce cavitation at the costotransverse joint of the sixth rib on the left (Fig. 9.41).

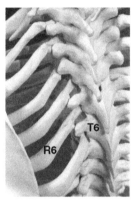

Figure 9.41

Key

✳ Stabilization

● Applicator

➡ Plane of thrust (operator)

⇨ Direction of body movement (patient)

Note: The dimensions for the arrows are not a pictorial representation of the amplitude or force of the thrust.

1. Contact points

a. Sixth rib on the left, just lateral to the transverse process of T6.
b. Patient's elbows and left forearm.

2. Applicators

a. Hypothenar eminence of the operator's right hand.
b. Operator's lower sternum or upper abdomen.

3. Patient positioning

Supine with the arms crossed over the chest and the hands passed around the shoulders. The left arm is placed over the right arm. The arms should be firmly clasped around the body as far as the patient can comfortably reach.

227

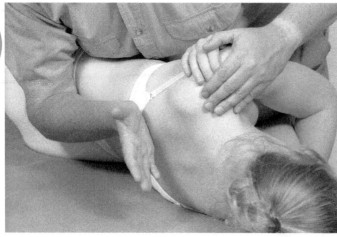

Figure 9.42

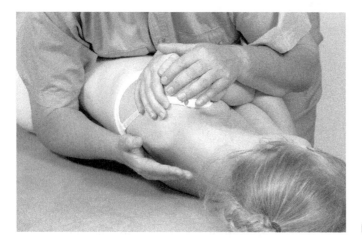

Figure 9.43

4. Operator stance

Stand on the right side of the patient, facing the couch.

5. Positioning for thrust

Reach over the patient with your left hand to take hold of the left shoulder and gently pull it towards you. With your right hand, locate the sixth rib on the left. Now place the hypothenar eminence of your right hand against the rib just lateral to the transverse process of T6 (Fig. 9.42).

Keeping contact with the rib, begin rolling the patient back to the supine position (Fig. 9.43). Continue until the patient's elbows are directly over your hypothenar eminence. This introduces additional rotation, which is a critical element in the technique.

Rest your lower sternum or upper abdomen on the patient's elbows and left forearm. Initially, a slow but firm pressure is applied with your lower sternum or upper abdomen downwards towards the couch. Maintaining this downwards leverage, introduce left rotation of the patient's upper thorax by directing forces towards the patient's left shoulder along the line of the

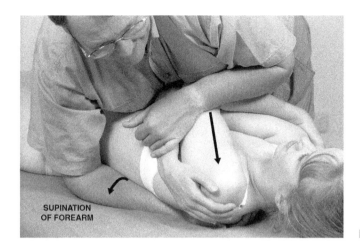

SUPINATION
OF FOREARM

Figure 9.44

patient's left upper arm. By balancing these different leverages, tension can be localized to the costotransverse joint of the sixth rib.

6. Adjustments to achieve appropriate prethrust tension

Ensure your patient remains relaxed. Maintaining all holds, make any necessary changes in flexion, extension, sidebending and rotation until you can sense a state of appropriate tension and leverage at the costotransverse joint of the sixth rib. The patient should not be aware of any pain or discomfort. Make these final adjustments by slight movements of the ankles, knees, hips and trunk. A common mistake is to lose the chest compression during the final adjustments.

7. Immediately prethrust

Relax and adjust your balance as necessary. Keep your head up and ensure that your contacts are firm and the patient's body weight is well controlled. An effective HVLA thrust technique is best achieved if the operator and patient are relaxed and not holding themselves rigid. This is a common impediment to achieving effective cavitation.

8. Delivering the thrust

This technique uses ligamentous myofascial positioning and not facet apposition locking. This approach generally requires a greater emphasis on the exaggeration of primary leverage than is the case with facet apposition locking techniques.

The shoulder girdles and thorax of the patient are now a solid mass against which a thrust may be applied. Apply an HVLA thrust downwards towards the couch and in the line of the patient's left upper arm via your lower sternum or upper abdomen. Simultaneously, apply an HVLA thrust with your right hypothenar eminence upwards against the sixth rib (Fig. 9.44). The force is produced by rapid supination of your right forearm.

A common fault is to emphasize the thrust via the patient's shoulder girdles at the expense of the thrust against the sixth rib. The hand contacting the rib must actively participate in the generation of thrust forces.

The thrust, although very rapid, must never be excessively forcible. The aim should be to use the absolute minimum force necessary to achieve joint cavitation. A common fault arises from the use of excessive amplitude with insufficient velocity of thrust.

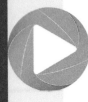

Summary

Ribs R4–10: Patient supine

Gliding thrust

Ligamentous myofascial positioning

- **Contact points:**
  - Sixth rib on the left, lateral to the transverse process
  - Patient's elbows and left forearm
- **Applicators:**
  - Hypothenar eminence of the operator's right hand
  - Operator's lower sternum or upper abdomen
- **Patient positioning:** Supine with arms crossed over the chest
- **Operator stance:** To the right side of the patient, facing the couch
- **Positioning for thrust:** Take hold of the patient's left shoulder, and pull it towards you. Place the hypothenar eminence of your right hand against the rib just lateral to the left transverse process of T6 (Fig. 9.42). Roll the patient back to the supine position (Fig. 9.43). Continue until the patient's elbows are directly over your hypothenar eminence. This is a critical element in the technique. Rest your lower sternum or upper abdomen on the patient's elbows and left forearm. Apply a slow firm pressure with your lower sternum or upper abdomen downwards towards the couch. Maintaining this downwards leverage, introduce left rotation of the patient's upper thorax by directing forces towards the patient's left shoulder along the line of the patient's left upper arm
- **Adjustments to achieve appropriate prethrust tension**
- **Immediately prethrust:** Relax and adjust your balance
- **Delivering the thrust:** The direction of thrust is downwards towards the couch and in the line of the patient's left upper arm via your lower sternum or upper abdomen. Simultaneously, apply a thrust with your right hypothenar eminence upwards against the sixth rib (Fig. 9.44). The force is produced by rapid supination of your right forearm. The hand contacting the rib must actively participate in the generation of thrust forces

9.7

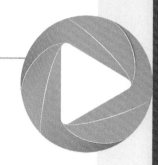

Ribs R4–10: Patient prone

Gliding thrust

Short-lever technique

Assume somatic dysfunction (S-T-A-R-T) is identified and you wish to produce cavitation at the costotransverse joint of the sixth rib on the left (Fig. 9.45).

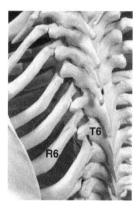

Figure 9.45

Key

✳ Stabilization

● Applicator

➡ Plane of thrust (operator)

⇨ Direction of body movement (patient)

Note: The dimensions for the arrows are not a pictorial representation of the amplitude or force of the thrust.

1. Contact points
Angle of left sixth rib (right applicator). Right transverse process of T6 (left applicator).

2. Applicators
Hypothenar eminence of left and right hands.

3. Patient positioning
Patient lying prone with the head and neck in a comfortable position and the arms hanging over the edge of the couch.

4. Operator stance
Stand at the left side of the patient, feet spread slightly and facing the patient. Stand

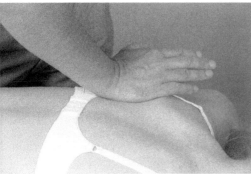

Figure 9.46

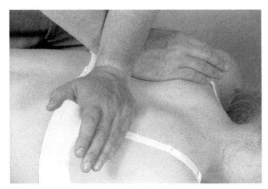

Figure 9.47

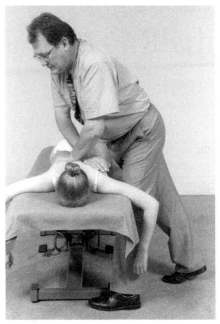

Figure 9.48

as erect as possible and avoid crouching, as this will limit the technique and restrict delivery of the thrust.

5. Palpation of contact points

There are many different ways to perform this technique. This is one approach. Locate the transverse processes of T6. Place the hypothenar eminence of your right hand against the angle of the patient's left sixth rib and establish a firm contact (Fig. 9.46). Place the hypothenar eminence of your left hand against the right transverse process of T6 (Fig. 9.47). Ensure that you have good contact and will not slip across the skin or superficial musculature.

6. Positioning for thrust

This is a short-lever technique, and as a consequence the velocity of the thrust is

critical. Move your centre of gravity over the patient by leaning your body weight forwards onto your arms and hypothenar eminences (Fig. 9.48). Shifting your centre of gravity forwards will direct a downwards pressure on both the transverse process of T6 and the sixth rib. You must apply an additional force directed cephalad with the right hand against the angle of the sixth rib. The final direction of thrust is influenced by the degree of thoracic kyphosis and any pre-existing scoliosis. This technique does not use facet apposition locking. The prethrust tension is achieved by positioning the costotransverse joint of the sixth rib towards the end-range of available joint gliding. Extensive practice is necessary to develop an appreciation of the required tension.

7. Adjustments to achieve appropriate prethrust tension

Ensure your patient remains relaxed. Maintaining all holds, make any necessary

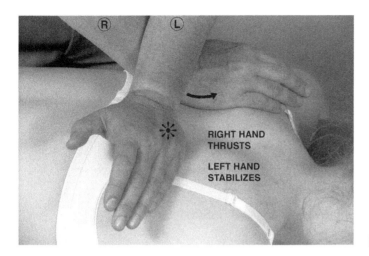

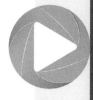

RIGHT HAND THRUSTS

LEFT HAND STABILIZES

Figure 9.49

changes in extension, sidebending and rotation until you sense a state of appropriate tension and leverage at the costotransverse joint of the sixth rib. The patient should not be aware of any pain or discomfort.

8. Immediately prethrust

Relax and adjust your balance as necessary. Keep your head up and ensure that your contacts are firm. An effective HVLA thrust technique is best achieved if the operator and patient are relaxed and not holding themselves rigid. This is a common impediment to achieving effective cavitation.

9. Delivering the thrust

Apply an HVLA thrust directed in a downwards and cephalad direction against the angle of the sixth rib. It is important to achieve fixation of T6 by maintaining a firm downwards pressure against the transverse process of T6 on the right. The thrust is generated by your right hand in contact with the sixth rib (Fig. 9.49).

The thrust, although very rapid, must never be excessively forcible. The aim should be to use the absolute minimum force necessary to achieve joint cavitation. A common fault arises from the use of excessive amplitude with insufficient velocity of thrust.

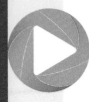

Summary

Ribs R4–10: Patient prone

Gliding thrust

Short-lever technique

- **Contact points:** Angle of left sixth rib (right applicator). Right transverse process of T6 (left applicator)

- **Applicators:** Hypothenar eminence of left and right hands

- **Patient positioning:** Prone with arms hanging over the edge of the couch

- **Operator stance:** To the left side of the patient, facing the couch

- **Palpation of contact points:** Place the hypothenar eminence of your right hand against the angle of the patient's left sixth rib and establish a firm contact (Fig. 9.46). Place the hypothenar eminence of left hand against the right transverse process of T6 (Fig. 9.47)

- **Positioning for thrust:** This is a short-lever technique and the velocity of the thrust is critical. Move your centre of gravity over the patient by leaning your body weight forwards onto your arms and hypothenar eminences (Fig. 9.48). Apply an additional force directed cephalad with the right hand against the angle of the sixth rib

- **Adjustments to achieve appropriate prethrust tension**

- **Immediately prethrust:** Relax and adjust your balance

- **Delivering the thrust:** The direction of thrust is in a downwards and cephalad direction against the angle of the sixth rib. It is important to achieve fixation of T6 by maintaining a firm downwards pressure against the transverse process of T6 on the right. The thrust is generated by your right hand in contact with the sixth rib (Fig. 9.49)

Ribs R4–10: Patient sitting

Gliding thrust

Ligamentous myofascial positioning

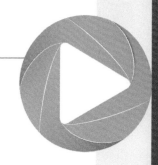

Assume somatic dysfunction (S-T-A-R-T) is identified and you wish to produce cavitation at the costotransverse joint of the right sixth rib (Fig. 9.50).

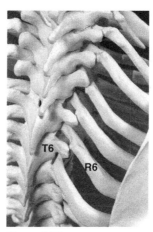

Figure 9.50

Key

✳ Stabilization

● Applicator

➡ Plane of thrust (operator)

⇨ Direction of body movement (patient)

Note: The dimensions for the arrows are not a pictorial representation of the amplitude or force of the thrust.

1. Contact point

Angle of right sixth rib.

2. Applicator

Hypothenar eminence of right hand.

3. Patient positioning

Sitting astride the treatment couch with the arms crossed over the chest and the hands passed around the shoulders. The arms should be firmly clasped around the body as far as the patient can comfortably reach.

4. Operator stance

Stand behind and slightly to the left of the patient with your feet spread. Pass your left arm across the front of the patient's chest to

235

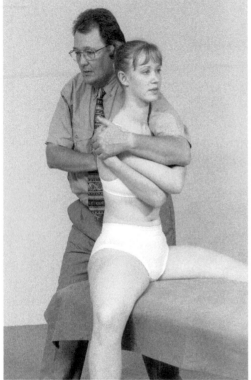

Figure 9.51

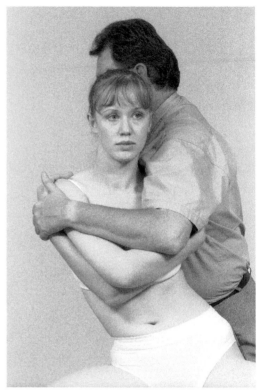

Figure 9.52

lightly grip over the patient's right shoulder region (Fig. 9.51).

5. Positioning for thrust

Translate the patient's trunk to the right and away from you. This opens up the intercostal space between the sixth and seventh ribs (Fig. 9.52) and allows better access to the inferior aspect of the sixth rib. Place your right hypothenar eminence on the inferior surface of the angle of the sixth rib. The thorax is now rotated to the left (Fig. 9.53). Sidebending to the right is introduced to localize tension at the costotransverse joint of the sixth rib. The operator maintains as erect a posture as possible. Keep your right hypothenar eminence firmly applied to the sixth rib with your right elbow held close to your body (Fig. 9.54).

6. Adjustments to achieve appropriate prethrust tension

Ensure your patient remains relaxed. Maintaining all holds, make any necessary changes in flexion, extension, sidebending or rotation until you can sense a state of appropriate tension and leverage at the costotransverse joint of the sixth rib on the right. The patient should not be aware of any pain or discomfort. Make these final adjustments by slight movements of the shoulders, trunk, ankles, knees and hips.

7. Immediately prethrust

Relax and adjust your balance as necessary. An effective HVLA thrust technique is best achieved if both the operator and patient are relaxed and not holding themselves rigid. This is a common impediment to achieving effective cavitation.

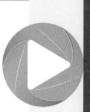

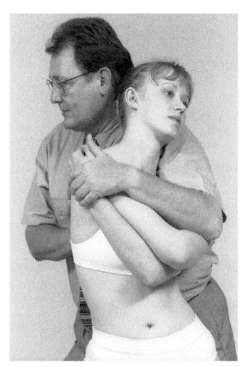

Figure 9.53

8. Delivering the thrust

This technique uses ligamentous myofascial positioning and not facet apposition locking. This approach generally requires a greater emphasis on the exaggeration of primary leverage than is the case with facet apposition locking techniques.

A degree of momentum is necessary to achieve a successful cavitation. Rock the patient into and out of rotation while maintaining the other leverages. When you sense a state of appropriate tension and leverage at the sixth rib, apply an HVLA thrust against the inferior aspect of the angle of the rib in a cephalad and anterior direction. Simultaneously, apply slight exaggeration of left trunk rotation (Fig. 9.55).

The thrust, although very rapid, must never be excessively forcible. The aim should be to use the absolute minimum force necessary to achieve joint cavitation. A common fault arises from the use of excessive amplitude with insufficient velocity of thrust.

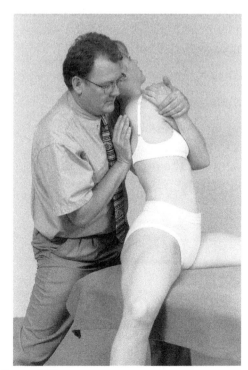

Figure 9.54

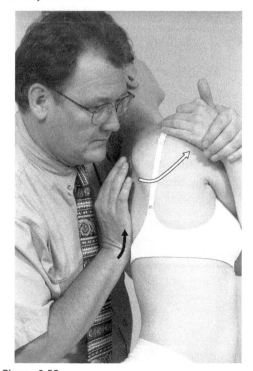

Figure 9.55

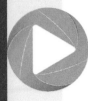

Summary

Ribs R4–10 Patient sitting

Gliding thrust

Ligamentous myofascial positioning

- **Contact point:** Angle of right sixth rib

- **Applicator:** Hypothenar eminence of right hand

- **Patient positioning:** Sitting astride the couch with the arms crossed over the chest and the hands passed around the shoulders

- **Operator stance:** Behind and slightly to the left of the patient with the feet spread. Pass your left arm across the front of the patient's chest to lightly grip over the patient's right shoulder region (Fig. 9.51)

- **Positioning for thrust:** Translate the patient's trunk to the right and away from you (Fig. 9.52). Place your right hypothenar eminence on the inferior surface of the angle of the sixth rib. The thorax is now rotated to the left (Fig. 9.53). Sidebending to the right is introduced to localize tension at the costotransverse joint of the sixth rib. The operator maintains as erect a posture as possible. Keep your right hypothenar eminence firmly applied to the sixth rib with your right elbow held close to your body (Fig. 9.54)

- **Adjustments to achieve appropriate prethrust tension**

- **Immediately prethrust:** Relax and adjust your balance

- **Delivering the thrust:** A degree of momentum is necessary to achieve a successful cavitation. The direction of thrust is in a cephalad and anterior direction against the inferior aspect of the angle of the rib. Simultaneously, apply slight exaggeration of left trunk rotation (Fig. 9.55)

10

Lumbar and thoracolumbar spine

UPPER BODY HOLDS FOR SIDELYING TECHNIQUES

All techniques in this manual are described with the operator taking up the axillary hold (Fig. 10.1). The hold selected for any particular technique is that which enables the operator to effectively localize forces to a specific segment of the spine and deliver a high-velocity low-amplitude (HVLA) force in a controlled manner. Patient comfort must be a major consideration in selecting the most appropriate hold.

Three alternative upper body holds are available:

- Pectoral hold (Fig. 10.2)
- Elbow hold (Fig. 10.3)
- Upper arm hold (Fig. 10.4).

LOWER BODY HOLDS FOR SIDELYING TECHNIQUES

There are a variety of lower body holds available (Figs. 10.5–10.9). The hold selected for any particular technique is that which enables the operator to effectively localize forces to a specific segment of the spine and deliver an HVLA force in a controlled manner. Patient comfort must be a major consideration in selecting the most appropriate hold.

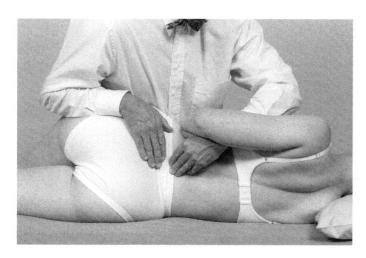

Figure 10.1

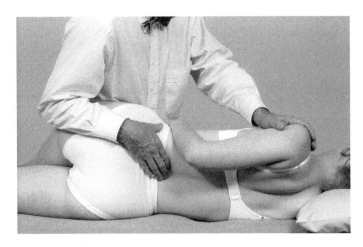

Figure 10.2

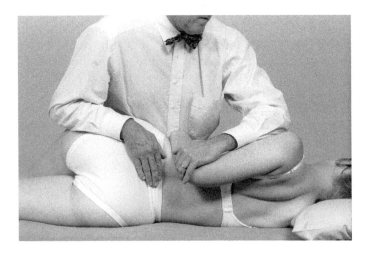

Figure 10.3

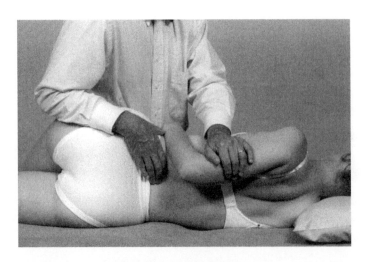

Figure 10.4

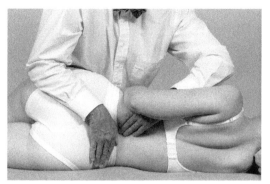

Figure 10.5

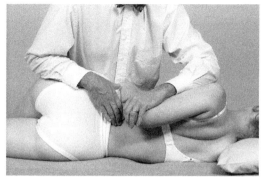

Figure 10.6

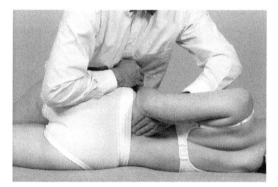

Figure 10.7

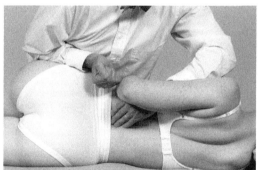

Figure 10.8

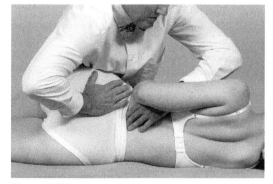

Figure 10.9

Thoracolumbar spine T10–L2:
Neutral positioning

Patient sidelying

Rotation gliding thrust

Assume somatic dysfunction (S-T-A-R-T) is identified and you wish to use a rotation gliding thrust to produce cavitation at T12–L1 on the left (Figs. 10.10, 10.11).

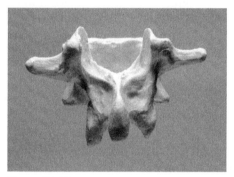

Figure 10.10

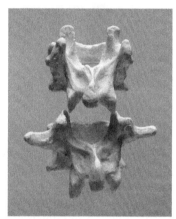

Figure 10.11

Key

✳ Stabilization

● Applicator

➡ Plane of thrust (operator)

⇨ Direction of body movement (patient)

Note: The dimensions for the arrows are not a pictorial representation of the amplitude or force of the thrust.

1. **Patient positioning**

Lying on the right side with a pillow to support the head and neck. The upper portion of the couch is raised 10° to 15° to introduce left sidebending in the lower thoracic and upper lumbar spine. Experienced practitioners may choose to achieve the left sidebending without raising the upper portion of the couch.

Lower body. Straighten the patient's lower (right) leg and ensure that the leg and spine are in a straight line, in a neutral position. Flex the patient's upper hip and knee slightly and place the upper leg just anterior to the lower leg. The lower leg and spine should form as near a straight line as possible, with no flexion at the lower hip or knee.

243

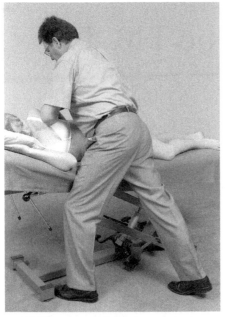

Figure 10.12

Upper body. Gently extend the patient's upper shoulder and place the patient's left forearm on the lower ribs. Using your right hand to palpate the T12–L1 interspinous space, introduce left rotation of the patient's upper body down to the T12–L1 segment. This is achieved by gently holding the patient's right elbow with your left hand and pulling it towards you, but also in a cephalad direction towards the head end of the couch. Be careful not to introduce any flexion to the spine during this movement. Left rotation is continued until your palpating hand at the T12–L1 segment begins to sense motion. Take up the axillary hold. This arm controls the upper body rotation.

2. Operator stance

Stand close to the couch with your feet spread and one leg behind the other (Fig. 10.12). Maintain an upright posture, facing slightly in the direction of the patient's upper body. Keep your right arm as close to your body as possible.

3. Positioning for thrust

Apply your right forearm to the region between the gluteus medius and the gluteus maximus. Your right forearm now controls lower body rotation. Your left forearm should be resting against the patient's upper pectoral and rib cage region and will control upper body rotation. First, rotate the patient's pelvis and lumbar spine towards you until motion is palpated at the T12–L1 segment. Rotate the patient's upper body away from you using your left arm until a sense of tension is palpated at the T12–L1 segment. Be careful to avoid undue pressure in the axilla. Finally, roll the patient about 10° to 15° towards you while maintaining the build-up of leverages at the T12–L1 segment.

4. Adjustments to achieve appropriate prethrust tension

Ensure your patient remains relaxed. Maintaining all holds, make any necessary changes in flexion, extension, sidebending or rotation until you can sense a state of appropriate tension and leverage at the T12–L1 segment. The patient should not be aware of any pain or discomfort. Make these final adjustments by slight movements of the shoulders, trunk, ankles, knees and hips.

5. Immediately prethrust

Relax and adjust your balance, as necessary. Keep your head up; looking down impedes the thrust. An effective HVLA thrust technique is best achieved if both the operator and patient are relaxed and not holding themselves rigid. This is a common impediment to achieving effective cavitation.

6. Delivering the thrust

Your left arm against the patient's pectoral region does not apply a thrust but acts as a stabilizer only. Keep the thrusting (right) arm as close to your body as possible. Apply an HVLA thrust with your right forearm

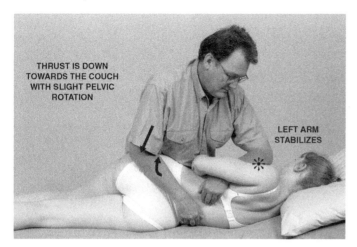

THRUST IS DOWN
TOWARDS THE COUCH
WITH SLIGHT PELVIC
ROTATION

LEFT ARM
STABILIZES

Figure 10.13

against the patient's buttock. The direction of force is down towards the couch accompanied by a slight exaggeration of pelvic rotation towards the operator (Fig. 10.13).

The thrust, although very rapid, must never be excessively forcible. The aim should be to use the absolute minimum force necessary to achieve joint cavitation. A common fault arises from the use of excessive amplitude with insufficient velocity of thrust.

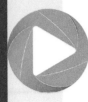

Summary

Thoracolumbar spine T10–L2: Neutral positioning

Patient sidelying

Rotation gliding thrust

- **Patient positioning:** Right sidelying with the upper portion of the couch raised 10° to 15° to introduce left sidebending in the lower thoracic and upper lumbar spine:

  - *Lower body.* Right leg and spine in a straight line. Left hip and knee flexed slightly and placed just anterior to the lower leg

  - *Upper body.* Introduce left rotation of the patient's upper body until your palpating hand at T12–L1 begins to sense motion. Do not introduce any flexion to the spine during this movement. Take up the axillary hold

- **Operator stance:** Stand close to the couch, feet spread and one leg behind the other. Maintain an upright posture, facing slightly in the direction of the patient's upper body (Fig. 10.12)

- **Positioning for thrust:** Place your right forearm in the region between the gluteus medius and the gluteus maximus. Rotate the patient's pelvis and lumbar spine towards you until motion is palpated at the T12–L1 segment. Rotate the patient's upper body away from you until a sense of tension is palpated at the T12–L1 segment. Roll the patient about 10° to 15° towards you

- **Adjustments to achieve appropriate prethrust tension**

- **Immediately prethrust:** Relax and adjust your balance

- **Delivering the thrust:** The direction of thrust is down towards the couch and is accompanied by exaggeration of pelvic rotation towards the operator (Fig. 10.13). Your left arm against the patient's axillary region does not apply a thrust but acts as a stabilizer only

10.2

Thoracolumbar spine T10–L2:
Flexion positioning

Patient sidelying

Rotation gliding thrust

Assume somatic dysfunction (S-T-A-R-T) is identified and you wish to use a rotation gliding thrust to produce cavitation at T12–L1 on the right (Figs. 10.14, 10.15).

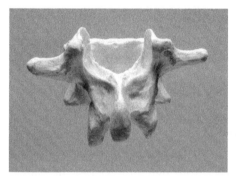

Figure 10.14

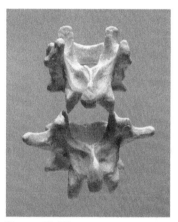

Figure 10.15

Key

✳ Stabilization

● Applicator

➡ Plane of thrust (operator)

⇨ Direction of body movement (patient)

Note: The dimensions for the arrows are not a pictorial representation of the amplitude or force of the thrust.

---

1. Patient positioning

Lying on the left side with a pillow to support the head and neck. A small pillow, or rolled towel, should be placed under the patient's waist to introduce left sidebending in the thoracolumbar spine. Experienced practitioners may choose to achieve the left sidebending without the use of a small pillow or rolled towel.

Lower body. Straighten the patient's lower (left) leg at the knee joint while keeping the left hip flexed. Flex the patient's upper hip and knee. Rest the upper flexed knee upon the edge of the couch, anterior to the left thigh, and place the patient's right foot behind the left calf. This position provides stability to the lower body.

Upper body. Gently extend the patient's upper shoulder and place the patient's right forearm on the lower ribs. Using your left hand to palpate the T12–L1 interspinous space, introduce right rotation of the patient's upper body down to the T12–L1 segment. Rotation with flexion positioning is achieved by gently holding the patient's left elbow with your right hand and pulling it towards you, but also in a caudad direction towards the foot end of the couch. Right rotation is continued until your palpating hand at the T12–L1 segment begins to sense motion. Take up the axillary hold. This arm controls the upper body rotation.

2. Operator stance

Stand close to the couch with your feet spread and one leg behind the other. Maintain an upright posture, facing slightly in the direction of the patient's upper body. Keep your left arm as close to your body as possible.

3. Positioning for thrust

Apply the palmar aspect of your left forearm to the sacrum and posterior superior iliac spine. Your left forearm now controls lower body rotation. Your right forearm should be resting against the patient's upper pectoral and rib cage region and will control upper body rotation. First, rotate the patient's pelvis and lumbar spine towards you until motion is palpated at the T12–L1 segment. Rotate the patient's upper body away from you using your right arm until a sense of tension is palpated at the T12–L1 segment. Be careful to avoid undue pressure in the axilla. Finally, roll the patient about 10° to 15° towards you while maintaining the build-up of leverages at the T12–L1 segment.

4. Adjustments to achieve appropriate prethrust tension

Ensure your patient remains relaxed. Maintaining all holds, make any necessary changes in flexion, extension, sidebending or rotation until you can sense a state of appropriate tension and leverage at the T12–L1 segment. The patient should not be aware of any pain or discomfort. Make these final adjustments by slight movements of the shoulders, trunk, ankles, knees and hips.

5. Immediately prethrust

Relax and adjust your balance as necessary. Keep your head up; looking down impedes the thrust. An effective HVLA thrust technique is best achieved if both the operator and patient are relaxed and not holding themselves rigid. This is a common impediment to achieving effective cavitation.

6. Delivering the thrust

Your right arm against the patient's pectoral region does not apply a thrust but acts as a stabilizer only. Keep the thrusting (left) arm as close to your body as possible. Apply an HVLA thrust with your left forearm against the patient's sacrum and posterior superior iliac spine. The direction of force is down towards the couch accompanied by slight exaggeration of pelvic rotation towards the operator (Fig. 10.16).

The thrust, although very rapid, must never be excessively forcible. The aim should be to use the absolute minimum force necessary to achieve joint cavitation. A common fault arises from the use of excessive amplitude with insufficient velocity of thrust.

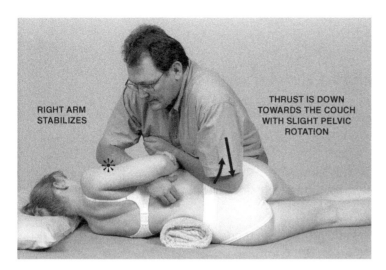

Figure 10.16

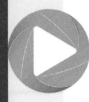

Summary

Thoracolumbar spine T10–L2: Flexion positioning

Patient sidelying

Rotation gliding thrust

- **Patient positioning:** Left sidelying with a small pillow or rolled towel placed under the patient's waist to introduce left sidebending in the thoracolumbar spine:

  - *Lower body.* Left hip flexed with knee extended. Right hip and knee flexed with patient's right foot behind the left calf

  - *Upper body.* Introduce right rotation of the patient's upper body until your palpating hand at T12–L1 begins to sense motion. Introduce flexion to the spine during this movement. Take up the axillary hold

- **Operator stance:** Stand close to the couch, feet spread and one leg behind the other. Maintain an upright posture, facing slightly in the direction of the patient's upper body

- **Positioning for thrust:** Place the palmar aspect of your left forearm against the patient's sacrum and posterior superior iliac spine. Rotate the patient's pelvis and lumbar spine towards you until motion is palpated at the T12–L1 segment. Rotate the patient's upper body away from you until a sense of tension is palpated at the T12–L1 segment. Roll the patient about 10° to 15° towards you

- **Adjustments to achieve appropriate prethrust tension**

- **Immediately prethrust:** Relax and adjust your balance

- **Delivering the thrust:** The direction of thrust is down towards the couch accompanied by exaggeration of pelvic rotation towards the operator (Fig. 10.16). Your right arm against the patient's axillary region does not apply a thrust but acts as a stabilizer only

Lumbar spine L1–5:
Neutral positioning

Patient sidelying

Rotation gliding thrust

Assume somatic dysfunction (S-T-A-R-T) is identified and you wish to use a rotation gliding thrust to produce cavitation at L3–4 on the right (Figs. 10.17, 10.18).

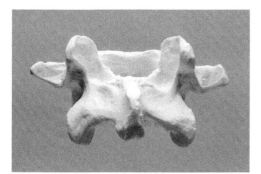

Figure 10.17

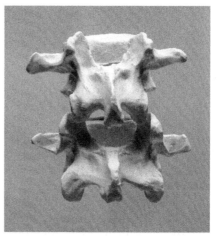

Figure 10.18

Key

✳ Stabilization

● Applicator

➡ Plane of thrust (operator)

⇨ Direction of body movement (patient)

Note: The dimensions for the arrows are not a pictorial representation of the amplitude or force of the thrust.

1. Patient positioning

Lying on the left side with a pillow to support the head and neck.

Lower body. Straighten the patient's lower leg and ensure that the leg and spine are in a straight line, in a neutral position. Flex the patient's upper hip and knee slightly and place the upper leg just anterior to the lower leg. The lower leg and spine should form as near a straight line as possible, with no flexion at the lower hip or knee.

Upper body. Gently extend the patient's upper shoulder and place the patient's right forearm on the lower ribs. Using your left hand to palpate the L3–4

251

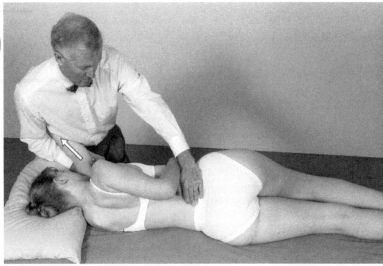

Figure 10.19

interspinous space, introduce right rotation of the patient's upper body down to the L3–4 segment. This is achieved by gently holding the patient's left elbow with your right hand and pulling it towards you, but also in a cephalad direction towards the head end of the couch (Fig. 10.19). Be careful not to introduce any flexion to the spine during this movement. Right rotation is continued until your palpating hand at the L3–4 segment begins to sense motion. Take up the axillary hold. This arm controls the upper body rotation.

2. **Operator stance**

Stand close to the couch with your feet spread and one leg behind the other (Fig. 10.20). Maintain an upright posture, facing slightly in the direction of the patient's upper body. Keep your left arm as close to your body as possible.

3. **Positioning for thrust**

Apply your left forearm to the region between the gluteus medius and the gluteus

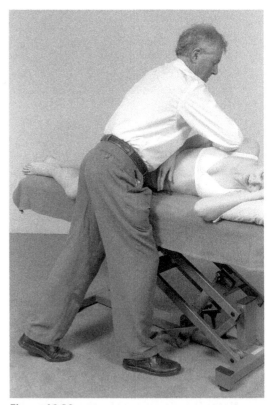

Figure 10.20

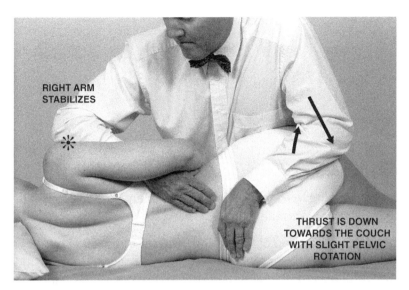

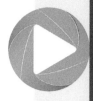

RIGHT ARM
STABILIZES

THRUST IS DOWN
TOWARDS THE COUCH
WITH SLIGHT PELVIC
ROTATION

Figure 10.21

maximus. Your left forearm now controls lower body rotation. Your right forearm should be resting against the patient's upper pectoral and rib cage region and will control upper body rotation. First, rotate the patient's pelvis and lumbar spine towards you until motion is palpated at the L3–4 segment. Rotate the patient's upper body away from you using your right arm until a sense of tension is palpated at the L3–4 segment. Be careful to avoid undue pressure in the axilla. Finally, roll the patient about 10° to 15° towards you while maintaining the build-up of leverages at the L3–4 segment.

4. Adjustments to achieve appropriate prethrust tension

Ensure your patient remains relaxed. Maintaining all holds, make any necessary changes in flexion, extension, sidebending or rotation until you can sense a state of appropriate tension and leverage at the L3–4 segment. The patient should not be aware of any pain or discomfort. Make these final adjustments by slight movements of the shoulders, trunk, ankles, knees and hips.

5. Immediately prethrust

Relax and adjust your balance as necessary. Keep your head up; looking down impedes the thrust. An effective HVLA thrust technique is best achieved if both the operator and patient are relaxed and not holding themselves rigid. This is a common impediment to achieving effective cavitation.

6. Delivering the thrust

Your right arm against the patient's pectoral region does not apply a thrust but acts as a stabilizer only. Keep the thrusting (left) arm as close to your body as possible. Apply an HVLA thrust with your left forearm against the patient's buttock. The direction of force is down towards the couch accompanied by slight exaggeration of pelvic rotation towards the operator (Fig. 10.21).

The thrust, although very rapid, must never be excessively forcible. The aim should be to use the absolute minimum force necessary to achieve joint cavitation. A common fault arises from the use of excessive amplitude with insufficient velocity of thrust.

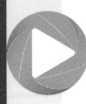

Summary

Lumbar spine L1–5: Neutral positioning

Patient sidelying

Rotation gliding thrust

- **Patient positioning:** Left sidelying:

  - *Lower body.* Left leg and spine in a straight line. Right hip and knee flexed slightly and placed just anterior to the lower leg

  - *Upper body.* Introduce right rotation of the patient's upper body until your palpating hand at L3–4 begins to sense motion. Do not introduce any flexion to the spine during this movement (Fig. 10.19). Take up the axillary hold

- **Operator stance:** Stand close to the couch, feet spread and one leg behind the other. Maintain an upright posture, facing slightly in the direction of the patient's upper body (Fig. 10.20)

- **Positioning for thrust:** Place your left forearm in the region between the gluteus medius and the gluteus maximus. Rotate the patient's pelvis and lumbar spine towards you until motion is palpated at the L3–4 segment. Rotate the patient's upper body away from you until a sense of tension is palpated at the L3–4 segment. Roll the patient about 10° to 15° towards you

- **Adjustments to achieve appropriate prethrust tension**

- **Immediately prethrust:** Relax and adjust your balance

- **Delivering the thrust:** The direction of thrust is down towards the couch accompanied by exaggeration of pelvic rotation towards the operator (Fig. 10.21). Your right arm against the patient's axillary region does not apply a thrust but acts as a stabilizer only

10.4

Lumbar spine L1–5:
Flexion positioning

Patient sidelying

Rotation gliding thrust

Assume somatic dysfunction (S-T-A-R-T) is identified and you wish to use a rotation gliding thrust to produce cavitation at L3–4 on the right (Figs. 10.22, 10.23).

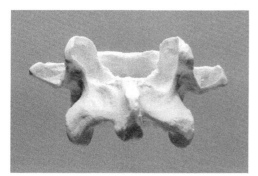

Figure 10.22

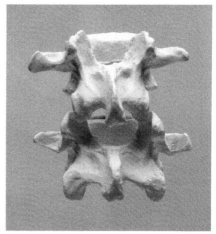

Figure 10.23

Key

✳ Stabilization

● Applicator

➡ Plane of thrust (operator)

⇨ Direction of body movement (patient)

Note: The dimensions for the arrows are not a pictorial representation of the amplitude or force of the thrust.

1. Patient positioning

Lying on the left side with a pillow to support the head and neck. A small pillow, or rolled towel, should be placed under the patient's waist to introduce left sidebending in the lumbar spine. Experienced practitioners may choose to achieve the left sidebending without the use of a small pillow or rolled towel.

Lower body. Straighten the patient's lower (left) leg at the knee joint while keeping the left hip flexed. Flex the patient's upper hip and knee. Rest the upper flexed knee upon the edge of the couch, anterior to the left thigh, and place the patient's right foot behind the left calf.

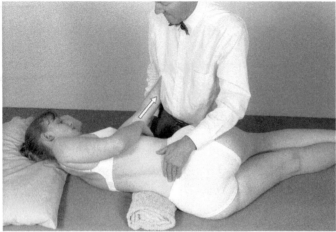

Figure 10.24

This position provides stability to the lower body.

Upper body. Gently extend the patient's upper shoulder and place the patient's right forearm on the lower ribs. Using your left hand to palpate the L3–4 interspinous space, introduce right rotation of the patient's upper body down to the L3–4 segment. Rotation with flexion positioning is achieved by gently holding the patient's left elbow with your right hand and pulling it towards you, but also in a caudad direction towards the foot end of the couch (Fig. 10.24). Right rotation is continued until your palpating hand at the L3–4 segment begins to sense motion. Take up the axillary hold. This arm controls the upper body rotation.

2. Operator stance

Stand close to the couch with your feet spread and one leg behind the other (Fig. 10.25). Maintain an upright posture, facing slightly in the direction of the patient's upper body. Keep your left arm as close to your body as possible.

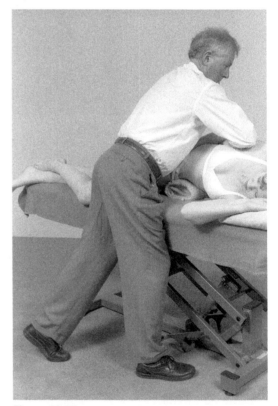

Figure 10.25

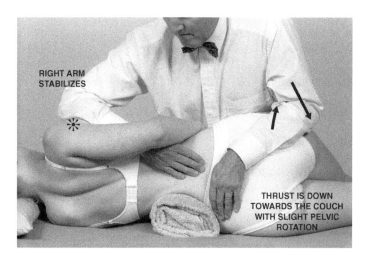

RIGHT ARM
STABILIZES

THRUST IS DOWN
TOWARDS THE COUCH
WITH SLIGHT PELVIC
ROTATION

Figure 10.26

3. Positioning for thrust

Apply your left forearm to the region
between the gluteus medius and the gluteus
maximus. Your left forearm now controls
lower body rotation. Your right forearm
should be resting against the patient's upper
pectoral and rib cage region and will control
upper body rotation. First, rotate the
patient's pelvis and lumbar spine towards
you until motion is palpated at the L3–4
segment. Rotate the patient's upper body
away from you using your right arm until a
sense of tension is palpated at the L3–4
segment. Be careful to avoid undue pressure
in the axilla. Finally, roll the patient about
10° to 15° towards you while maintaining
the build-up of leverages at the L3–4
segment.

4. Adjustments to achieve appropriate prethrust tension

Ensure your patient remains relaxed.
Maintaining all holds, make any necessary
changes in flexion, extension, sidebending
or rotation until you can sense a state of
appropriate tension and leverage at the
L3–4 segment. The patient should not be
aware of any pain or discomfort. Make these
final adjustments by slight movements of
the shoulders, trunk, ankles, knees and hips.

5. Immediately prethrust

Relax and adjust your balance as necessary.
Keep your head up; looking down impedes
the thrust. An effective HVLA thrust
technique is best achieved if both the
operator and patient are relaxed and not
holding themselves rigid. This is a common
impediment to achieving effective
cavitation.

6. Delivering the thrust

Your right arm against the patient's pectoral
region does not apply a thrust but acts as a
stabilizer only. Keep the thrusting (left) arm
as close to your body as possible. Apply an
HVLA thrust with your left forearm against
the patient's buttock. The direction of force
is down towards the couch accompanied by
a slight exaggeration of pelvic rotation
towards the operator (Fig. 10.26).

The thrust, although very rapid, must
never be excessively forcible. The aim
should be to use the absolute minimum
force necessary to achieve joint cavitation.
A common fault arises from the use of
excessive amplitude with insufficient
velocity of thrust.

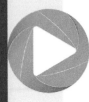

Summary

Lumbar spine L1–5: Flexion positioning

Patient sidelying

Rotation gliding thrust

- **Patient positioning:** Left sidelying with a small pillow or rolled towel placed under the patient's waist to introduce left sidebending in the lumbar spine:

  - *Lower body.* Left hip flexed with knee extended. Right hip and knee flexed with the patient's right foot behind the left calf

  - *Upper body.* Introduce right rotation of the patient's upper body until your palpating hand at L3–4 begins to sense motion. Introduce flexion to the spine during this movement (Fig. 10.24). Take up the axillary hold

- **Operator stance:** Stand close to the couch, feet spread and one leg behind the other. Maintain an upright posture, facing slightly in the direction of the patient's upper body (Fig. 10.25)

- **Positioning for thrust:** Place your left forearm in the region between the gluteus medius and the gluteus maximus. Rotate the patient's pelvis and lumbar spine towards you until motion is palpated at the L3–4 segment. Rotate the patient's upper body away from you until a sense of tension is palpated at the L3–4 segment. Roll the patient about 10° to 15° towards you

- **Adjustments to achieve appropriate prethrust tension**

- **Immediately prethrust:** Relax and adjust your balance

- **Delivering the thrust:** The direction of thrust is down towards the couch accompanied by exaggeration of pelvic rotation towards the operator (Fig. 10.26). Your right arm against the patient's axillary region does not apply a thrust but acts as a stabilizer only

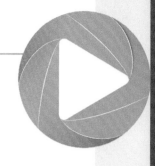

10.5

Lumbar spine L1–5:
Neutral positioning

Patient sitting

Rotation gliding thrust

Assume somatic dysfunction (S-T-A-R-T) is identified and you wish to use a rotation gliding thrust to produce cavitation at L3–4 on the left (Figs. 10.27, 10.28).

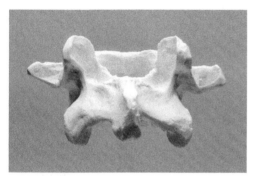

Figure 10.27

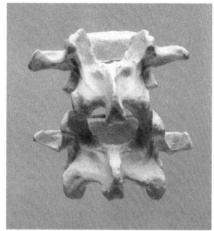

Figure 10.28

Key

❋ Stabilization

● Applicator

➡ Plane of thrust (operator)

⇨ Direction of body movement (patient)

Note: The dimensions for the arrows are not a pictorial representation of the amplitude or force of the thrust.

1. Patient positioning
Sitting on the treatment couch with the arms folded. The patient should be encouraged to maintain an erect posture.

2. Operator stance
Stand behind and slightly to the right of the patient with your feet spread. Pass your right arm across the front of the patient's chest to lightly grip the patient's left thorax (Fig. 10.29).

3. Positioning for thrust
Place your left hypothenar eminence to the right side of the spinous process of L3, and introduce right sidebending to the patient's

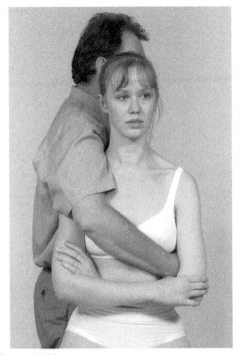

Figure 10.29

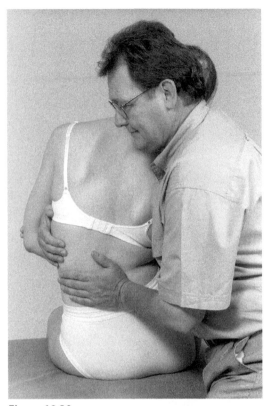

Figure 10.30

thoracic and upper lumbar spine
(Fig. 10.30). The thoracic and upper lumbar
spine is now rotated to the right to lock
the spine down to but not including L3–4.
The operator maintains as erect a posture
as possible. Keep your left hypothenar
eminence firmly applied to the spinous
process of L3 with your left arm held close
to your body.

4. Adjustments to achieve appropriate prethrust tension

Ensure your patient remains relaxed.
Maintaining all holds, make any necessary
changes in flexion, extension, sidebending
or rotation until you can sense a state of
appropriate tension and leverage at the
L3–4 segment. The patient should not be
aware of any pain or discomfort. Make these
final adjustments by slight movements of
the shoulders, trunk, ankles, knees and hips.

5. Immediately prethrust

Relax and adjust your balance as necessary.
An effective HVLA thrust technique is best
achieved if both the operator and patient
are relaxed and not holding themselves
rigid. This is a common impediment to
achieving effective cavitation.

6. Delivering the thrust

A degree of momentum is necessary to
achieve a successful cavitation. It is desirable
for the momentum component of the thrust
to be restricted to one plane of motion, and
this should be rotation. Rock the patient
into and out of rotation while maintaining
the sidebending and flexion/extension
positioning. When close to full rotation,
you will sense a state of appropriate tension

and leverage at the L3–4 segment, at which point you apply an HVLA thrust against the spinous process of L3. The thrust is directed to the spinous process of L3 and accompanied by a slight exaggeration of right rotation (Fig. 10.31).

The thrust, although very rapid, must never be excessively forcible. The aim should be to use the absolute minimum force necessary to achieve joint cavitation. A common fault arises from the use of excessive amplitude with insufficient velocity of thrust.

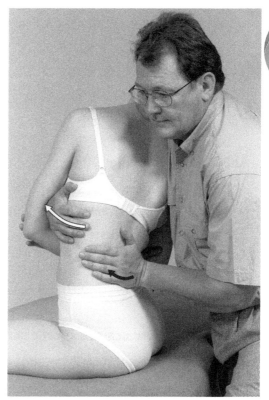

Figure 10.31

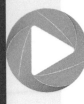

Summary

Lumbar spine L1–5: Neutral positioning

Patient sitting

Rotation gliding thrust

- **Patient positioning:** Sitting erect

- **Operator stance:** Behind and slightly to the right of the patient with your right arm across the front of the patient's chest (Fig. 10.29)

- **Positioning for thrust:** Place your left hypothenar eminence to the right side of the spinous process of L3, and introduce right sidebending to the patient's thoracic and upper lumbar spine (Fig. 10.30). The thoracic and upper lumbar spine is now rotated to the right to lock the spine down to but not including L3–4

- **Adjustments to achieve appropriate prethrust tension**

- **Immediately prethrust:** Relax and adjust your balance

- **Delivering the thrust:** The thrust is directed to the spinous process of L3 and accompanied by exaggeration of right rotation (Fig. 10.31). A degree of momentum is necessary to achieve a successful cavitation. The momentum component of the thrust should be in the direction of rotation

10.6

Lumbosacral joint (L5–S1):
Neutral positioning

Patient sidelying

Thrust direction is dependent on apophysial joint plane*

Assume somatic dysfunction (S-T-A-R-T) is identified and you wish to use a gliding thrust to produce cavitation at L5–S1 on the right (Figs. 10.32, 10.33).

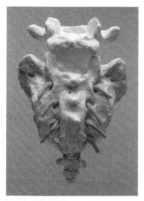

Figure 10.32

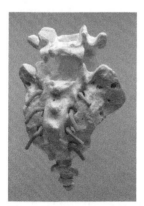

Figure 10.33

Key

❋ Stabilization

● Applicator

➡ Plane of thrust (operator)

⇨ Direction of body movement (patient)

Note: The dimensions for the arrows are not a pictorial representation of the amplitude or force of the thrust.

---

*The condition where joints are asymmetrically orientated is referred to as articular tropism. The lumbosacral zygapophysial joints would normally be orientated at approximately 45° with respect to the sagittal plane. There is considerable individual variation, and you will encounter patients with lumbosacral apophysial joint planes that range between sagittal and coronal orientation. The variation in apophysial joint plane means that considerable palpatory skill is required to localize forces accurately at the lumbosacral joint and to determine the most suitable direction of thrust.

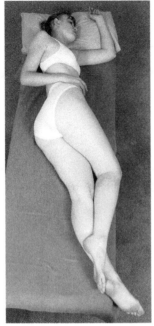

Figure 10.34

1. **Patient positioning**

Lying on the left side with a pillow to support the head and neck.

Lower body. Straighten the patient's lower (left) leg at the knee joint while placing the left hip in approximately 20° of flexion. Flex the patient's upper knee, and place the patient's right foot behind the left lower leg (Fig. 10.34). This position provides stability to the lower body.

Upper body. Gently extend the patient's upper shoulder and place the patient's right forearm on the lower ribs. Using your left hand to palpate the L5–S1 interspinous space, introduce right rotation of the patient's upper body down to the L5–S1 segment. This is achieved by gently holding the patient's left elbow with your right hand and pulling it towards you, but also in a cephalad direction towards the head end of the couch. Be careful not to introduce any flexion to the spine during this movement. Right rotation is continued until your palpating hand at the L5–S1 segment begins to sense motion. Take up the axillary hold. This arm controls the upper body rotation.

2. **Operator stance**

Stand close to the couch with your feet spread and one leg behind the other. Maintain an upright posture, facing slightly in the direction of the patient's upper body. Keep your left arm as close to your body as possible.

3. **Positioning for thrust**

Apply your left forearm to the region between the gluteus medius and the gluteus maximus. Your left forearm now controls lower body rotation. Your right forearm rests on the patient's right axillary area. This will control upper body rotation. First, apply pressure to the patient's pelvis until motion is palpated at the L5–S1 segment. Rotate the patient's upper body away from you using your right arm until a sense of tension is palpated at the L5–S1 segment. Finally, roll the patient about 10° to 15° towards you while maintaining the build-up of leverages at the L5–S1 segment.

4. **Adjustments to achieve appropriate prethrust tension**

Ensure your patient remains relaxed. Maintaining all holds, make any necessary changes in flexion, extension, sidebending or rotation until you can sense a state of appropriate tension and leverage at the L5–S1 segment. The patient should not be aware of any pain or discomfort. Make these final adjustments by slight movements of the shoulders, trunk, ankles, knees and hips.

5. **Immediately prethrust**

Relax and adjust your balance as necessary. Keep your head up; looking down impedes the thrust. An effective HVLA thrust technique is best achieved if both the operator and patient are relaxed and not

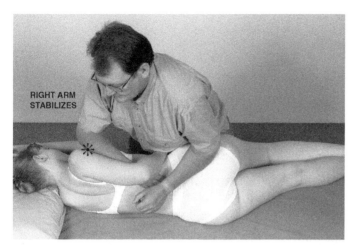

RIGHT ARM
STABILIZES

Figure 10.35

holding themselves rigid. This is a common impediment to achieving effective cavitation.

6. Delivering the thrust

Your right arm against the patient's axillary region does not apply a thrust but acts as a stabilizer only (Fig. 10.35). Keep the thrusting (left) arm as close to your body as possible. Apply an HVLA thrust with your left forearm against the patient's buttock. The direction of thrust is variable depending on the apophysial joint plane. Commonly the direction of thrust approximates to a line along the long axis of the patient's right femur (Fig. 10.36).

The thrust, although very rapid, must never be excessively forcible. The aim should be to use the absolute minimum force necessary to achieve joint cavitation. A common fault arises from the use of excessive amplitude with insufficient velocity of thrust.

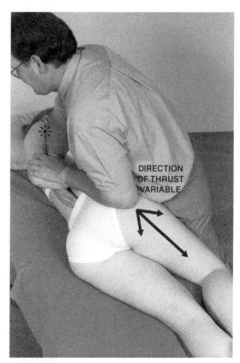

DIRECTION
OF THRUST
VARIABLE

Figure 10.36

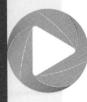

Summary

Lumbosacral Joint (L5–S1): Neutral positioning

Patient sidelying

Thrust direction is dependent on apophysial joint plane

- **Patient positioning:** Left sidelying:
  - *Lower body.* Left hip in approximately 20° of flexion with knee extended. Right hip and knee flexed (Fig. 10.34)
  - *Upper body.* Introduce right rotation of the patient's upper body until your palpating hand at the L5–S1 segment begins to sense motion. Do not introduce any flexion to the spine during this movement. Take up the axillary hold

- **Operator stance:** Stand close to the couch, feet spread and one leg behind the other. Maintain an upright posture, facing slightly in the direction of the patient's upper body

- **Positioning for thrust:** Place your left forearm in the region between the gluteus medius and the gluteus maximus. Apply pressure to the patient's pelvis until motion is palpated at the L5–S1 segment. Rotate the patient's upper body away from you until a sense of tension is palpated at the L5–S1 segment. Roll the patient about 10° to 15° towards you

- **Adjustments to achieve appropriate prethrust tension**

- **Immediately prethrust:** Relax and adjust your balance

- **Delivering the thrust:** Your right arm against the patient's axillary region does not apply a thrust but acts as a stabilizer only (Fig. 10.35). The direction of thrust is variable depending on the apophysial joint plane. Commonly, the thrust is along the long axis of the patient's right femur (Fig. 10.36)

10.7

Lumbosacral joint (L5–S1):
Flexion positioning

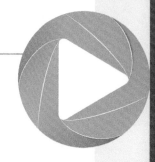

Patient sidelying

Thrust direction is dependent on apophysial joint plane*

Assume somatic dysfunction (S-T-A-R-T) is identified and you wish to use a gliding thrust to produce cavitation at L5–S1 on the right (Figs. 10.37, 10.38).

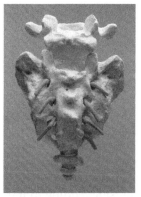

Figure 10.37

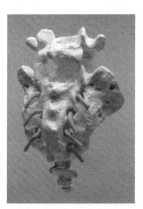

Figure 10.38

Key

☀ Stabilization

● Applicator

➡ Plane of thrust (operator)

⇨ Direction of body movement (patient)

Note: The dimensions for the arrows are not a pictorial representation of the amplitude or force of the thrust.

---

*The condition where joints are asymmetrically orientated is referred to as articular tropism. The lumbosacral zygapophysial joints would normally be orientated at approximately 45° with respect to the sagittal plane. There is considerable individual variation, and you will encounter patients with lumbosacral apophysial joint planes that range between sagittal and coronal orientation. The variation in apophysial joint plane means that considerable palpatory skill is required to localize forces accurately at the lumbosacral joint and to determine the most suitable direction of thrust.

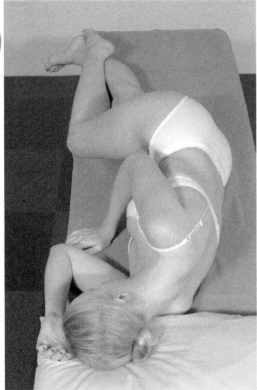

Figure 10.39

1. Patient positioning

Lying on the left side with a pillow to support the head and neck.

Lower body. Straighten the patient's lower (left) leg at the knee joint while placing the left hip in approximately 20° of flexion. Flex the patient's upper knee and place the patient's right foot behind the left lower leg (Fig. 10.39). This position provides stability to the lower body.

Upper body. Gently extend the patient's upper shoulder and place the patient's right forearm on the lower ribs. Using your left hand to palpate the L5–S1 interspinous space, introduce right rotation of the patient's upper body down to the L5–S1 segment. Rotation with flexion positioning is achieved by gently holding the patient's left elbow with your right hand and pulling it

towards you, but also in a caudad direction towards the foot end of the couch. Right rotation is continued until your palpating hand at the L5–S1 segment begins to sense motion. Take up the axillary hold. This arm controls the upper body rotation.

2. Operator stance

Stand close to the couch with your feet spread and one leg behind the other. Maintain an upright posture, facing slightly in the direction of the patient's upper body. Keep your left arm as close to your body as possible.

3. Positioning for thrust

Apply your left forearm to the region between the gluteus medius and the gluteus maximus. Your left forearm now controls lower body rotation. Your right forearm rests on the patient's right axillary area. This will control upper body rotation. First, apply pressure to the patient's pelvis until motion is palpated at the L5–S1 segment. Introduce left sidebending to lumbar spine by applying pressure with the left forearm to the patient's pelvis in a caudad direction (Fig. 10.40). Now rotate the patient's upper body away from you using your right arm until a sense of tension is palpated at the L5–S1 segment. Finally, roll the patient about 10° to 15° towards you while maintaining the build-up of leverages at the L5–S1 segment.

4. Adjustments to achieve appropriate prethrust tension

Ensure your patient remains relaxed. Maintaining all holds, make any necessary changes in flexion, extension, sidebending or rotation until you can sense a state of appropriate tension and leverage at the L5–S1 segment. The patient should not be aware of any pain or discomfort. Make these final adjustments by slight movements of the shoulders, trunk, ankles, knees and hips.

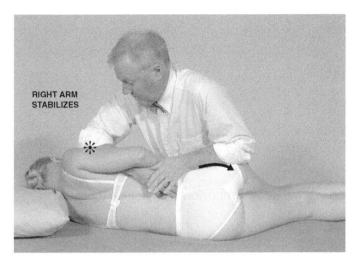

RIGHT ARM
STABILIZES

Figure 10.40

5. Immediately prethrust

Relax and adjust your balance as necessary. Keep your head up; looking down impedes the thrust. An effective HVLA thrust technique is best achieved if both the operator and patient are relaxed and not holding themselves rigid. This is a common impediment to achieving effective cavitation.

6. Delivering the thrust

Your right arm against the patient's axillary region does not apply a thrust but acts as a stabilizer only. Keep the thrusting (left) arm as close to your body as possible and maintain the left lumbar sidebending leverage. Apply an HVLA thrust with your left forearm against the patient's buttock. The direction of thrust is variable depending on the apophysial joint plane. Commonly the direction of thrust approximates to a line along the long axis of the patient's right femur (Fig. 10.41).

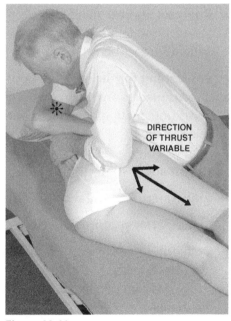

DIRECTION
OF THRUST
VARIABLE

Figure 10.41

The thrust, although very rapid, must never be excessively forcible. The aim should be to use the absolute minimum of force necessary to achieve joint cavitation. A common fault arises from the use of excessive amplitude with insufficient velocity of thrust.

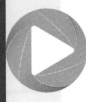

Summary

Lumbosacral joint (L5–S1): Flexion positioning

Patient sidelying

Thrust direction is dependent on apophysial joint plane

- **Patient positioning:** Left sidelying:

  - *Lower body.* Left hip in approximately 20° of flexion with knee extended. Right hip and knee flexed (Fig. 10.39)

  - *Upper body.* Introduce right rotation of the patient's upper body until your palpating hand at the L5–S1 segment begins to sense motion. Introduce flexion to the spine during this movement. Take up the axillary hold

- **Operator stance:** Stand close to the couch, feet spread and one leg behind the other. Maintain an upright posture, facing slightly in the direction of the patient's upper body

- **Positioning for thrust:** Place your left forearm in the region between the gluteus medius and the gluteus maximus. Apply pressure to the patient's pelvis until motion is palpated at the L5–S1 segment. Sidebend the lumbar spine to the left (Fig. 10.40), and then rotate the patient's upper body away from you until a sense of tension is palpated at the L5–S1 segment. Roll the patient about 10° to 15° towards you

- **Adjustments to achieve appropriate prethrust tension**

- **Immediately prethrust:** Relax and adjust your balance

- **Delivering the thrust:** Your right arm against the patient's axillary region does not apply a thrust but acts as a stabilizer only. It is critical to maintain left lumbar sidebending when delivering the thrust. The direction of thrust is variable depending on the apophysial joint plane. Commonly, the thrust is along the long axis of the patient's right femur (Fig. 10.41)

Pelvis

INTRODUCTION

The sacroiliac joint (SIJ) as a source of pain and dysfunction is a subject of controversy.[1-8] Many authors implicate the SIJ as a cause of low back pain,[6-22] but there is disagreement as to the exact prevalence of SIJ pain within the population with low back pain. It is estimated that 5% to 25% of chronic low back pain may involve the SIJ.[7,16,18,23] The pain referral patterns of the SIJ are extremely variable.[24] Pain originating in the SIJ is predominantly perceived in the gluteal region, although pain is often referred into the upper and lower lumbar region, groin, abdomen and lower limbs.[22] Dysfunctional upper segments of the SIJ have been reported to be associated with pain in the upper buttock and lower segments with pain in the lower buttock.[25] Evidence supports both intraarticular and extraarticular causes for SIJ pain.[24] However, no single historical, physical examination or radiological feature can definitively establish a diagnosis of SIJ pain.[7,24] Radiological imaging is important to exclude red flags but contributes little to the diagnosis of mechanical low back pain arising from the SIJ. Diagnostic blocks have been reported to be the diagnostic gold standard but must be interpreted with caution because false-positive as well as false-negative results occur frequently.[22] Although many practitioners believe the SIJ is a source of

pain and dysfunction and treat perceived sacroiliac lesions, there is no general agreement concerning the different diagnostic tests and their validity in determining somatic dysfunction of the pelvis (Fig. 11.1).[18,26-38] Assessment of the SIJ in the male population may be confounded by joint fusion, which is present in 5.8% of males up to the age of 39 years increasing to 46.7% of males over 80 years of age.[39]

A large number of diagnostic tests exist to evaluate the SIJ. Motion tests and static palpation of bony landmarks have generally shown poor interobserver reliability. The absence of objective indicators of mechanical dysfunction of the SIJ and poor reliability of motion dysfunction tests used to detect it make sacroiliac dysfunction difficult to validate.[8] Pain provocation tests

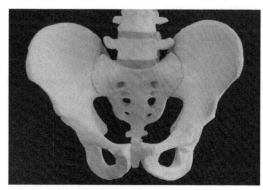

Figure 11.1 The pelvic girdle.

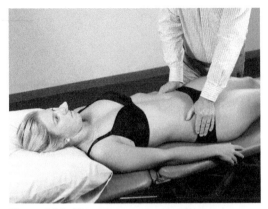

Figure 11.2 Distraction provocation SIJ test.

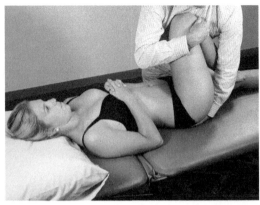

Figure 11.3 Right-sided thigh thrust provocation SIJ test.

have shown better reliability,[40] with clusters of pain provocation tests showing even greater reliability.[40-44] Arab et al[45] suggested that composites of motion palpation and provocation tests may be useful in clinical practice. Laslett[46] suggested that the combination of noncentralization of pain on repeated trunk movements with three or more SIJ provocation tests that reproduce the patient's familiar pain might help differentiate SIJ pain from other painful conditions. Laslett[46] also commented that centralization of symptoms with repeated movement testing in the lumbar spine is highly specific to discogenic pain and positive provocation SIJ tests in these patients should be ignored.

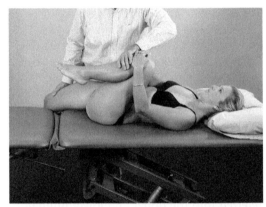

Figure 11.4 Right-sided Gaenslen's provocation SIJ test.

SACROILIAC PAIN PROVOCATION TESTS

The patient lies supine for the distraction provocation SIJ test (Fig. 11.2). The operator applies a vertically oriented, posteriorly directed force to both the anterior superior iliac spines. The test is positive if it reproduces the patient's familiar symptoms.

The patient lies supine for the right-sided thigh thrust provocation SIJ test. The operator stands on the left side of the patient. The operator flexes the patient's right hip and knee to 90 degrees and places

one hand under the sacrum (Fig. 11.3). The operator then applies axial pressure along the length of the patient's right femur in a posterior direction. The test is positive if it reproduces the patient's familiar symptoms.

The patient lies supine with the leg of the painful side resting on the edge of the treatment table for the right-sided Gaenslen's provocation SIJ test. The operator stands on the right side of the patient. The operator flexes the patient's left hip and knee and the patient is requested to hold the leg in this position with both hands (Fig. 11.4). The operator applies a downwards force to the right leg putting it into hyperextension at the hip, while a

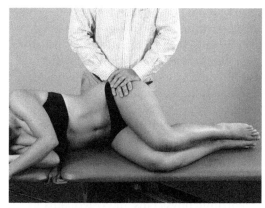

Figure 11.5 Compression provocation SIJ test.

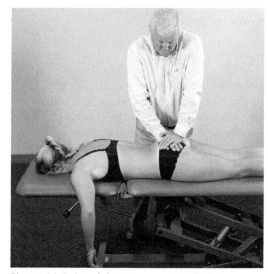

Figure 11.6 Sacral thrust provocation SIJ test.

flexion counterforce is applied to the patient's left hip. The test is positive if it reproduces the patient's familiar symptoms.

The patient is in the sidelying position with both hips and knees flexed for the compression provocation SIJ test (Fig. 11.5). The operator stands behind the patient. The operator places both hands over the upper part of the iliac crest and applies a force on the uppermost iliac crest vertically downwards towards the floor. The test is positive if it reproduces the patient's familiar symptoms.

The patient lies prone for the sacral thrust provocation SIJ test (Fig. 11.6). The operator places one hand directly over the centre of the sacrum and reinforces with the other hand. A force vertically downwards towards the floor is applied on the centre of the sacrum. The test is positive if it reproduces the patient's familiar symptoms.

In a study of 46 patients in whom SIJ arthropathy had been confirmed by infiltration of the SIJ under fluoroscopic guidance, Werner et al[47] reported that a new posterior superior iliac spine (PSIS) distraction provocation test was found to be of high sensitivity, specificity and accuracy. The test consisted of a medial to lateral impulse with the operator's thumb against the medial border of the PSIS and is performed with the patient standing or prone. The test was described as positive if the patient reported the production of new or aggravation of pain. Further clinical and research exploration needs to occur before the clinical utility of this test can be evaluated.

Some authors[21,48] have questioned whether the SIJ pain provocation tests can accurately identify a painful SIJ because forces are transmitted to a range of pain generating structures other than the SIJ, including the lateral branches of the dorsal sacral rami and the posterior sacrococcygeal plexus.

Various models of sacroiliac motion have been proposed, and there have been a number of studies relating to mobility in the SIJ,[49-56] but the precise nature of normal motion remains unclear.[1,4,19,57,58] There is significant variation in SIJ movement both between individuals and within individuals when mobility of one SIJ is compared with the other side.[51] Mobility alters with age and can increase during pregnancy.

At our present state of knowledge, what model should guide our clinical decision making to incorporate high-velocity low-amplitude (HVLA) thrust techniques within a treatment regimen for somatic dysfunction

---

Box 11.1 Pelvic girdle dysfunctions

PUBIS
- Superior
- Inferior

SACROILIAC
- Bilaterally nutated anteriorly
- Bilaterally nutated posteriorly
- Unilaterally nutated anteriorly (sacrum flexed)
- Unilaterally nutated posteriorly (sacrum extended)
- Torsioned anteriorly (left on left or right on right)
- Torsioned posteriorly (left on right or right on left)

ILIOSACRAL
- Rotated anteriorly
- Rotated posteriorly
- Superior (cephalic) shear
- Inferior (caudad) shear
- Rotated medially (inflare)
- Rotated laterally (outflare)

Reproduced with permission from Greenman.[62]

---

of the pelvis? There are a number of different biomechanical models used to determine the nature of any pelvic dysfunction.[59-63] These vary from very complex to less complex, with no research evidence as to their clinical utility. Greenman[62] described a number of possible pelvic girdle dysfunctions, which are listed in Box 11.1.

Web-based surveys in the United Kingdom and the United States revealed that both osteopaths and osteopathic physicians used a wide range of manual treatment techniques in the management of sacroiliac somatic dysfunction. In the survey of osteopathic physicians in the United States, Fryer et al[64] reported that the most commonly used treatment techniques were muscle energy (70%), myofascial release (67%), patient self-stretches (66%), osteopathy in the cranial field (59%),

muscle strengthening exercises (58%), soft tissue technique (58%) and articulatory technique (53%). In the survey of British osteopaths, Fryer et al[65] found a higher use of HVLA thrust techniques for sacroiliac somatic dysfunction and reported that the most commonly used treatment techniques by British osteopaths were joint articulation (91%), soft tissue technique (91%), patient self-stretches (76%) and HVLA thrust techniques (74%).

If HVLA thrust techniques are used by osteopathic physicians and osteopaths to treat pelvic pain and dysfunction, they are usually combined with other nonthrust osteopathic techniques in a multimodal treatment approach.

COCCYDYNIA

Coccydynia is the term used to describe pain in the coccygeal region. Despite its small size, the coccyx has several important functions. It serves as one leg of the tripod – along with the ischial tuberosities – that provides weight-bearing support in the sitting position along with being the insertion site for the anterior and posterior sacrococcygeal ligaments, the anococcygeal ligaments and the levator ani muscles. The most common cause of coccydynia is trauma as a result of falling on the buttocks, repetitive microtrauma or childbirth,[66-69] but in up to 30% of patients the cause is unknown.[69] Coccydynia is almost three times more common in patients with ankylosing spondylitis than in patients with nonspecific chronic low back pain.[69]

The diagnosis of coccydynia is based on patient history (Box 11.2) and clinical examination (Box 11.3).

Lateral sacral radiographs and dynamic radiographs may also aid in the diagnosis of coccydynia by examining the shape and movement of the coccyx.[70]

Some cases of coccydynia resolve without treatment, but for refractory cases treatments include nonsteroidal antiinflammatory

Box 11.2 Coccydynia: History

- History of direct coccygeal trauma
- Localized and persistent pain in sacrococcygeal region without significant low back pain or pain radiation
- Local pain on sitting
- Pain may be exacerbated rising from sitting
- Local pain on passing stool and/or sexual intercourse

Box 11.3 Coccydynia: Examination findings

- Localized coccygeal tenderness
- May be aberrant position of coccyx
- May be reproduction of symptoms on springing coccyx externally

drugs, ring-shaped cushions, pelvic floor rehabilitation, intrarectal massage and manipulation, transcutaneous electrical nerve stimulation, injections, psychotherapy, nerve blocks, spinal cord stimulation and surgery.[71,72]

Coccydynia can be treated by manual therapists either externally or internally. A number of cases of coccydynia are nonresponsive to external techniques and may benefit from the use of an intrarectal approach.

There is limited research evidence regarding the effectiveness of intrarectal mobilization or manipulation in the treatment of coccydynia. The following studies have examined the use of intrarectal manipulation for coccydynia: intrarectal manipulation with massage,[73] intrarectal manipulation with massage and diathermy,[74] intrarectal manipulation with phonophoresis, transcutaneous electrical nerve stimulation and analgesics.[75] All these studies reported a significant decrease in pain. Howard et al[76] undertook a systematic review of conservative interventions and

their effectiveness for coccydynia. They reported that more high-quality research is needed to determine the effectiveness and applicability of manipulation and mobilization in the treatment of coccydynia.

A number of manual medicine texts[60,62,77–82] refer to the use of HVLA thrust techniques to the SIJs, but there is little evidence that cavitation is uniformly associated with these procedures. When an audible release does occur, its site of origin remains open to speculation. Studies undertaken to measure the effects of manipulation upon the SIJs provide contradictory findings. Roentgen stereophotogrammetric analysis was unable to detect altered position of the SIJ postmanipulation despite normalization of different types of clinical tests.[83] However, an alteration in pelvic tilt was identified postmanipulation in one study of patients with low back pain[84] and a further study demonstrated an immediate improvement in iliac crest symmetry immediately after manipulation.[85] A review of the literature does not reveal any randomized controlled trials investigating the use of HVLA thrust techniques for sacroiliac pain and dysfunction.

However, many practitioners believe that HVLA thrust techniques applied to the SIJ can be associated with good clinical outcomes. As a result, many clinicians continue to use HVLA thrust techniques to treat somatic dysfunction of the SIJ.

Somatic dysfunction is identified by the S-T-A-R-T of diagnosis:
- **S** relates to symptom reproduction.
- **T** relates to tissue tenderness.
- **A** relates to asymmetry.
- **R** relates to range of motion.
- **T** relates to tissue texture changes.

The remainder of Chapter 11 describes in detail four HVLA thrust techniques for the SIJ and one mobilization/thrust technique for the sacrococcygeal joint. All the techniques are described using a variable-height manipulation couch.

After making a diagnosis of somatic dysfunction and before proceeding with a mobilization or thrust, it is recommended the following checklist be used for each of the techniques described in this chapter:

- Have I excluded all contraindications?
- Have I explained to the patient what I am going to do?
- Do I have informed consent?
- Is the patient well positioned and comfortable? (minimal leverage positioning)
- Am I in a comfortable and balanced position?
- Do I need to modify any prethrust physical or biomechanical factors? (Refer to Box C3, Part C)
- Have I achieved appropriate prethrust tissue tension? (not end-range)
- Am I relaxed and confident to proceed?
- Is the patient relaxed and willing for me to proceed?

References

1 Alderink GJ. The sacroiliac joint: Review of anatomy, mechanics, and function. J Orthop Sports Phys Ther 1991;13:71–84.

2 Bernard TN, Cassidy JD. The sacroiliac joint syndrome – pathophysiology, diagnosis and management. In: Frymoyer JW ed. The adult spine: Principles and practice. New York, NY: Raven Press; 1991 2107–30.

3 Walker JM. The sacroiliac joint: A critical review. Phys Ther 1992;72:903–16.

4 Dreyfuss P, Cole AJ, Pauza K. Sacroiliac joint injection techniques. Phys Med Rehabil Clin North Am 1995;6(4):785–813.

5 Cibulka M. Understanding sacroiliac joint movement as a guide to the management of a patient with unilateral low back pain. Man Ther 2002;7(4):215–21.

6 Brolinson P, Kozar A, Cibor G. Sacroiliac joint dysfunction in athletes. Curr Sports Med Rep 2003;2(1):47–56.

7 Simopoulos TT, Manchikanti L, Singh V, et al. A systematic evaluation of prevalence and diagnostic accuracy of sacroiliac joint interventions. Pain Physician 2012;15(3): E305–44.

8 Fryer G. Muscle energy technique: An evidence-informed approach. Int J Osteopath Med 2011;14(1):3–9.

9 Grieve G. The sacroiliac joint. Physiotherapy 1976;62:384–400.

10 Weismantel A. Evaluation and treatment of sacroiliac joint problems. J Am Phys Ther Assoc 1978;3(1):1–9.

11 Mitchell F. The muscle energy manual, vol. 1. East Lansing, MI: MET Press; 1995.

12 DonTigny RL. Function and pathomechanics of the sacroiliac joint. Phys Ther 1985;65:35–43.

13 Bernard TN, Kirkaldy-Willis WH. Recognizing specific characteristics of nonspecific low back pain. Clin Orthop 1987;217:266–80.

14 Bourdillon JF, Day EA. Boohhout MR. Spinal manipulation, 5th edn. Avon: Bath Press; 1995.

15 Shaw JL. The role of the sacroiliac joint as a cause of low back pain and dysfunction. First Interdisciplinary World Congress on Low Back Pain and its Relation to the Sacroiliac Joint. Rotterdam: ECO; 1992.

16 Schwarzer AC, Aprill CN, Bogduk N. The sacroiliac joint in chronic low back pain. Spine 1995;20:31–7.

17 Herzog W. Clinical biomechanics of spinal manipulation. New York: Churchill Livingstone; 2000.

18 Maigne JY, Aivaliklis A, Pfefer F. Results of sacroiliac joint double block and value of sacroiliac pain provocation tests in 54 patients with low back pain. Spine 1996;21(16):1889–92.

19 Foley B, Buschbacher R. Sacroiliac joint pain: Anatomy, biomechanics, diagnosis, and treatment. Am J Phys Med Rehabil 2006;85(12):997–1006.

20 Forst S, Wheeler M, Fortin J, et al. The sacroiliac joint: Anatomy, physiology and clinical significance. Pain Physician 2006;9(1):61–7.

21 Hansen H, McKenzie-Brown A, Cohen S, et al. Sacroiliac joint interventions: A systematic review. Pain Physician 2007;10(1):165–84.

22 Vanelderen P, Szadek K, Cohen SP, et al. Sacroiliac joint pain. Pain Pract 2010;10(5): 470–8.

23 Hansen H, Helm S. Sacroiliac joint pain and dysfunction. Pain Physician 2003;6(2): 179–89.

24 Cohen SP, Chen Y, Neufeld NJ. Sacroiliac joint pain: A comprehensive review of epidemiology, diagnosis and treatment. Expert Rev Neurother 2013;13(1):99–116.

25 Kurosawa D, Murakami E, Aizawa T. Referred pain location depends on the affected segment of the sacroiliac joint. Eur Spine J 2014;24(3): 521–7.

26 Speed C. ABC of rheumatology. Low back pain. BMJ 2004;328:1119–21.

27 Carmichael JP. Inter and intra-examiner reliability of palpation for sacroiliac joint dysfunction. J Manipulative Physiol Ther 1987;10:164–71.

28 Dreyfuss P, Dreyer S, Griffin J, et al. Positive sacroiliac screening tests in asymptomatic adults. Spine 1994;19:1138–43.

29 Dreyfuss P, Michaelsen M, Pauza K, et al. The value of medical history and physical examination in diagnosing sacroiliac joint pain. Spine 1996;21:2594–602.

30 Herzog W, Read L, Conway P, et al. Reliability of motion palpation procedures to detect sacro-iliac joint fixations. J Manipulative Physiol Ther 1988;11:151–7.

31 Laslett M, Williams M. The reliability of selected pain provocation tests for sacroiliac joint pathology. Spine 1994;19:1243–9.

32 Van Deursen LLJM, Patijn J, Ockhuysen AL, et al. The value of some clinical tests of the sacro-iliac joint. Man Med 1990;5:96–9.

33 Riddle D, Freburger J. Evaluation of the presence of sacroiliac joint region dysfunction using a combination of tests: A multicenter intertester reliability study. Phys Ther 2002;82(8): 772–81.

34 Young S, Aprill C, Laslett M. Correlation of clinical examination characteristics with three sources of chronic low back pain. Spine 2003;3(6):460–5.

35 Meijne W, van Neerbos K, Aufdemkampe G, et al. Intraexaminer and interexaminer reliability of the Gillet test. J Manipulative Physiol Ther 1999;22(1):4–9.

36 Sturesson B, Uden A, Vleeming A. A radiostereometric analysis of the movements of the sacroiliac joints during the standing hip flexion test. Spine 2000;25(3):364–8.

37 Vincent-Smith B, Gibbons P. Inter-examiner and intra-examiner reliability of palpatory findings for the standing flexion test. Man Ther 1999;4(2):87–93.

38 O'Haire C, Gibbons P. Inter-examiner and intra-examiner agreement for assessing sacro-iliac anatomical landmarks using palpation and observation: A pilot study. Man Ther 2000;5(1): 13–20.

39 Dar G, Khamis S, Peleg S, et al. Sacroiliac joint fusion and the implications for manual therapy diagnosis and treatment. Man Ther 2008;13(2): 155–8.

40 Laslett M, Aprill C, McDonald B, et al. Diagnosis of sacroiliac joint pain: Validity of individual provocation tests and composites of tests. Man Ther 2005;10(3):207–18.

41 Kokmeyer D, van der Wurff P, et al. The reliability of multitest regimens with sacroiliac pain provocation tests. J Manipulative Physiol Ther 2002;25(1):42–8.

42 van der Wurff P, Buijs E, Groen G. A multitest regimen of pain provocation tests as an aid to reduce unnecessary minimally invasive sacroiliac joint procedures. Arch Phys Med Rehabil 2006;87(1):10–14.

43 Robinson H, Brox J, Robinson R, et al. The reliability of selected motion and pain provocation tests for the sacroiliac joint. Man Ther 2007;12(1):72–9.

44 Hancock MJ, Maher CG, Latimer J, et al. Systematic review of tests to identify the disc, SIJ or facet joint as the source of low back pain. Eur Spine J 2007;16(10):1539–50.

45 Arab A, Abdollahi I, Joghataei T, et al. Inter- and intra-examiner reliability of single and composites of selected motion palpation and pain provocation tests for sacroiliac joint. Man Ther 2009;14(2):213–21.

46 Laslett M. Pain provocation tests for diagnosis of sacroiliac joint pain. Aust J Physiother 2006;52(3):229.

47 Werner CM, Hoch A, Gautier L, et al. Distraction test of the posterior superior iliac spine (PSIS) in the diagnosis of sacroiliac arthropathy. BMC Surg 2013;13:52.

48 McGrath MC. Composite sacroiliac joint pain provocation tests: A question of clinical significance. Int J Osteopath Med 2010;13(1): 24–30.

49 Colachis SC, Worden RE, Brechtol CO, et al. Movement of the sacroiliac joint in the adult male: A preliminary report. Arch Phys Med Rehabil 1963;44:490–8.

50 Egund N, Olsson TH, Schmid H, et al. Movements in the sacroiliac joints demonstrated with Roentgen stereophotogrammetry. Acta Radiol Diagn 1978;19:833–46.

51 Sturesson B, Selvik G, Uden A. Movements of the sacroiliac joints. A Roentgen stereophotogrammetric analysis. Spine 1989;14:162–5.

52 Jacob H, Kissling R. The mobility of the sacroiliac joints in healthy volunteers between 20 and 50 years of age. Clin Biomechanics 1995;10(7):352–61.

53 Kissling R, Jacob H. The mobility of the sacroiliac joint in healthy subjects. Bull Hosp Jt Dis 1996;54(3):158–64.

54 Lund P, Krupinski E, Brooks W. Ultrasound evaluation of sacroiliac motion in normal volunteers. Acad Radiol. 1996;3(3):192–6.

55 Wang M, Dumas G. Mechanical behavior of the female sacroiliac joint and influence of the anterior and posterior sacroiliac ligaments under sagittal loads. Clin Biomechanics 1998;13(4/5): 293–9.

56 Sturesson B, Uden A, Vleeming A. A radiostereometric analysis of the movements of the sacroiliac joints in the reciprocal straddle position. Spine 2000;25(2):214–17.

57 Beal MC. The sacroiliac problem: Review of anatomy, mechanics, and diagnosis. J Am Osteopath Assoc 1982;81:667–79.

58 McGrath MC. Clinical considerations of sacroiliac joint anatomy: A review of function, motion and pain. J Osteopath Med 2004;7(1): 16–24.

59 Kaltenborn F. The spine. Basic evaluation and mobilization techniques, 2nd edn. Oslo, Norway: Olaf Norlis Bokhandel; 1993.

60 DiGiovanna EL, Schiowitz S, Dowling DJ. An osteopathic approach to diagnosis and treatment, 3rd edn. Philadelphia, PA: Lippincott Williams & Wilkins; 2005.

61 Mitchell F, Mitchell P. Muscle Energy Manual, vol. 3. Evaluation and treatment of the pelvis and sacrum. East Lansing, MI: MET; 1999.

62 DeStephano L. Greenman's principles of manual medicine, 4th edn. Philadelphia, PA: Wolters Kluwer Health / Lippincott Williams & Wilkins; 2010.

63 Heinking K, Kappler R. Pelvis and Sacrum. In: Chila A. Foundations of osteopathic medicine, 3rd edn. Philadelphia, PA: Wolters Kluwer Health/Lippincott Williams & Wilkins; 2010: Ch. 41.

64 Fryer G, Morse CM, Johnson JC. Spinal and sacroiliac assessment and treatment techniques used by osteopathic physicians in the United States. Osteopath Med Prim Care 2009;3:4.

65 Fryer G, Johnson JC, Fussum C. The use of spinal and sacroiliac joint procedures within the British Osteopathic profession. Part 2: Treatment. Int J Osteopath Med 2010;13(4): 152–9.

66 Fogel GR, Cunningham PY, Esses SI. Coccygodynia: Evaluation and management. J Am Acad Orthop Surg 2004;12:49–54.

67 Patijn J, Janssen M, Hayek S, et al. Coccygodynia. Pain Pract 2010;10(6):554–9.

68 Emerson SS, Speece AJ. Manipulation of the coccyx with anaesthesia for the management of coccydynia. J Am Osteopath Assoc 2012;112(12):805–7.

69 Deniz R, Ozen G, Yilmaz-Oner S, et al. Ankylosing Spondylitis and a diagnostic dilemma: Coccydynia. Clin Exp Rheumatol 2014;32(2):194–8.

70 Karadimas EJ, Trypsiannis G, Giannoudis PV. Surgical treatment of coccygodynia: An analytic review of the literature. Eur Spine J 2011;20(5): 698–705.

71 Lirette LS, Chaiban G, Tolba R, et al. Coccydynia: An overview of the anatomy, aetiology and treatment of coccyx pain. Ochsner J 2014;14(1):84–7.

72 Nathan ST, Fisher BE, Roberts CS. Coccydynia: A review of pathoanatomy, aetiology, treatment and outcome. J Bone Joint Surg Br 2010;92(12): 1622–7.

73 Maigne J, Chatellier G, Faou ML, et al. The treatment of chronic coccydynia with intrarectal manipulation: A randomised controlled study. Spine 2006;31(18):E621–7.

74 Wu C, Yu K, Chuang H, et al. The application of infrared thermography in the assessment of patients with coccydynia before and after manual therapy combined with diathermy. J Manipulative Physiol Ther 2009;32: 287–93.

75 Khatri SM, Nitsure P, Jatti RS. Effectiveness of coccygeal manipulation in coccydynia: A randomized controlled trial. Indian J Physiother Occup Ther 2011;5(3):110–12.

76 Howard PD, Dolan AN, Falco AN, et al. A comparison of conservative interventions and their effectiveness for coccydynia: A systematic review. J Man Manip Ther 2013;21(4): 213–19.

77 Stoddard A. Manual of osteopathic technique, 2nd edn. London: Hutchinson Medical; 1972.

78 Walton WJ. Textbook of osteopathic diagnosis and technique procedures, 2nd edn. St. Louis, MO: Matthews; 1972.

79 Kimberly PE. Outline of osteopathic manipulative procedures, 2nd edn. Kirksville, MO: Kirksville College of Osteopathic Medicine; 1980.

80 Downing HD. Principles and Practice of Osteopathy. London: Tamor Pierston; 1981.

81 Hartman L. Handbook of osteopathic technique, 3rd edn. London: Chapman & Hall; 1997.

82 Hohner JG, Cymet TC. Thrust (high velocity / low amplitude) approach: "The pop". In: Chila

A ed. Foundations of osteopathic medicine, 3rd edn. Philadelphia, PA: Wolters Kluwer Health/Lippincott Williams & Wilkins; 2010: Ch. 45.

83 Tullberg T, Blomberg S, Branth B, et al. Manipulation does not alter the position of the sacroiliac joint: A Roentgen stereophotogrammetric analysis. Spine 1998;23(10):1124–9.

84 Cibulka MT, Delitto A, Koldehoff RM. Changes in innominate tilt after manipulation of the sacroiliac joint in patients with low back pain. Phys Ther 1988;68(9):1359–63.

85 Childs J, Piva S, Erhard R. Immediate improvements in side-to-side weight bearing and iliac crest symmetry after manipulation in patients with low back pain. J Manipulative Physiol Ther 2004;27(5):306–13.

11.1

Sacroiliac joint:
Left innominate posterior

Patient prone

Ligamentous myofascial positioning

Assume somatic dysfunction (S-T-A-R-T) is identified and you wish to thrust the left innominate anteriorly.

Key

❋ Stabilization

● Applicator

➡ Plane of thrust (operator)

⇨ Direction of body movement (patient)

Note: The dimensions for the arrows are not a pictorial representation of the amplitude or force of the thrust.

1. Contact points
a. Left posterior superior iliac spine (PSIS).
b. Anterior aspect of left lower thigh.

2. Applicators
a. Hypothenar eminence of right hand.
b. Palmar aspect of left hand.

3. Patient positioning
Patient lying prone in a comfortable position.

4. Operator stance
Stand at the right side of the patient, feet spread slightly and facing the patient. Stand as erect as possible and avoid crouching, as this will limit the technique and restrict delivery of the thrust.

5. Palpation of contact points
Place the hypothenar eminence of your right hand against the inferior aspect of the left PSIS. Ensure that you have good contact and will not slip across the skin or superficial musculature. Place the palmar aspect of your left hand gently under the anterior aspect of the left thigh just proximal to the knee.

6. Positioning for thrust
Lift the patient's left leg into extension and slight adduction (Fig. 11.7). Avoid introducing extension into the lumbar spine. Apply a force directed downwards towards the couch and slightly cephalad to fix your right hand against the inferior aspect of the PSIS.

Move your centre of gravity over the patient by leaning your body weight forwards onto your right arm and hypothenar eminence. Shifting your centre of gravity forwards assists firm contact point pressure on the PSIS.

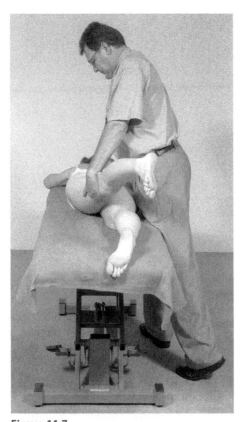

Figure 11.7

7. Adjustments to achieve appropriate prethrust tension

Ensure your patient remains relaxed. Maintaining all holds, make any necessary changes in hip extension, adduction and rotation. Simultaneously, adjust the direction of pressure applied to the PSIS until applicator forces are balanced and you sense a state of appropriate tension and leverage at the left sacroiliac joint. The patient should not be aware of any pain or discomfort. Make these final adjustments by slight movements of the shoulders, trunk, ankles, knees and hips.

8. Immediately prethrust

Relax and adjust your balance as necessary. Keep your head up and ensure that your contacts are firm. An effective HVLA thrust technique is best achieved if the operator and patient are relaxed and not holding themselves rigid. This is a common impediment to achieving effective cavitation.

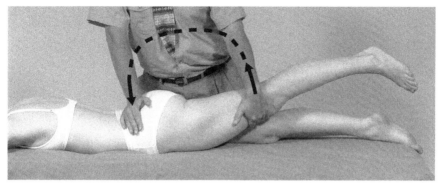
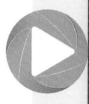

Figure 11.8

9. Delivering the thrust

This technique uses ligamentous myofascial positioning and not facet apposition locking. This approach generally requires a greater emphasis on the exaggeration of primary leverage than is the case with facet apposition locking techniques.

Apply an HVLA thrust with your right hand directed against the PSIS in a curved plane towards the couch. Simultaneously, apply slight exaggeration of hip extension with your left hand (Fig. 11.8). It is important that you do not overemphasize hip extension at the time of thrust. The aim of this technique is to achieve anterior rotation of the left innominate and movement at the left sacroiliac joint. The direction of thrust will alter from patient to patient as a result of the wide variation in sacroiliac anatomy and biomechanics.

The thrust, although very rapid, must never be excessively forcible. The aim should be to use the absolute minimum force necessary.

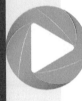

Summary

Sacroiliac joint: Left innominate posterior

Patient prone

Thrust anteriorly

Ligamentous myofascial positioning

- **Contact points:**
  - Left PSIS
  - Anterior aspect of left lower thigh

- **Applicators:**
  - Hypothenar eminence of right hand
  - Palmar aspect of left hand

- **Patient positioning:** Prone in a comfortable position

- **Operator stance:** To right side of patient, facing the couch

- **Palpation of contact points:** Place the hypothenar eminence of your right hand against the inferior aspect of the left PSIS. Place the palmar aspect of your left hand under the anterior aspect of the left thigh proximal to the knee

- **Positioning for thrust:** Lift left leg into extension and slight adduction (Fig. 11.7). Avoid introducing extension into the lumbar spine. Apply a force directed downwards towards the couch and slightly cephalad to fix your right hand against the inferior aspect of the PSIS

- **Adjustments to achieve appropriate prethrust tension:** Make any necessary changes in hip extension, adduction and rotation. Simultaneously, adjust the direction of pressure applied to the PSIS

- **Immediately prethrust:** Relax and adjust your balance

- **Delivering the thrust:** The thrust against the PSIS is in a curved plane towards the couch and accompanied by slight exaggeration of hip extension (Fig. 11.8)

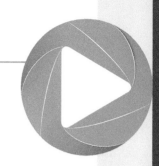

Sacroiliac joint:
Right innominate posterior

Patient sidelying

Assume somatic dysfunction (S-T-A-R-T) is identified and you wish to thrust the right innominate anteriorly.

Key

✳ Stabilization

● Applicator

➡ Plane of thrust (operator)

⇨ Direction of body movement (patient)

Note: The dimensions for the arrows are not a pictorial representation of the amplitude or force of the thrust.

1. Patient positioning

Lying on the left side with a pillow to support the head and neck. The upper portion of the couch is raised 30° to 35° to introduce right sidebending in the lower thoracic and upper lumbar spine.

Lower body. Straighten the patient's lower leg and ensure that the leg and spine are in a straight line, in a neutral position. Flex the patient's upper hip to approximately 90°. Flex the patient's upper knee and place the heel of the foot just anterior to the knee of the lower leg. The lower leg and spine should form as near a straight line as possible with no flexion at the lower hip or knee.

Upper body. Gently extend the patient's upper shoulder and place the patient's right forearm on the lower ribs. Using your left hand to palpate the L5–S1 interspinous space, introduce right rotation of the patient's trunk, down to and including the L5–S1 segment. This is achieved by gently holding the patient's left elbow with your right hand and pulling it towards you, but also in a cephalad direction towards the head end of the couch. Be careful not to introduce any flexion to the spine during this movement. Now modify the pectoral hold by positioning the patient's upper arm behind the thorax.

2. Operator stance

Stand close to the couch with your feet spread and one leg behind the other. Ensure that the patient's upper knee is placed between your legs. This will enable you to make the necessary adjustments to achieve the appropriate prethrust tension (Fig. 11.9). Maintain an upright posture, facing in the direction of the patient's upper body.

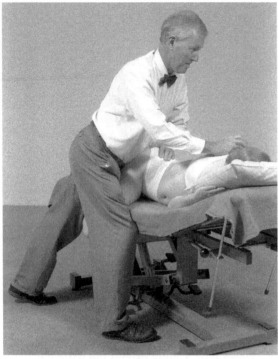

Figure 11.9

3. Positioning for thrust

Apply the heel of your left hand to the inferior aspect of the posterior superior iliac spine (PSIS). Your right hand should be resting against the patient's upper pectoral and rib cage region. Gently rotate the patient's trunk away from you using your right hand until you achieve spinal locking. Avoid applying direct pressure to the glenohumeral joint. Finally, roll the patient about 10° to 15° towards you while maintaining the build-up of leverages.

4. Adjustments to achieve appropriate prethrust tension

Ensure your patient remains relaxed. Maintaining all holds, make any necessary changes in hip flexion and adduction. Simultaneously, adjust the direction of pressure applied to the PSIS until the forces are balanced and you sense a state of appropriate tension and leverage at the right sacroiliac joint. The patient should not be aware of any pain or discomfort. Make these final adjustments by slight movements of the shoulders, trunk, ankles, knees and hips.

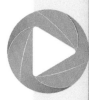

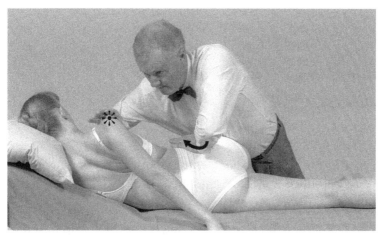

Figure 11.10

5. Immediately prethrust

Relax and adjust your balance as necessary. Keep your head up and ensure your contacts are firm. An effective HVLA thrust technique is best achieved if the operator and patient are relaxed and not holding themselves rigid. This is a common impediment to achieving effective cavitation.

6. Delivering the thrust

Apply an HVLA thrust with the heel of your left hand directed against the PSIS in a curved plane towards you (Fig. 11.10).

Your right arm against the patient's pectoral region does not apply a thrust but acts as a stabilizer only. The aim of this technique is to achieve anterior rotation of the right innominate and movement at the right sacroiliac joint. The direction of thrust will alter between patients as a result of the wide variation in sacroiliac anatomy and biomechanics.

The thrust, although very rapid, must never be excessively forcible. The aim should be to use the absolute minimum force necessary.

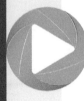

Summary

Sacroiliac joint: Right innominate posterior

Patient sidelying

Thrust anteriorly

- **Patient positioning:** Left sidelying with the upper portion of the couch raised 30° to 35° to introduce right sidebending in the lower thoracic and upper lumbar spine:

  - *Lower body.* Left leg and spine in a straight line. Right hip flexed to approximately 90°. Right knee flexed and heel of right foot placed just anterior to knee of lower leg

  - *Upper body.* Introduce right rotation of the patient's upper body down to and including L5–S1. Do not introduce any flexion to the spine during this movement. Modify the pectoral hold by positioning the patient's upper arm behind the thorax

- **Operator stance:** Stand close to the couch, feet spread and one leg behind the other. Ensure that the patient's upper knee is placed between your legs (Fig. 11.9). Maintain an upright posture facing in the direction of the patient's upper body

- **Positioning for thrust:** Apply the heel of your left hand to the inferior aspect of the PSIS. Rotate the patient's upper body away from you until spinal locking is achieved. Roll the patient about 10° to 15° towards you

- **Adjustments to achieve appropriate prethrust tension:** Make any necessary changes in hip flexion and adduction. Simultaneously, adjust direction of pressure applied to the PSIS

- **Immediately prethrust:** Relax and adjust your balance

- **Delivering the thrust:** The thrust against the PSIS is in a curved plane towards you (Fig. 11.10). Your right arm against the patient's pectoral region does not apply a thrust but acts as a stabilizer only

11.3

Sacroiliac joint:
Left innominate anterior

Patient supine

Assume somatic dysfunction (S-T-A-R-T) is identified and you wish to thrust the left innominate posteriorly.

Key

 Stabilization

● Applicator

➡ Plane of thrust (operator)

⇨ Direction of body movement (patient)

Note: The dimensions for the arrows are not a pictorial representation of the amplitude or force of the thrust.

1. Contact points
a. Left anterior superior iliac spine (ASIS).
b. Posterior aspect of left shoulder girdle.

2. Applicators
a. Palm of right hand.
b. Palmar aspect of left hand and wrist.

3. Patient positioning
Patient lying supine in a comfortable position. Move the patient's pelvis towards his/her right. Move the feet and shoulders in the opposite direction to introduce left sidebending of the trunk. Place the patient's left foot and ankle on top of the right ankle. Ask the patient to clasp his/her fingers behind the neck (Fig. 11.11).

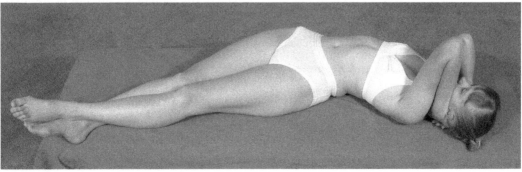

Figure 11.11

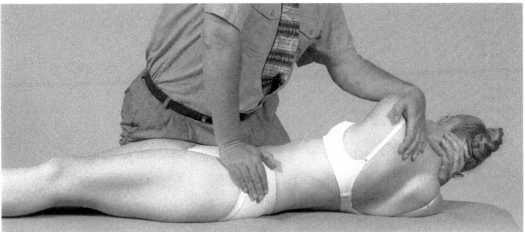

Figure 11.12

4. Operator stance

Stand at the right side of the patient, feet spread slightly and facing the couch. Stand as erect as possible and avoid crouching, as this will limit the technique and restrict delivery of the thrust.

5. Palpation of contact points

Place the palm of your right hand over the ASIS. Ensure that you have good contact and will not slip across the skin or superficial musculature. Place the palmar aspect of your left hand and wrist gently over the posterior aspect of the left shoulder girdle.

6. Positioning for thrust

Rotate the patient's trunk to the right and towards you. It is critical to maintain the left trunk sidebending introduced during initial positioning. Apply a force directed downwards towards the couch and slightly cephalad to fix your right hand against the inferior aspect of the ASIS (Fig. 11.12).

Move your centre of gravity over the patient by leaning your body weight forwards onto your right arm and hand. Shifting your centre of gravity forwards assists firm contact point pressure on the ASIS.

7. Adjustments to achieve appropriate prethrust tension

Ensure your patient remains relaxed. Maintaining all holds, make any necessary changes in trunk rotation, flexion and sidebending. Simultaneously, adjust the direction of pressure applied to the ASIS until applicator forces are balanced and you sense a state of appropriate tension and leverage. The patient should not be aware of any pain or discomfort. Make these final adjustments by slight movements of the shoulders, trunk, ankles, knees and hips.

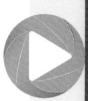

8. Immediately prethrust

Relax and adjust your balance as necessary. Keep your head up and ensure that your contacts are firm. An effective HVLA thrust technique is best achieved if the operator and patient are relaxed and not holding themselves rigid. This is a common impediment to achieving effective cavitation.

9. Delivering the thrust

Apply an HVLA thrust with your right hand directed against the ASIS in a curved plane towards the couch (Fig. 11.13). Your left forearm, wrist and hand over the patient's shoulder girdle do not apply a thrust but act as stabilizers only. The aim of this technique is to achieve posterior rotation of the left innominate and movement at the left sacroiliac joint. The direction of thrust will alter between patients as a result of the wide variation in sacroiliac anatomy and biomechanics.

The thrust, although very rapid, must never be excessively forcible. The aim should be to use the absolute minimum force necessary.

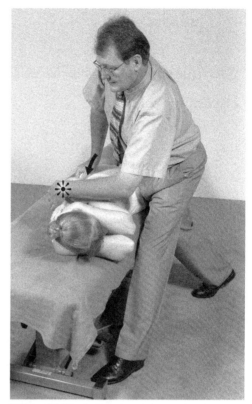

Figure 11.13

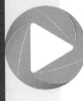

Summary

Sacroiliac joint: Left innominate anterior

Patient supine

Thrust posteriorly

- **Contact points:**
  - Left ASIS
  - Posterior aspect of left shoulder girdle

- **Applicators:**
  - Palm of right hand
  - Palmar aspect of left hand and wrist

- **Patient positioning:** Supine. Move patient's pelvis towards the right. Move feet and shoulders in the opposite direction to introduce left sidebending of the trunk. Place the patient's left foot and ankle on top of the right ankle. Ask the patient to clasp fingers behind the neck (Fig. 11.11)

- **Operator stance:** To the right side of the patient, facing the couch

- **Palpation of contact points:** Place the palm of your right hand over the ASIS. Place the palmar aspect of your left hand and wrist over the posterior aspect of the left shoulder girdle

- **Positioning for thrust:** Rotate the patient's trunk to the right. Maintain left trunk sidebending. Apply a force directed downwards towards the couch and slightly cephalad to fix your right hand against the inferior aspect of the ASIS (Fig. 11.12)

- **Adjustments to achieve appropriate prethrust tension:** Make any necessary changes in trunk rotation, flexion and sidebending. Simultaneously, adjust direction of pressure applied to the ASIS

- **Immediately prethrust:** Relax and adjust your balance

- **Delivering the thrust:** The thrust against the ASIS is in a curved plane towards the couch (Fig. 11.13). Your left forearm, wrist and hand over the patient's shoulder girdle do not apply a thrust but act as stabilizers only

Sacroiliac joint:
Sacral base anterior

Patient sidelying

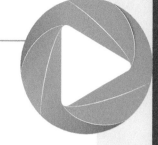

Assume somatic dysfunction (S-T-A-R-T) is identified and you wish to thrust the apex of the sacrum anteriorly.

Key

❋ Stabilization

● Applicator

➡ Plane of thrust (operator)

⇨ Direction of body movement (patient)

Note: The dimensions for the arrows are not a pictorial representation of the amplitude or force of the thrust.

---

1. Patient positioning

Lying on the right side with a pillow to support the head and neck.

Lower body. Straighten the patient's lower leg and ensure that the leg and spine are in a straight line, in a neutral position. Flex the patient's upper hip and knee slightly and place the upper leg just anterior to the lower leg. The lower leg and spine should form as near a straight line as possible with no flexion at the lower hip or knee.

Upper body. Gently extend the patient's upper shoulder and place the patient's left forearm on the lower ribs. Using your right hand to palpate the L5–S1 interspinous space, introduce left rotation of the patient's trunk down to and including the L5–S1 segment. This is achieved by gently holding the patient's right elbow with your left hand and pulling it towards you, but also in a cephalad direction towards the head end of the couch. Be careful not to introduce any flexion to the spine during this movement. Take up the axillary hold. This arm controls and maintains trunk rotation.

2. Operator stance

Stand close to the couch with your feet spread and one leg behind the other. Maintain an upright posture, facing slightly in the direction of the patient's upper body.

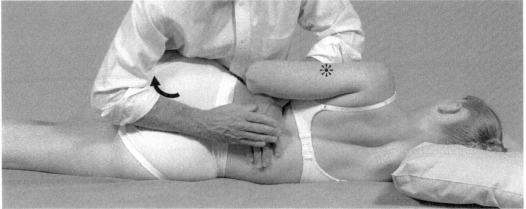

Figure 11.14

3. Positioning for thrust

Apply the palmar aspect of your right forearm to the apex of the sacrum. Ensure that contact is below the second sacral segment. Your left forearm should be resting against the patient's upper pectoral and rib cage region and will control and maintain trunk rotation. Gently rotate the patient's trunk away from you using your left forearm until you achieve spinal locking. Be careful to avoid undue pressure in the axilla. Finally, roll the patient about 10° to 15° towards you while maintaining the build-up of leverages.

4. Adjustments to achieve appropriate prethrust tension

Ensure your patient remains relaxed. Maintaining all holds, make any necessary changes in flexion, extension, sidebending or rotation until you are confident that full spinal locking is achieved. The patient should not be aware of any pain or discomfort. Make these final adjustments by slight movements of your shoulders, trunk, ankles, knees and hips.

5. Immediately prethrust

Relax and adjust your balance as necessary. Keep your head up and ensure contacts are firm. An effective HVLA thrust technique is best achieved if both the operator and patient are relaxed and not holding themselves rigid. This is a common impediment to achieving effective cavitation.

6. Delivering the thrust

Apply an HVLA thrust with your right forearm against the apex of the sacrum in a curved plane towards you (Fig. 11.14). Your left arm against the patient's pectoral region does not apply a thrust but acts as a stabilizer only. The aim of this technique is to achieve a counternutation movement of the sacrum.

The thrust, although very rapid, must never be excessively forcible. The aim should be to use the absolute minimum force necessary.

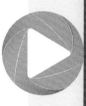

Summary

Sacroiliac joint: Sacral base anterior

Patient sidelying

Thrust apex anteriorly

- **Patient positioning:** Right sidelying:

  - *Lower body.* Right leg and spine in a straight line. Left hip and knee flexed slightly and placed just anterior to the lower leg

  - *Upper body.* Introduce left rotation of the patient's trunk down to and including the L5–S1 segment. Do not introduce any flexion to the spine during this movement. Take up the axillary hold

- **Operator stance:** Stand close to the couch, feet spread and one leg behind the other. Maintain an upright posture, facing slightly in the direction of the patient's upper body

- **Positioning for thrust:** Apply the palmar aspect of your right forearm to the apex of the sacrum. Ensure that contact is below the second sacral segment. Your left forearm should be resting against the patient's upper pectoral and rib cage region. Rotate the patient's trunk away from you using your left forearm until you achieve spinal locking. Roll the patient about 10° to 15° towards you

- **Adjustments to achieve appropriate prethrust tension**

- **Immediately prethrust:** Relax and adjust your balance

- **Delivering the thrust:** The thrust against the apex of the sacrum is in a curved plane towards you (Fig. 11.14). Your left arm against the patient's pectoral region does not apply a thrust but acts as a stabilizer only

11.5

Sacrococcygeal joint:
Coccyx anterior

Patient sidelying

Assume somatic dysfunction (S-T-A-R-T) is identified and you wish to mobilize or thrust the coccyx posteriorly.

Key

✳ Stabilization

● Applicator

➡ Plane of mobilization or thrust (operator)

⇨ Direction of body movement (patient)

Note: The dimensions for the arrows are not a pictorial representation of the amplitude or force of the mobilization or thrust.

The operator must exercise care and attention to ensure that the patient is fully informed as to the nature of this procedure. This technique involves both assessment and treatment via a rectal approach. It is assumed that the operator will examine the anal and rectal region to determine whether there are any contraindications to performing this procedure. This technique can be used either as a means of gently mobilizing the sacrococcygeal joint or applying a high-velocity low-amplitude (HVLA) thrust to the coccyx. Coccydynia can be severe, and the choice of technique depends as much upon patient comfort as perceived efficacy of approach. Practitioners should become familiar with mobilizing the sacrococcygeal joint before attempting a thrust to the coccyx.

1. Contact points
a. Anterior aspect of the coccyx through the posterior wall of the rectum.
b. Posterior aspect of the coccyx.

2. Applicators
a. Lubricated index finger of operator's gloved right hand.
b. Thumb of operator's gloved right hand.

3. Patient positioning
Lying in the left lateral position with the maximal amount of flexion of the hips, knees and spine consistent with patient comfort. The patient should be fully undressed so that access to the anal canal is possible. The buttocks should be at the edge of the couch.

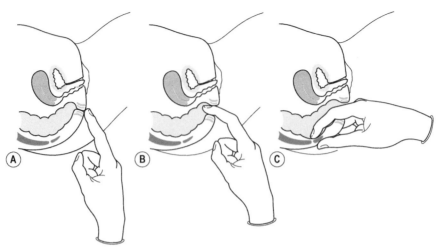

Figure 11.15 Sacrococcygeal joint. A: The index finger is placed against the anal margin. B: The finger is inserted as shown. C: After examination of the rectum, the coccyx is held between the index finger internally and the thumb externally.

4. Operator stance

Stand behind the patient, approximately at the level of the patient's hip joints, facing the couch and patient's back.

5. Palpation of contact points

The operator should be wearing a pair of suitable gloves with lubricant smeared over the right index finger. The patient must be informed that a finger within the rectum will cause a sensation similar to that of opening the bowels. Ask the patient to relax, and place the index finger of your right hand against the anal margin (Fig. 11.15A). With steady pressure, insert your right index finger into the patient's anal canal in a cephalic and slightly anterior direction (Fig. 11.15B). The finger will pass through the anal sphincter and into the rectum. If the patient has difficulty relaxing, ask him / her to bear down as if opening the bowels and gently slip your finger past the anal sphincter and into the rectum. Once through the anal sphincter, the direction of the rectum is cephalic and posteriorly along the curve of the coccyx and sacrum.

The palpating right index finger identifies the sacrum and coccyx through the posterior wall of the rectum. Place the distal phalanx of the right index finger against the anterior surface of the coccyx immediately below the sacrococcygeal joint. Use the thumb of your right hand externally to identify the posterior aspect of the coccyx between the buttocks. The coccyx is now gently held between your index finger internally and the thumb externally (Fig. 11.15C). Gentle pressure is applied in a number of directions to determine undue tenderness or any reproduction of the patient's familiar symptoms. The mobility and position of the coccyx relative to the sacrum is also noted.

6. Fixation of contact points

Keep your right index finger on the anterior aspect of the coccyx while applying pressure against the posterior aspect of the coccyx with your right thumb. The fixation is gentle but firm with less pressure against the anterior surface of the coccyx.

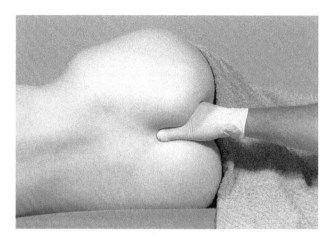

Figure 11.16

7. Adjustments to achieve appropriate prethrust tension

The operator should be in a position to move the coccyx through a range of motion and in different planes. Ensure your patient remains relaxed. Maintaining all holds, make any necessary changes in flexion, extension, sidebending and rotation of the coccyx until you sense a state of appropriate tension and leverage at the sacrococcygeal joint.

8. Immediately prethrust

Relax and adjust your balance as necessary. Ensure that your contacts are firm. An effective HVLA thrust technique is best achieved if the operator and patient are relaxed and not holding themselves rigid. This is a common impediment to achieving effective cavitation.

9. Delivering the thrust

Apply an HVLA thrust towards you in a curved plane (Fig. 11.16).

The thrust, although very rapid, must never be excessively forcible. The aim should be to use the absolute minimum force necessary.

Summary

Sacrococcygeal joint: Coccyx anterior

Patient sidelying

Mobilization or thrust posteriorly

- **Contact points:**
  - Anterior aspect of the coccyx
  - Posterior aspect of the coccyx
- **Applicators:**
  - Lubricated index finger of operator's gloved right hand
  - Thumb of operator's gloved right hand
- **Patient positioning:** Left lateral position with flexion of the hips, knees and spine
- **Operator stance:** Behind the patient
- **Palpation of contact points:** Place the index finger of right hand against the anal margin (Fig. 11.15A). Insert your right index finger into the anal canal in a cephalic and anterior direction (Fig. 11.15B). The palpating index finger identifies the sacrum and coccyx through the posterior wall of the rectum. Place the distal phalanx of the right index finger against the anterior surface of the coccyx. Identify the posterior aspect of the coccyx between the buttocks. The coccyx is now gently held between your right index finger internally and the thumb externally (Fig. 11.15C)
- **Fixation of contact points:** Keep right index finger on the anterior aspect of the coccyx while applying pressure against the posterior aspect of the coccyx with your right thumb
- **Adjustments to achieve appropriate prethrust tension**
- **Immediately prethrust:** Relax and adjust your balance
- **Delivering the thrust:** The direction of thrust is towards you in a curved plane (Fig. 11.16)

Technique failure and analysis

Techniques in this manual have been described in a structured format. This format allows flexibility so that each technique can be modified to suit both the patient and practitioner.

Competence and expertise in the use of high-velocity low-amplitude (HVLA) thrust techniques increase with practice and experience. Development of a high level of skill in the use of HVLA thrust techniques is predicated upon critical reflection of performance. When an HVLA thrust technique does not produce cavitation with minimal force, the practitioner should reflect upon how the technique might have been modified and improved. Even the experienced practitioner should review each HVLA thrust technique to identify factors that might improve technique delivery.

Inability to achieve cavitation with minimal force may arise for a number of reasons and can be reviewed under three broad headings:

- General technique analysis
  - Incorrect selection of technique
  - Inadequate localization of forces
  - Ineffective thrust
- Practitioner and patient variables
  - Patient comfort and cooperation
  - Patient positioning
  - Practitioner comfort and confidence
  - Practitioner posture
- Physical and biomechanical modifying factors
  - Primary leverage
  - Secondary leverages
  - Contact point pressure
  - Identification of appropriate prethrust tension
  - Direction of thrust
  - Velocity of thrust
  - Amplitude of thrust
  - Force of thrust
  - Arrest of technique.

If you have experienced technique failure, follow the process of review outlined below:

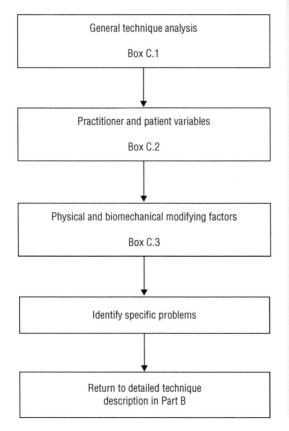

General technique analysis

Box C.1

↓

Practitioner and patient variables

Box C.2

↓

Physical and biomechanical modifying factors

Box C.3

↓

Identify specific problems

↓

Return to detailed technique description in Part B

Box C.1 General technique analysis

INCORRECT SELECTION OF TECHNIQUE
- Practitioner too small and patient too large
- Practitioner has physical limitations that limit effective delivery of technique
- Practitioner inexperienced with selected technique
- Inability to position patient due to pain, discomfort or physical limitations
- Patient apprehension

INADEQUATE LOCALIZATION OF FORCES
- Incorrect application of primary leverage
- Incorrect application of secondary leverages
- Inability to recognize appropriate prethrust tension

INEFFECTIVE THRUST
- Loss of contact point pressure
- Poor bimanual coordination
- Incorrect direction of thrust
- Inadequate velocity of thrust
- Incorrect amplitude of thrust
- Incorrect force of thrust
- Loss of leverage at time of thrust
- Poor practitioner posture
- Practitioner not relaxed
- Failure to arrest thrust and leverage adequately
- Lack of practitioner confidence

Box C.2 Practitioner and patient variables

COMMON FAULTS
- Patient not comfortably positioned
- Patient not relaxed
- Rough patient handling
- Rushing technique
- Poor practitioner posture
- Lack of practitioner confidence

CHECKLIST
Patient comfort and cooperation
Dependent upon:
- Confidence and trust in practitioner
- Patient experience of previous successful HVLA thrust technique
- Slow, firm and gentle patient handling
- Confident and reassuring approach by practitioner
- Explanation of technique and informed consent
- Optimal patient positioning

Patient positioning
Dependent upon:
- Appropriate positioning to match patient's physical and medical condition
- Correct identification of primary leverage and secondary leverages

- Pain-free positioning
- Appropriate use of pillows and treatment couch adjustment

Practitioner comfort and confidence
Dependent upon:
- Establishing a working diagnosis
- Selecting a technique to match patient's physical and medical condition
- Confidence that the technique will improve and not worsen the patient's symptoms
- Previous experience and success with the selected HVLA thrust technique
- Optimal practitioner posture

Practitioner posture
Dependent upon:
- Using as wide a base as possible
- Not relying solely upon arm strength and speed
- Using your body where possible to generate thrust force
- Not stooping or bending over the patient
- Keeping your own spine erect
- Optimal treatment couch height

Box C.3 Physical and biomechanical modifying factors

COMMON FAULTS
- Insufficient primary leverage
- Too much secondary leverage – locking often results from the over-application of secondary leverages. This can occur during the build-up of leverages or at the point of thrust
- Loss of contact point pressure immediately prethrust
- Not identifying appropriate prethrust tension and leverage before thrust – if in doubt about optimum prethrust tension, attempt multiple light thrusts
- Incorrect direction of thrust – the thrust should be in a direction that is comfortable for the patient. Multiple light thrusts can assist in the identification of the appropriate direction of thrust
- Insufficient velocity of thrust

- Too much amplitude – this is often a consequence of too much force and/or poor control
- Too much force
- Insufficient arrest of technique – this is often a consequence of poor practitioner coordination and control

CHECKLIST
- Primary leverage
- Secondary leverages
- Contact point pressure
- Identification of appropriate prethrust tension
- Direction of thrust
- Velocity of thrust
- Amplitude of thrust
- Force of thrust
- Arrest of technique

Index

Page numbers followed by *"f"* indicate figures, *"b"* indicate boxes, and *"t"* indicate tables.